T0179256

Structural Equation Modeling
for Health and Medicine

Chapman & Hall/CRC Biostatistics Series

Series Editors:

Shein-Chung Chow, Duke University School of Medicine, USA
Byron Jones, Novartis Pharma AG, Switzerland
Jen-pei Liu, National Taiwan University, Taiwan
Karl E. Peace, Georgia Southern University, USA
Bruce W. Turnbull, Cornell University, USA

Recently Published Titles

Bayesian Applications in Pharmaceutical Development
Mani Lakshminarayanan, Fanni Natanegara

Innovative Statistics in Regulatory Science
Shein-Chung Chow

Geospatial Health Data: Modeling and Visualization with R-INLA and Shiny
Paula Moraga

Artificial Intelligence for Drug Development, Precision Medicine, and Healthcare
Mark Chang

Bayesian Methods in Pharmaceutical Research
Emmanuel Lesaffre, Gianluca Baio, Bruno Boulanger

Biomarker Analysis in Clinical Trials with R
Nusrat Rabbee

Interface between Regulation and Statistics in Drug Development
Demissie Alemayehu, Birol Emir, Michael Gaffney

Innovative Methods for Rare Disease Drug Development
Shein-Chung Chow

Medical Risk Prediction Models: With Ties to Machine Learning
Thomas A Gerds, Michael W. Kattan

Real-World Evidence in Drug Development and Evaluation
Harry Yang, Binbing Yu

Cure Models: Methods, Applications, and Implementation
Yingwei Peng, Binbing Yu

Bayesian Analysis of Infectious Diseases: COVID-19 and Beyond
Lyle D. Broemeling

Statistical Meta-Analysis Using R and Stata, Second Edition
Ding-Geng (Din) Chen and Karl E. Peace

Advanced Survival Models
Catherine Legrand

Structural Equation Modeling for Health and Medicine
Douglas D. Gunzler, Adam T. Perzynski and Adam C. Carle

For more information about this series, please visit: https://www.routledge.com/ Chapman--Hall-CRC-Biostatistics-Series/book-series/CHBIOSTATIS

Structural Equation Modeling for Health and Medicine

Douglas D. Gunzler
Population Health Research Institute
Center for Health Care Research and Policy
The MetroHealth System and Case Western Reserve University
Cleveland, Ohio

Adam T. Perzynski
Population Health Research Institute
Center for Health Care Research and Policy
The MetroHealth System and Case Western Reserve University
Cleveland, Ohio

Adam C. Carle
James M. Anderson Center for Health Systems Excellence
Department of Pediatrics
Cincinnati Children's Hospital Medical Center
University of Cincinnati College of Medicine
Cincinnati, Ohio
and
Department of Psychology
University of Cincinnati College of Arts and Sciences
Cincinnati, Ohio

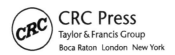

CRC Press
Taylor & Francis Group
Boca Raton London New York

CRC Press is an imprint of the
Taylor & Francis Group, an **informa** business
A CHAPMAN & HALL BOOK

First edition published 2021
by CRC Press
6000 Broken Sound Parkway NW, Suite 300, Boca Raton, FL 33487-2742

and by CRC Press
2 Park Square, Milton Park, Abingdon, Oxon, OX14 4RN

ISBN: 9781138574250 (hbk)
ISBN: 9780367742331 (pbk)
ISBN: 9780203701133 (ebk)

Typeset in Palatino
by codeMantra

Contents

Part I Introduction to Concepts and Principles of Structural Equation Modeling for Health and Medical Research

Part II   Theory of Structural Equation Modeling

Preface

The book came about due to a series of workshops and panels on structural equation modeling (SEM) we presented at national health services research and medical decision-making meetings. Our initial workshop goal was to satisfy the curiosity of graduate students, faculty, industry professionals and other attendees and help them gain a solid understanding of the introductory principles of SEM. However, it became clear to us during both question and answer portions and informal post-lecture discussion that many attendees still needed a deeper understanding of how to apply these techniques with particular health and medical studies in mind. The problems and questions from our health science audience did not follow "linearly" from the typical introductory SEM examples for the social sciences. A classic example [1] that appears often in SEM introductions, manuals and tutorials describes the relationships between alienation and background variables such as education and occupation. While concepts such as alienation are familiar to many sociologists and other social scientists, they may be less helpful at the introductory stage for researchers studying health and medicine.

Health and medical researchers use a wide variety of data sources, including complex and messy real-world data. Study designs are also highly variable. Translating a conceptual model into a formal structural equation model under the boundaries of a study can be difficult in practice. Likewise, output from software for the analysis of structural equation models (SEMs) commonly requires thorough review and interpretation. Careful consideration of theory, logic and prior literature is mandatory (as with all SEM research). Thus, our workshops and panels over time became adapted to showcase the methods for more nuanced examples in health and medicine.

We, ourselves, learned SEM in traditional graduate school programs in biostatistics, sociology and psychology. However, countless hours thinking about how to analyze data with SEM as faculty in departments in schools of medicine over the past decade have shaped our views and presentation of SEM for this textbook. This collaboration between the three authors of this textbook is reflective of our recommended usages of SEM for health and medicine. Most of our applications of SEM have been done using a *team science* approach.

Team science is a collaborative effort from a group of researchers to address a scientific challenge. In team science a research group leverages the strengths and expertise of each of the individuals trained in different fields. In a *cross-disciplinary* (e.g. *interdisciplinary, multidisciplinary, transdisciplinary*) approach within team science a research group with expertise in different fields work together to combine or integrate their perspectives with a purpose in mind (e.g. addressing the research aims of a study). In a multidisciplinary approach, researchers draw from multiple disciplines to redefine problems and reach solutions. However, the researchers remain within the boundaries of the different disciplines. An interdisciplinary approach integrates separate disciplines into a coordinated and coherent whole. A transdisciplinary approach transcends the pre-conceived boundaries of the different disciplines and refers to learning that is authentic and relevant to the real world [2]. Rather than being confined by traditional ways of thinking about research problems, learning in the transdisciplinary approach is supported and enriched by them. For example, a non-clinician could take part in a comprehensive clinical observership of patients with a condition under study (e.g. multiple sclerosis or lung cancer), under the supervision of a clinician, to better understand the emotional, mental and physical symptoms of the condition. The training activity is useful for the later development of a transdisciplinary conceptual model for persons with the condition under study as well as recommendations for implementing the analytic results in clinical application [3].

More generally, researchers using SEM in health and medicine can benefit from a team science approach. The team can work together in designing the study under appropriate boundaries and make suitable study assumptions. Further, the experts of different disciplines under the guidance of a primary investigator (or investigators) can collaboratively develop conceptual models, specify measurement and structural models, interpret output and draw fitting study conclusions. In the SEM examples presented throughout this book, answering difficult research questions required the integration of perspectives and expertise across disciplines.

Our goal with this textbook is to both introduce SEM and then present illustrative applications with software that can be used for the analysis of SEMs (e.g. Mplus, AMOS). We use the nomenclature SEM in this textbook for a diverse set of methods incorporating a combination of continuous and categorical latent variables.

This textbook presents both a nontechnical overview of topics with introductory examples and a more intermediate level technical description of SEM with more detailed examples. We envision this textbook can work on its own to cover topics ranging from introductory and above for SEM students and researchers in a range of health and medical departments. Thus we hope that a reader, similar to our course and panel participants, comes away with an understanding of how to effectively use SEM for their own research in health and medicine. An understanding, in this sense, includes grasping (1) basic principles of SEM and recommended strategies for application in health and medicine and (2) a sense of how to flexibly and creatively use SEM. We've written this book in three parts.

Part I (Chapters 1 and 2) presents a basic overview of SEM for health and medicine. These chapters introduce the history, vocabulary, concepts and usages of SEM.

Part II (Chapters 3–5) presents the basic theory of SEM using illustrative examples in health and medicine. These chapters include material on the graphical and mathematical forms of SEMs and model specification, estimation, evaluation, identification and equivalence.

Part III (Chapters 6–15) presents applications and examples of SEM for health and medical studies. In these chapters, there is material on confirmatory factor analysis, exploratory factor analysis, mediation and moderation analysis, model modification, comparison and specification searches, multiple indicator multiple cause and multigroup analysis, mixture modeling and longitudinal modeling. These chapters include illustrative examples involving patient reported outcomes data and other health-related outcomes, large observational studies, randomized controlled trials, clinical risk factors, disease progression and other commonly occurring phenomena in health and medicine. The book ends with Chapter 15 on a series of special topics relevant for SEM health and medical researchers.

Several of the applied examples in this book focus on depression screening and individuals studied have comorbid conditions (e.g. depression and multiple sclerosis, depression and HIV). We particularly use the patient health questionnaire (PHQ-9) as a short-item self-report depression screening tool [4]. As one reads the book, it should be noted that these are some of the study samples and measures used in our research. The reader should envision applying the methods for their own research which may involve vastly different study samples and measures.

It has been a truly rewarding experience in completing this textbook. This achievement marks an important path traveled in the longer journey to make SEM more accessible for health and medical researchers. This field will continue to evolve as funders, research institutions and companies alike dedicate more resources to population health research.

REFERENCES

1. Wheaton, B., et al., Assessing reliability and stability in panel models. *Sociological Methodology*, 1977. **8**: pp. 84–136.
2. Choi, B.C. and A.W. Pak, Multidisciplinarity, interdisciplinarity and transdisciplinarity in health research, services, education and policy: 1. Definitions, objectives, and evidence of effectiveness. *Clinical and Investigative Medicine*, 2006. **29**(6): pp. 351–364.
3. Gunzler, D., et al., Training a nonclinician to become a leader in transdisciplinary clinical research: Clinical observerships. *International Journal of Clinical Biostatistics and Biometrics*, 2015. **1**(5).
4. Kroenke, K., R.L. Spitzer, and J.B. Williams, The PHQ-9. *Journal of General Internal Medicine*, 2001. **16**(9): pp. 606–613.

Acknowledgments

This book represents collaborative work by the three authors. Financial support for this study was provided by grants from NIH/NIDDK 1R01DK112905-01A1 (Sehgal and Gunzler), NIH/NCATS UL1 TR 002548-01 (Konstan), NIH/NIA, R01AG055480 (Dalton and Perzynski), NIH/NIA R01AG022459 (Sudano), NIH/NIA R01AG024206 (Sudano), Health Resources and Services Administration H97HA27429-01-00 (Avery), NIH NCI/FDA R01CA190130 (Flocke), NIH/NIAAA R01AA013302 (Dawson) and NIH/NIMH R01MH085665 (Dawson and Sajatovic).

The funding agreement ensured the authors' independence in conceptualizing, designing, writing and publishing this textbook.

We appreciate the contributions from five independent and anonymous reviewers and Drs. Neal Dawson, Ann Avery, Jarrod Dalton, Farren Briggs, Susan Flocke, Karen Ishler, Kristen Berg, Nathan Morris, Martha Sajatovic, Richard McCormick and Joseph Sudano. We are grateful to Rob Hamm and other leaders at the Society for Medical Decision Making for choosing to offer our SEM short course for many years, to the learners in those courses who shared their questions and ideas with us, and to Dana Alden who (together with Kristen Berg and Joseph Sudano) has co-taught with us on many occasions.

We thank Rob Calver, Vaishali Singh and Iris Fahrer from Chapman & Hall and Vijay Shanker at CodeMantra. We would like to thank all others heavily involved in this process as well from both the editing and production side.

From author Dr. Douglas D. Gunzler: To my thesis advisor Dr. Xin M. Tu for your friendship, wisdom and ardent introduction to SEM and mediation analysis. On a personal note, I would like to specially thank my wonderful wife, Meredith, and children, Paige and Jacob, for their all-around patience, love, support and understanding throughout this process.

From Dr. Adam T. Perzynski: To my peers Tanetta Andersson, Chris Burant, Katy Abbott, Heather Menne, Joshua Terchek and Noah Webster: if not for your friendship and inspiring scholarship, I would not have had anything to offer this book. Thanks to Kyle Kercher for his enthusiastic (and at times relentless) introduction to SEM in Sociology 509 which set me on a pathway to contributing to this book. Most of all thanks to my loving family Maureen, Holly, Sophie and Eddie.

From Dr. Adam C. Carle: I would like to thank Tara J. Carle, Lyla S. B. Carle and Margaret Carle for their love and unending support. I would also like to thank the sheep and the dogs for being, well, sheep and dogs.

Authors

Dr. Douglas D. Gunzler is a tenured Associate Professor of Medicine and Population and Quantitative Health Sciences in the Population Health Research Institute at the Center for Health Care Research and Policy, MetroHealth and Case Western Reserve University. He is a biostatistician with specialties in structural equation modeling (SEM) and longitudinal data analysis. His research interests lie in the areas of mediation analysis, factor analysis, mixture modeling, psychometrics, age-period-cohort analysis and their application to both clinical trials and observational studies in health and medicine. In his research, he is using SEM for analysis of overlapping symptoms in co-occurring conditions. Dr. Gunzler earned his PhD from the Department of Biostatistics & Computational Biology at the University of Rochester in 2011.

Dr. Adam T. Perzynski is a tenured Associate Professor of Medicine and Sociology in the Population Health Research Institute at the Center for Health Care Research and Policy, MetroHealth and Case Western Reserve University. He is also the Founding Director of the Patient Centered Media Lab. His doctoral degree is in sociology, and his current research interests include novel strategies to eliminate health disparities, outcomes measurement over the life course and research methods. His methodologic expertise spans the continuum from focus groups and ethnography to psychometrics and structural equation modeling. His publications span many disciplines and stand out against the backdrop of a career-long effort to infuse the study of biomedical scientific problems with the knowledge, theories and methods of social science.

Dr. Adam C. Carle is a clinically and quantitatively trained investigator. He is nationally recognized as an expert in pediatric patient reported outcomes and measurement. He uses structural equation models (SEM), multilevel models (MLM) and contemporary test theory (e.g. item response theory – IRT) to advance the methodological science used to measure health and health-related outcomes from the family and child's perspective, investigate the correlates of children and their families' well-being, and investigate and eliminate health disparities. Additionally, his work seeks to better understand individual and contextual variables' influences on health and health disparities at individual, local, system, state and national levels. He is a PI, Co-PI or Co-I on numerous federal grants and has served as a reviewer for federal granting agencies and national foundations. He has published more than 80 peer-reviewed manuscripts. Most important, he thinks his family is amazing (including the dogs and sheep).

Table of Greek Symbols

Name	Uppercase	Lowercase
alpha	A	α
beta	B	β
gamma	Γ	γ
delta	Δ	δ
epsilon	E	ε
zeta	Z	ζ
eta	H	η
theta	Θ	θ
iota	I	ι
kappa	K	κ
lambda	Λ	λ
mu	M	μ
nu	N	ν
xi	Ξ	ξ
omicron	O	o
pi	Π	π
rho	P	ρ
sigma	Σ	σ
tau	T	τ
upsilon	Υ	υ
phi	Φ	ϕ
chi	X	χ
psi	Ψ	ψ
omega	Ω	ω

Part I

Introduction to Concepts and Principles of Structural Equation Modeling for Health and Medical Research

1

Introduction and Brief History of Structural Equation Modeling for Health and Medical Research

1.1 An Overview of the Material in This Textbook

Structural equation modeling (SEM) has its roots in the social sciences [1]. In writing this textbook, we look to make SEM accessible to a wider audience of researchers across many disciplines, addressing issues unique to health and medicine. As SEM enthusiasts situated among clinicians and multidisciplinary researchers in medical settings we provide a broad, current, on the ground understanding of the issues faced by clinical and health services researchers and decision scientists.

For the past several years we have given short courses, written statistical tutorials and authored applied research articles in the field of SEM. We have noticed in feedback from students, readers and editors a serious gap in the medical and bioscientific literature that makes this type of book fundamental for the fields of SEM, medicine and public health. Readers will be introduced to a full range of SEM methods within the context of health and medicine. Prior knowledge of SEM is not required. Readers with an understanding of the fundamentals of traditional regression analysis will benefit from this book. More seasoned SEM researchers with a focus on health and medicine will also benefit from it for the particular applications to health and medical research.

We present an overview of SEM principles, common nomenclature, diagrams and many real-world examples. We also present some more advanced latent variable approaches applicable to health and medicine, such as modeling to establish measurement invariance, latent variable mixture modeling and latent growth curve modeling. These techniques are very useful with a wide range of practical applications. For example, we will cover how to use SEM with patient-reported outcomes (PROs) and clinician ratings scales as found in both clinical trial data and electronic health records. Readers of this book will be able to understand the theory behind SEM, understand modeling guidelines, interpret SEM analyses and understand advantages and limitations of SEM relative to more traditional analytic techniques.

In brief:

- The book covers basic, intermediate and advanced SEM topics.
- Applications are detailed and relevant for health and medical scientists.
- Topics and examples are relevant to both new SEM researchers as well as more seasoned SEM researchers.
- Substantive issues in health and medicine in the context of SEM are discussed.
- Chapters are referenced with both methodological and applied examples.
- Illustrative figures and diagrams are included for the examples used.

1.2 Introduction to Structural Equation Modeling

Defining *structural equation modeling* is a great task in itself. There is no straightforward manner for us to describe SEM to a novice user that will encompass all that it is or allow one to thoroughly understand what it does and does not do. Metaphorically speaking, we take the approach of immersing the reader in the water rather than merely getting their feet wet first. We provide here a broad view of SEM and focus on the big picture and then get more and more nuanced throughout the chapters in this textbook. In this context, this is likely the more comprehensible approach.

Let us begin our general description of SEM with a short segue for clarity to distinguish between "multivariable" and "multivariate" analysis. *Multivariable analysis* refers to statistical techniques used to evaluate multiple variables. *Multivariate analysis*, more specifically, refers to statistical techniques that can be used to evaluate multiple dependent variables simultaneously. "Multivariate" and "multivariable" analysis are somewhat synonymous terms (both types of analysis can include multiple dependent variables and multiple independent variables). However, the terminology "multivariable" is typically used in the context of a multiple regression model with a single dependent variable and multiple independent variables. Meanwhile, the terminology "multivariate" analysis is commonly used as defined for analysis with multiple dependent variables at the same time. With that explanation, we can now provide a broad definition of SEM.

Definition: SEM is a very general and flexible multivariate technique that allows relationships among variables to be examined.

Structural equation models (SEMs) are multi-equation models that commonly involve multiple dependent and independent variables. Variables may play the role of both a dependent and independent variable in different equations within a structural equation model (Chapter 2). In practical settings, SEM, among many applications, includes a diverse set of methods equipped to handle *measurement error* and evaluate the hypothesized causal relations among observed and unobserved variables [2]. SEM researchers must differentiate between observed and unobserved variables and understand the concept of measurement error.

Observed variables are variables which are measured and recorded in the data (e.g. sex, age, height and weight). Unobserved variables are variables that are not directly measured. Unobserved variables are also called *latent variables*, *latent traits* or *latent constructs*. Phenomena such as depression, intelligence, perceived pain and happiness may be treated as latent variables in research studies. In SEM, multiple observed variables are commonly used as surrogates of a latent variable(s). For example, responses to multiple observed items from a questionnaire about mental health (multiple observed variables) can be used to measure a hypothetical construct of mental health (unobserved variable).

Most typically and as theoretically appropriate, an SEM researcher hypothesizes that multiple observed items influence the manifestation of the latent variable(s) rather than the other way around. These causal assumptions will be elaborated on in an illustrative example in this chapter regarding a latent construct for pain behavior. Causal assumptions are strong assumptions. Given that one makes these assumptions about the hypothesized directionality between a set of observed items and latent variable(s), SEM uses the latent variable(s) to account for measurement error.

Measurement error is the difference between the underlying true values (e.g. mental health) and the actual values (e.g. a score based on responses to multiple items from a questionnaire about mental health). Observed measurements, being influenced by latent variables, have measurement error. Latent variables themselves do not have measurement error associated with them. Measurement error is accounted for in the model of relationships between a latent variable and its indicator variables. Refer to Chapter 2 for more details about different forms of measurement error.

We have now provided a very basic description of how one typically views a latent variable in SEM. As we have defined it, in summary, SEM is an approach that can model latent variables and then conduct multivariate regression of latent variables on each other (as well as observed variables).

1.2.1 Path Diagrams, Confirmatory Factor Analysis and Path Analysis

Latent variables are treated as continuous in what we shall refer to as conventional SEM (or what are sometimes called *first-generation SEM* [3,4]). Later we discuss *second-generation SEM* which includes more advanced, related techniques and uses a combination of continuous and categorical latent variables [3,4]. In this section, we fundamentally describe the methods included in conventional SEM as a basis.

One way SEM deals with continuous latent variables in practice is through *confirmatory factor analysis (CFA)*. *Factor analyses* are approaches to represent the relationships among multiple observed variables in terms of a smaller number of hypothesized latent variables. In the context of factor analysis, latent variables are commonly also referred to as *factors*. *Exploratory factor analysis (EFA)* is a data-driven method used to help identify the underlying latent variable or variables from a set of observed variables. CFA is used to verify hypothesized relationships between the latent variables and the set of observed variables. EFA can also be viewed as a special case of CFA and vice versa. Both EFA and CFA employ the same common mathematical model under different constraints (Chapter 8).

Exploratory data analysis, such as EFA, is data-driven, while confirmatory data analysis, such as CFA, is hypothesis-driven (relies on a priori hypothesis). In connection, EFA can be used to help determine the number of factors to retain and then CFA can be used to evaluate prespecified relationships between factors and their indicators. These techniques (EFA and CFA) can be successively applied on the same set of indicators in different data (to prevent overfitting of the CFA model). We will introduce latent variables and factor analysis in some more detail in Chapter 2 and then dedicate full chapters to CFA and EFA (Chapters 7 and 8) in the context of health and medicine.

Full SEM [5] emphasizes not just the measuring of continuous latent variables but the regression of these latent variables on each other. The term "full" is used in the sense that in the hypothesized model every observed variable is an indicator of a latent variable and every variable in the regression analysis is a latent variable. Hypothesized relationships amongst latent and observed variables in a structural equation model can be illustrated with a *path diagram*. A path diagram is a visualization of the *conceptual model*. A conceptual model is a general idea of the relationships under study. Another way to think about the distinction is that path diagrams are usually a reduction or elaboration of a conceptual model to something that can be both represented and tested in the SEM framework. We will construct path diagrams for illustrative examples later in this chapter.

Path diagrams can be used to represent full SEMs. Path diagrams can also be used to represent many special cases of SEMs that are not full including a CFA model or a hypothesized structural equation model in which only observed variables are examined. *Path analysis* is a form of regression and multivariate statistical analysis most often used to evaluate hypothesized causal relationships between observed variables. The SEM framework links together conceptual models, path diagrams, CFA and path analysis.

1.2.2 How Do Classic Approaches to SEM Analysis Work?

A researcher may theorize a causal model making use of strong causal assumptions. In the process of *model specification,* a researcher translates the conceptual model into a formal structural equation model and indicates causal paths and directionality between variables (latent or observed) under study. The plausibility of the hypothesized model under the model specification can be tested using observed data in the SEM framework. Much emphasis is given in SEM to examining the fit of the model to the data.

There is no statistical methodology in and of itself that can uncover casual relationships among variables. The classic approaches to SEM analysis use the covariance matrix of the data to estimate the *free parameters* (e.g. causal path estimates) in a hypothesized model under the model specification. A free parameter is unknown and of interest to estimate. Thus, free parameters are also referred to as *unknown parameters.*

Essentially, the researcher can either supply the raw data itself or covariance matrix data in available software for conducting these classic approaches to SEM analysis. SEM then estimates the unknown parameters with the aim of most closely reproducing the covariance matrix. Additionally, a researcher can analyze means in SEM. We will provide details regarding model estimation in Chapter 4.

A full structural equation model consists of two models [6–8]. These two models are the *measurement model* (i.e. CFA) that measures latent variables using multiple observed variables and a *structural model* (i.e. path analysis incorporating latent variables) that evaluates the relationships between latent variables. Each regression equation in the structural model has an error term referred to as a *disturbance term.* Disturbance terms reflect the residual error in regressing an outcome variable on a predictor (or set of predictors).

In a full structural equation model every variable in the structural model is latent. Most typically in our own health and medical research a structural equation model is not full, but still consists of a measurement and structural model. That is, we use a structural model in which at least one of the variables is latent and at least one of the variables is observed [9]. Many different models are also a special case of a structural equation model (e.g. linear regression, ANOVA, CFA and path analysis).

We discuss in more detail the basic vocabulary, history, concepts and usages of SEM for health and medicine in these first two chapters of this textbook to help clarify this broad description of SEM. In Part II of this book we provide more technical details that allow the reader to represent and evaluate a structural equation model. In Part III, we build off these fundamentals to apply both first- and second-generation SEM to address problems in health and medicine.

1.2.3 First- and Second-Generation SEM

Some researchers (possibly unintentionally) will use the term SEM as an umbrella term for an extensive list of techniques involving latent variables. Other researchers prefer to distinguish between SEM as it was originally developed and the larger set of latent variable models that now coexist with SEM. In this setting, first-generation SEM applies to continuous latent variables. However, different approaches described later in this textbook will use continuous latent variables (e.g. CFA), categorical latent variables (e.g. latent class analysis and latent profile analysis) or both (e.g. growth mixture modeling). Second-generation SEM uses a combination of continuous *and* categorical latent variables [3]. Second-generation SEM is an expansion of the capacity of first-generation SEM [10]. If the first- and second-generation distinction and the particular methods mentioned are not clear as of yet, these nuances and approaches will become more evident throughout this textbook.

There are many other extensions of SEM that were developed during the first- and second-generations of SEM. SEM was originally derived to only consider continuous observed variables. We will present many applications of SEM with ordered-categorical observed variables and/or missing data. Applications of SEM can also involve other types of data such as count and survival time data. SEM has been extended for analysis with these other types of variables and data. Applications of SEM can involve either cross-sectional or longitudinal data. For example, latent growth curve modeling (Chapter 13) is an application of CFA for longitudinal data. Multilevel modeling (Chapter 13) and multi-group analysis (Chapters 9 and 10) have also been integrated for use with SEM. Further, Bayesian approaches have been adapted for SEM in parallel with the development of the first- and second-generation of SEM [4].

Beyond just using the methods in a straightforward manner, one has the opportunity to extend these methods and flexibly and creatively apply them to address specific research questions. For example, in applying latent growth curve modeling, one can analyze the antecedents and consequences of change, higher-order models and multiple growth trajectories related to each other. *We will use the term SEM hereafter in this textbook, unless denoting otherwise, as an umbrella term in reference to these extensions and first- and second-generation SEM.*

One necessitates a very broad framework to represent and flexibly and creatively apply the different latent variable methods commonly used in studies in health and medicine. These approaches (e.g. conventional linear SEM, conventional SEM with nonmetric data, factor analysis, latent class analysis, growth mixture modeling) can be described as belonging to a family of statistical techniques referred to as *general latent variable modeling (GLVM)*. When one defines SEM as broadly as we have in this textbook, the terminology GLVM and SEM can be viewed as synonymous. GLVM is a unified latent variable framework that uses a combination of continuous and categorical latent variables for statistical analysis [11]. The vision of GLVM is to provide a unified an organized set of tools for conducting many different types of statistical analysis. The interested reader should refer to Muthén [11] for an introduction to GVLM.

SEM techniques have many advantages in practice including:

- acknowledging and modeling forms of measurement error;
- modeling of hypothesized causal relationships for analyses of direct and indirect effects;
- modeling latent variable relationships;
- evaluating multiple equation models in a single analysis;
- flexible techniques for model selection and comparison;
- evaluating measurement equivalence in scales based on group differences by variables such as sex, race/ethnicity, age, area-level deprivation, language and cross-cultural factors;
- flexible techniques for understanding longitudinal relationships and subpopulation structures.

These advantages are well-suited to address research questions and theory development in the medical and health sciences.

1.3 Introduction to Causal Assumptions and Path Diagrams

Researchers using SEM for the purpose of evaluating causal relationships among latent and observed variables make strong causal assumptions. Causality is a much stronger assumption and more difficult to support than association. To illustrate this point, we lead the reader through an example in Figure 1.1.

Here we present a simplified, hypothesized model of how disease duration presumably affects pain behavior in people with rheumatoid arthritis. Pain behavior encompasses behaviors that commonly suggest to others that an individual is experiencing pain [12]. In the model, we implement the hypothesis that in people with rheumatoid arthritis, a longer disease duration leads to an increase in pain behavior via an increase in inflammation. The amount of inflammation present can be measured by the erythrocyte sedimentation rate.

Figure 1.1 consists of two path diagrams (A and B) to illustrate the hypothesized relationships between variables. Recall, path diagrams are commonly used to visualize a conceptual model and represent a structural equation model. Observed variables are represented by squares/rectangles and latent variables by circles/ovals.

We depict in Figure 1.1a a latent pain behavior variable as the underlying cause of four observed indicators of pain behavior describing level of movement, facial expressions, protected body and stopped activity. Figure 1.1b shows the hypothesized cause and effect relationships between disease duration (an observed variable), inflammation (an observed variable) and pain behavior (a latent variable). Figure 1.1a is a representation of a measurement model, and Figure 1.1b is a representation of a structural model.

The type of model hypothesizing cause and effect relationships among variables relies on strong causal assumptions that a researcher must make a priori. The researcher ideally makes these causal assumptions based on logic, theory and prior knowledge before performing empirical analyses. Between any two measures, causal assumptions imply both cause and effect and temporal order. A predictor occurs first in time and

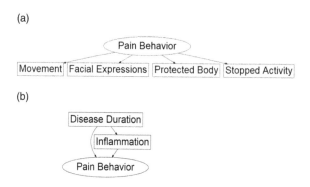

FIGURE 1.1
Path diagrams representing hypothesized model in people with rheumatoid arthritis. (a) Hypothesized latent variable for *pain behavior* and (b) Hypothesized causal relationships.

Disease duration and inflammation are observed variables while pain behavior is a latent variable. The amount of inflammation present can be measured by the erythrocyte sedimentation rate. Pain behavior is hypothesized as the underlying cause of observed indicators describing the level of movement (moved slower), facial expressions, protected body (protected the part of the body that was hurt) and stopped activity.

is hypothesized to be the cause of an outcome that occurs subsequently in time and is the effect.

Figure 1.1 provides a causal assumption every time an arrow points from one variable (the cause) in the direction of another variable (the effect). One in general assumes for any one-way arrow; the variable at the end of the arrow is explained in terms of the variable at the beginning of the arrow. For example, we are making a causal assumption about the relationship between disease duration, the cause, and inflammation, the effect. Thus this model has been specified to assume that a longer disease duration leads to an increase in inflammation. We could also make a temporal assumption: first the participant had the disease and then as time progresses the participant experiences an increase in inflammation. Since the relationship between disease duration and inflammation is just one causal path in our hypothesized model, we make a causal assumption in every causal path, seven total, in Figure 1.1. Note that a two-way arrow (instead of a one-way arrow) is used on a path diagram when one assumes association or correlation between two variables.

Philosophically, making causal assumptions may be viewed as an idealized process that is never quite obtainable in practice. In health and medicine as in other sciences, causal considerations nearly always depend on context. Thus, a causal assumption in one setting does not necessarily hold in other settings. For example, a causal assumption in a basic science application may involve a simple linear relationship between cause and effect, while in an epidemiological context the same assumption may involve a host, an environment and an organism as contributors to causation and be interactive and nonlinear. In practice, researchers rarely expect to observe the "true" relationships between causes and effects. There may be a single cause or there may be multiple causes, each partially influencing the effect of interest.

1.3.1 A Note about Error Terms in Path Diagrams

We did not explicitly show any error terms (i.e. measurement error and disturbance terms) in the path diagrams in Figure 1.1. In Figure 1.1, there is measurement error associated with every observed indicator (movement, facial expressions, protected body, stopped activity) of the latent variable of pain behavior. Disturbance terms are associated with inflammation and pain behavior in the structural model. Error terms are implicit in the path diagrams in this chapter. We will explicitly show error terms in the path diagrams in Chapter 2 as we provide more details about measurement error and the symbols commonly used in SEM research.

1.3.2 Path Analysis Model

In Figure 1.1, we represented using a path diagram a measurement model and a structural model with both observed and latent variables. We represent a path analysis model in the path diagram in Figure 1.2. All variables are observed.

We hypothesize increased intensity of current smoking and sugar consumption cause a spike in the inflammatory marker C-reactive protein (CRP). Elevated CRP levels are then hypothesized to lead to an increase in the number of hospitalizations. Further, increased intensity of current smoking and sugar consumption are hypothesized to lead to an increase in the number of hospitalizations. We again make strong causal assumptions for every causal pathway specified in Figure 1.2. An implicit assumption we made in Figure 1.2 is that there is no relationship between current

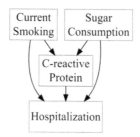

FIGURE 1.2
Path analysis model for hospitalization example.

smoking and sugar consumption (i.e. there is no arrow linking current smoking and sugar consumption).

1.3.3 Full Structural Equation Model

In Figure 1.3, we represent a full structural equation model in the path diagram.

In the measurement model, hypothesized relationships are examined between latent variables for emotional intelligence, career adaptability and happiness and their associated observed items. In the structural model, hypothesized relationships between the three latent variables are evaluated. Once again, we make strong causal assumptions in the model represented in Figure 1.3.

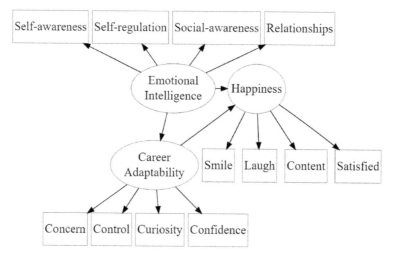

FIGURE 1.3
Full structural equation model for happiness example.

Emotional intelligence, career adaptability and happiness are latent variables. Emotional intelligence is hypothesized as the underlying, or latent, cause of scores on observed indicators for self-awareness, self-regulation, social-awareness and success in relationships. Career adaptability is hypothesized as the underlying cause of scores on career concern, control, curiosity and confidence. This latent variable of career adaptability was adapted from Nilforooshan, P. and S. Salimi, Career adaptability as a mediator between personality and career engagement. *Journal of Vocational Behavior*, 2016. 94: pp. 1–10. Happiness is hypothesized as the underlying cause of scores on observed indicators for smile, laugh, content and satisfied.

1.4 Brief History of SEM

Figures 1.1 involves two components in the measurement and structural models. In one component (A), we use multiple indicators to measure a continuous latent variable. In the other component (B), we model hypothesized causal relationships among latent and observed variables. These two main components of the conventional SEM framework have origins, respectively, within factor analysis and path analysis (see Box 1.1).

Following these origins, SEM has grown due to social scientists and other academics looking to understand the structure of latent phenomena and relationships among latent and observed phenomena [1]. As latent variable models have become more complex, the advancement of latent variable software has played a prominent role in the accessibility of SEM.

The first widely distributed latent variable software was LISREL (linear structural relations; Scientific Software International, Inc., Skokie, IL, USA) and was developed by Karl Jöreskog in the 1970s [6,8]. Other specialized software came about in the 1980s such as EQS (Multivariate Software, Inc., Encino, CA, USA) [15] and LISCOMP, which was later developed into MPlus [16].

As SEM has become more widely used, many more specialized packages have been developed such as AMOS [17], in addition to the availability of procedures for fitting SEM in general-purpose statistical packages such as R (i.e. LAVAAN, OpenMX), SAS (i.e. PROC CALIS), STATA and Statistica. Many of these software packages are versatile modeling packages which extend the basic SEM framework to include new types of observed and unobserved traits, such as categorical traits and time to event traits, and include many different model estimation methods. Another feature of some of these packages is the ability to draw a model to run analysis (AMOS is notable in this regard) rather than write programming syntax.

Kline [9] has written an influential introductory text on the topic of SEM, accessible to applied researchers. Bollen [7] provides a comprehensive and thorough overview of the theoretical underpinnings of SEM. Bollen [7] describes general structure equation systems, commonly known as the LISREL model as developed by Jöreskog [4]. Brown [18] has provided an in-depth introduction of CFA. Brown describes the theoretical

BOX 1.1

ORIGIN OF FACTOR ANALYSIS

Charles Spearman [13] is credited with constructing the first factor model, which laid the foundations for measuring latent variables within the SEM framework [1]. In his work he proposed a general ability factor, which he called g, that influences the performance on disparate cognitive ability measures [1].

ORIGIN OF PATH ANALYSIS (AND PATH DIAGRAMS)

Sewell Wright [14], a geneticist, was the originator of path analysis. In his work, he laid out an analytical strategy for imposing a causal structure for describing causal relationships between measures [1]. He developed path diagrams to graphically depict the relationships between measures in these types of analyses [1].

framework used for CFA while providing many timely, illustrative examples. In SEM computing, Byrne [5,17–21] has provided useful resources for researchers for using SEM in MPlus, EQS (Multivariate Software, Inc., Encino, CA, USA), LISREL, PRELIS (Scientific Software International), SIMPLIS (SIMPLIS Technologies, Inc., Portland, OR, USA) and AMOS (IBM Corporation, Armonk, NY, USA). Further, the MPlus website, Statmodel.com [16] is filled with manuals and examples to assist an applied researcher in conducting SEM analysis.

1.5 Health and Medical Research Studies

In this section, we will briefly provide an overview of the different types of research studies using participants in health and medicine. Then, we go on to describe more generally the foundation of SEM in health and medicine.

In a research study in health and medicine, a common objective is to acquire information that helps support or disprove a hypothesis. We describe three common types of studies in health and medicine: *experimental, non-experimental (observational)* and *quasi-experimental*. The type of study, as we will explain, determines the structure in which a researcher approaches this objective.

In conducting *experimental research*, the researcher maintains control over the environment (i.e. design and setting of the study) and is able to manipulate the boundaries on the primary independent variable. Experimental research is performed prospectively, and an intervention is tested in a regulated environment. For example, in a randomized, controlled clinical trial of a new sodium chloride tablet for patients with low sodium level, each patient is randomly assigned to receive the tablet or a placebo (a binary independent variable). The patients could be randomized into the treatment arm using stratification or minimization as well as a block design. As a result of the study design (and given a large enough sample), potential confounders such as age, gender and race should be approximately evenly distributed at least in theory between tablet and placebo group.

In *non-experimental (observational) research* (e.g. case-control studies, cohort studies), the researcher has limited to no control over the study environment and variables under study. This research can be conducted retrospectively or prospectively from an existing database.

A *quasi-experimental* study typically involves intervention research or the collection of multiple measures prospectively, but study participants are not randomly assigned. Survey studies or clinical research studies with treatment and control groups but no randomization (non-equivalent groups) could be categorized as a quasi-experiment. We summarize these three main types of studies in Table 1.1.

TABLE 1.1

Common Types of Research Studies in Health and Medicine

Study Type	Experimental	Quasi-experimental	Observational
Boundaries/limits	Control of environment and random assignment to intervention or control	No random assignment to intervention or control	Limited to no control over environment or variables
Examples	Randomized controlled trial	Survey research, non-equivalent group research	Cohort study, case-control study

Under ideal circumstances, experimental research might allow a researcher to draw cause and effect conclusions. Based on our prior example for experimental research, given strong background knowledge and study results, we might be comfortable stating that these sodium chloride tablets lead to higher levels of sodium in the population under study.

Experimental designs often entail high costs to implement for researcher and participant time and lab facilities. This often limits the number of participants enrolled in an experimental study. Finding eligible participants meeting inclusion criteria can also be difficult. Further, with limited resources and imperfect knowledge, collecting information about all study confounders and maintaining total control over study conditions are rarely feasible in practice. Under these limitations, researchers using an experimental design in practice are often limited in their ability to draw conclusions about causality.

In observational research (and quasi-experiments), multiple strategies are available that attempt to mitigate the bias of the non-random sample in a comparison study. For example, propensity matching [22], an approach to balance treatment and control group observations across covariates, can be used for this purpose. Observational studies, due to the high possibility of confounding, often have poor internal validity. Similarly, due to possible confounding and lack of control over the study conditions, researchers conducting observational studies must confront challenges in establishing causality and poor external validity.

1.5.1 SEM in Health and Medicine

Causality assumptions are made by a researcher through a synthesis of logic, theory and prior knowledge. Causal relationships among latent and observed variables can therefore be conceptually hypothesized with clinical expert judgment. Experimental, quasi-experimental and observational studies can all make use of SEM analyses.

Traditionally, in health and medicine, SEM researchers have used survey data or randomized trial data for measuring latent variables and evaluating causal relationships among the latent and observed variables under study. Clinical trial data has given rise to *mediation* studies using SEM. In mediation, we consider an intermediate variable, called the *mediator*, that helps explain how or why an independent variable influences an outcome [7,9,23–25]. Mediation can further our understanding of the pathology of a disease and the workings behind an effective treatment. Mediation studies may also help us identify alternative, more efficient intervention strategies. In the protocol of a RCT, mediation is often a secondary aim. As a result, a common limitation of mediation studies in this context is that RCTs are randomized for the intervention, but not for the levels of the mediator in each treatment arm.

Health services researchers have increasingly seen the potential for using SEM for observational studies of large existing electronic registries and cohort studies. Technology has evolved to where many hospitals and institutions routinely collect clinical information on large and diverse populations. These observational databases hold important advantages to decision scientists in the availability of big data with extensive demographic and clinical information on a diverse range of patients. Many such large retrospective cohort studies do not involve hypotheses revolving around any intervention. Instead, these types of studies evaluate complex relationships between clinical factors, sociodemographic characteristics, disease states and health outcomes for a population under study.

In Figure 1.4, a path diagram depicts a web of observed and unobserved variables for the relationship between risk factors (heath-related and demographic variables and social determinants) and cardiovascular events. This complex model involves many hypothesized causal relations, each of which should be supported by sound logic, theory and prior evidence, as well as other statistical considerations. Competent scientists could disagree about which paths should be included, and how the model should be specified. In this respect, SEM can be seen as creating a practical scientific dialogue that engages researchers in processes of specifying and testing models. Models like the one shown in Figure 1.4 are not intended to intimidate a novice SEM researcher. This is an advanced example for learning to apply SEM to complex problems in health and medicine. In this book, we work our way through a series of smaller examples intended to launch readers into investigating ever more complex and interesting questions and relationships.

It is important to recognize that there are many applications of SEM that do not involve performing regression to evaluate hypothesized causal relationships in confirmatory data analysis. Exploratory factor analysis (Chapter 8) and latent class analysis (Chapter 11) are both techniques commonly used in health and medicine for more exploratory data analysis. Many researchers also use SEM to revise a model. That is, they use quantitative and subjective criteria to test an initial specified model against alternative modified models with the intentions of developing the "best" model for the data (Chapter 6). Hypothesized associations are also commonly evaluated using SEM.

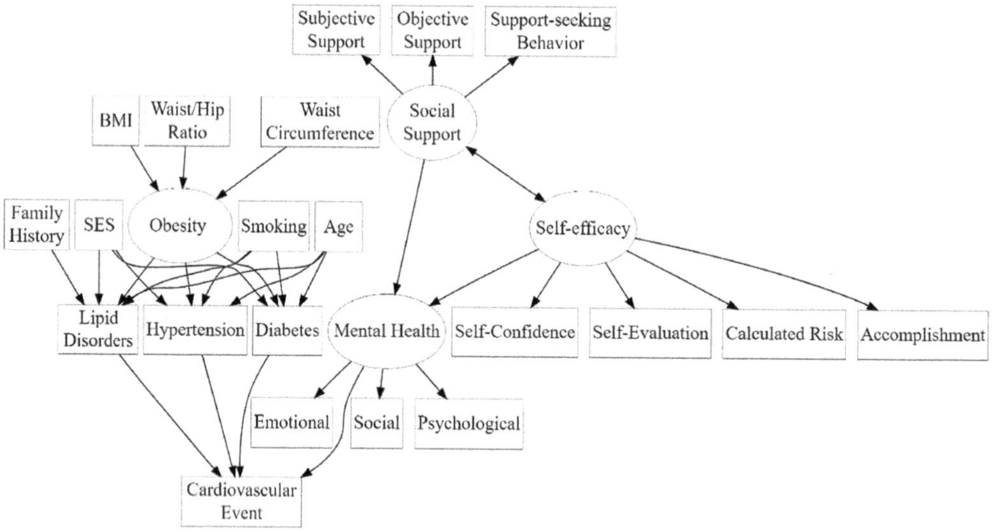

FIGURE 1.4
Hypothesized relationships between risk factors and cardiovascular event.

Obesity, mental health, social support and *self-efficacy* are latent variables. *Mental health* is hypothesized as the underlying, or latent, cause of scores on observed indicators for emotional, psychological and social well-being. *Social support* is hypothesized as the underlying cause of scores on objective support, subjective support and support-seeking behavior. These three domains can be measured using the Social Support Self-Rating Scale developed by Xiao (Reference: Xiao, S., The theoretical basis and research applications of "Social Support Rating Scale". *Journal of Clinical Psychiatry*, 1994. 4(2): pp. 98–100). *Self-efficacy* is hypothesized as the underlying cause of scores on observed indicators for self-confidence, accuracy of self-evaluation, taking calculated risks and accomplishment. Here, *obesity* is hypothesized as the underlying, or latent, effect of scores on observed indicators of waist circumference, waist/hip ratio and body mass index (BMI). We have not specified all potential paths of interest, including correlations, in this diagram due to visual complexity. For example, in practice many implied pairwise correlations would be reasonable like SES and smoking. SES, socioeconomic status.

Conducting analyses of SEMs in health and medicine often does not go strictly according to "rules of thumb" or follow linearly from "textbook" examples. The researcher should carefully take account of prior expert knowledge, make reasonable assumptions, weigh in on oftentimes conflicting empirical evidence from multiple tests and indices, and draw reasonable conclusions. Throughout this book, we describe examples and the SEM decision-making involved in this type of research.

1.5.2 A Contrarian View of SEMs: Can Causal Claims Be Justified When Using SEM Approaches?

We have explicitly stated that researchers necessitate strong, a priori theories to substantiate causal relations. We have mentioned that the classic approaches to SEM analysis use the covariance matrix of the data to estimate the unknown parameters (e.g. causal path estimates) in a model. A criticism of SEM that it cannot avoid is that some claim the sample covariance matrix may not be a sufficient statistic to capture causal relations. There is nothing magical about the multivariate statistical techniques used in SEM that allow one to evaluate causal relations. Carefully reasoned, referenced and tested assumptions are necessary foundations for hypotheses and theories of causality. Aforementioned, one does not have to make causal assumptions when using SEM. One can make assumptions about associative relationships. Even for the SEM contrarian, the statistical techniques used in the SEM framework can be used for a wide range of univariate and multivariate analysis tasks.

1.6 Conclusions

In this chapter, we provided an overview of the material covered in this book. Briefly, we defined and described SEM and the components of SEM. The strong implications when one makes causal assumption were stressed in this chapter. We discussed the roots and history of SEM including the history of latent variable software and recommendations of classic introductory textbooks depending on the needs of a reader. We provided a background of three common types of health and medical studies, experimental, observational and quasi-experimental, and a foundation for the use of SEM in health and medicine.

References

1. Tarka, P., An overview of structural equation modeling: Its beginnings, historical development, usefulness and controversies in the social sciences. *Quality and Quantity*, 2017. **52**(1): pp. 1–42.
2. Bollen, K.A. and M.D. Noble, Structural equation models and the quantification of behavior. *Proceedings of the National Academy of Sciences*, 2011. **108**(Supplement 3): pp. 15639–15646.
3. Muthén, B., Second-generation structural equation modeling with a combination of categorical and continuous latent variables: New opportunities for latent class–latent growth modeling. 2001.
4. Kaplan, D. and S. Depaoli, Bayesian structural equation modeling, in Handbook of structural equation modeling, R.H. Hoyle, Editor. 2012, New York: The Guilford Press, pp. 650–673.

5. Byrne, B.M., *Structural equation modeling with Mplus: Basic concepts, applications, and programming*. 2013, Abingdon: Routledge.
6. Joreskog, K. and D. Sorbom, *LISREL 8 user's reference guide*. 1996, Chicago, IL: Scientific Software Chicago.
7. Bollen, K., *Structural equations with latent variables*. 1989, New York: Wiley.
8. Jöreskog, K.G. and M. Thiilo, Lisrel: A general computer program for estimating a linear structural equation system involving multiple indicators of unmeasured variables. ETS Research Report Series, 1972.
9. Kline, R.B., *Principles and practice of structural equation modeling, fourth edition*. 2016, New York: Guilford Press.
10. Fan, Y., et al., Applications of structural equation modeling (SEM) in ecological studies: An updated review. *Ecological Processes*, 2016. **5**(1): p. 19.
11. Muthén, B.O., Beyond SEM: General latent variable modeling. *Behaviormetrika*, 2002. **29**(1): pp. 81–117.
12. Cunningham, N.R., et al., Development and validation of the self-reported PROMIS pediatric pain behavior item bank and short form scale. *Pain*, 2017. **158**(7): p. 1323.
13. Spearman, C., "General Intelligence," objectively determined and measured. *The American Journal of Psychology*, 1904. **15**(2): pp. 201–292.
14. Wright, S., Correlation and causation. *Journal of Agricultural Research*, 1921. **20**(7): pp. 557–585.
15. Bentler, P.M., *EQS structural equations program manual*, 1989. Los Angeles, CA: BMDP Statistical Software Pages.
16. Muthén, L.K. and B.O. Muthén, *Mplus: The comprehensive modeling program for applied researchers: User's guide*. Eighth edition. 1998–2017, Los Angeles, CA: Muthén & Muthén.
17. Arbuckle, J., *Amos 6.0 user's guide*. 2005, Chicago, IL: Marketing Department, SPSS Incorporated.
18. Brown, T.A., *Confirmatory factor analysis for applied research*. 2014, New York: Guilford Publications.
19. Byrne, B.M., *Structural equation modeling with AMOS: Basic concepts, applications, and programming*. 2013, Abingdon: Routledge.
20. Byrne, B.M., *Structural equation modeling with EQS: Basic concepts, applications, and programming*. 2013, Abingdon: Routledge.
21. Byrne, B.M., *Structural equation modeling with LISREL, PRELIS, and SIMPLIS: Basic concepts, applications, and programming*. 2013, Hove: Psychology Press.
22. Rosenbaum, P.R. and D.B. Rubin, The central role of the propensity score in observational studies for causal effects. *Biometrika*, 1983. **70**(1): pp. 41–55.
23. Gunzler, D., et al., Introduction to mediation analysis with structural equation modeling. *Shanghai Archives of Psychiatry*, 2013. **25**(6): pp. 390–394.
24. Baron, R.M. and D.A. Kenny, The moderator–mediator variable distinction in social psychological research: Conceptual, strategic, and statistical considerations. *Journal of Personality and Social Psychology*, 1986. **51**(6): p. 1173.
25. MacKinnon, D., *Introduction to statistical mediation analysis*. 2012, Abingdon: Routledge.

2

Vocabulary, Concepts and Usages of Structural Equation Modeling

2.1 Introduction to the Vocabulary, Concepts and Usages of Structural Equation Modeling

We view conventional SEM as a framework consisting of three core components: *conceptual model*, *path diagram* and *system of linked regression-type equations* to capture the relationships among observed and unobserved variables [1,2]. We will present these three core components in an illustrative example below. However, before discussing the form of conventional SEMs in technical detail (i.e. path diagrams and mathematical representation of SEMs) (Chapter 3), we introduce vocabulary, concepts and usages of SEM in this chapter.

In Figure 2.1, we hypothesize in a conceptual model the manner in which a wellness program lowers anxiety and body mass index (BMI) based on prior scientific knowledge.

In the example in Figure 2.1, the conceptual model, path diagram and mathematical equations interrelate for evaluating a wellness program in study participants. The mathematical equations in SEM can also be referred to as *structural equations*.

Traditional regression models, conducted sequentially, allow for testing associations between the wellness program and different outcomes. However, the SEM approach is used since (1) we are interested in examining *both if and how this program works* and (2) our analyses involve a latent variable *anxiety*. Conclusions drawn from the results of the more nuanced SEMs could have broad implications for refining the program and/or implementing the program in different settings.

We are interested in evaluating hypothesized causal relationships in our model corresponding to Figure 2.1. These causal paths were hypothesized via logic, theory and prior evidence. For some associated or correlated measures, we may not make causal assumptions. In our example, calorie intake and weekly exercise are not specified as causally related. We hypothesize that they are associated.

One consequence of the nature of hypothesized causal relationships in the SEM framework is that a single variable can act as both a cause and an effect. For example, in Figure 2.1, *calorie intake* and *weekly exercise* are both causes of *anxiety* and *BMI*. *Calorie intake* and *weekly exercise* are also both effects in relation to the *wellness program*. Standard statistical language to describe a variable as solely an independent or dependent variable is inadequate. *Calorie intake* and *weekly exercise* are both independent variables in relation to *anxiety* and *BMI* and dependent variables in relation to *wellness program*. In SEM, variables may be divided into two classes: *exogenous* and *endogenous* [1].

Endogenous variables act as a dependent variable in at least one of the equations in a structural equation model, while exogenous variables are always independent variables.

<u>**Conceptual Model**</u>
A researcher runs a year long randomized controlled trial to study the effect of a wellness program given to participants with a high level of anxiety and a high body mass index (BMI). The program is hypothesized to work by decreasing the number of calories a participant consumes as well as increasing the weekly time a participant spends on physical exercise, which will lead to lower anxiety and BMI. The number of calories a participant consumes is hypothesized to be associated with weekly time a participant spends on physical exercise.

<u>**Path Diagram to Represent the Conceptual Model**</u>

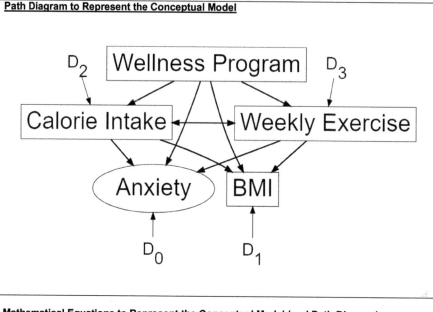

<u>**Mathematical Equations to Represent the Conceptual Model (and Path Diagram)**</u>

Anxiety $= \alpha_0 + \beta_1 Weekly\ Exercise + \beta_2 Calorie\ Intake + \gamma_1 Wellness\ Program + D_0$,

BMI $= \alpha_1 + \beta_3 Weekly\ Exercise + \beta_4 Calorie\ Intake + \gamma_2 Wellness\ Program + D_1$,

Calorie Intake $= \alpha_2 + \gamma_3 Wellness\ Program + D_2$,

Weekly Exercise $= \alpha_3 + \gamma_4 Wellness\ Program + D_3$

FIGURE 2.1
Model of wellness program.

The covariance between calorie intake and weekly exercise is represented in the model-implied covariance matrix and does not appear in the mathematical equations in this figure. See Chapter 4 for more details about the model-implied covariance matrix. In this figure we have omitted the measurement model (model of the influence of *anxiety* on the observed indicators of *anxiety*) and focused on the structural model. While left out of the model, a covariance between *anxiety* and BMI might be theoretically reasonable and could potentially be added at the discretion of a research team. See Chapter 3 for more details regarding the mathematical equations. Briefly, here $\alpha_0, \alpha_1, \alpha_2$ and α_3 are intercepts, $\beta_1, \beta_2, \beta_3$ and β_4 are slopes relating endogenous variables to each other, and $\gamma_1, \gamma_2, \gamma_3$ and γ_4 are slopes relating the endogenous variables to the sole exogenous variable (*wellness program*). D_0, D_1, D_2 and D_3 are error terms.

In other words, an endogenous variable is an effect in relation to at least one other variable, while an exogenous variable is always the cause and never an effect. Another way to phrase this is that the values of exogenous variables are determined by things outside/not within the model, whereas the values of endogenous variables are determined by things within the model. In Figure 2.1, *anxiety, BMI, calorie intake* and *weekly exercise* are all endogenous variables while *wellness program* is an exogenous variable. In the path diagram in Figure 2.1, the sole exogenous variable is the variable with no arrows pointing into it, and thus, its variation is not explained by other variables in the model.

Researchers commonly use simple sets of symbols from SEM notation to translate a conceptual model into a path diagram (as in Figure 2.1). Table 2.1 displays some of the most commonly used symbols and vocabulary, as well as the meaning, for researchers using SEM. We will use these symbols and vocabulary throughout this book.

The reader should take Table 2.1 with some flexibility. Throughout the SEM literature, there are sometimes variations in the general nomenclature.

TABLE 2.1

Commonly Used Symbols and Vocabulary for SEM Researchers

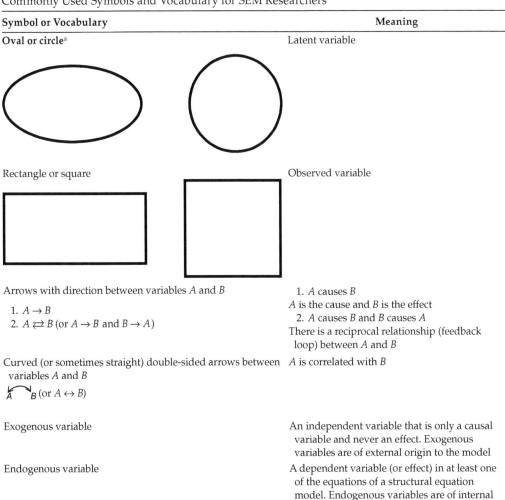

Symbol or Vocabulary	Meaning
Oval or circle[a]	Latent variable
Rectangle or square	Observed variable
Arrows with direction between variables *A* and *B* 1. $A \rightarrow B$ 2. $A \rightleftarrows B$ (or $A \rightarrow B$ and $B \rightarrow A$)	1. *A* causes *B* *A* is the cause and *B* is the effect 2. *A* causes *B* and *B* causes *A* There is a reciprocal relationship (feedback loop) between *A* and *B*
Curved (or sometimes straight) double-sided arrows between variables *A* and *B* A ⌒ B (or $A \leftrightarrow B$)	*A* is correlated with *B*
Exogenous variable	An independent variable that is only a causal variable and never an effect. Exogenous variables are of external origin to the model
Endogenous variable	A dependent variable (or effect) in at least one of the equations of a structural equation model. Endogenous variables are of internal origin to the model

(Continued)

TABLE 2.1 (*Continued*)

Commonly Used Symbols and Vocabulary for SEM Researchers

Symbol or Vocabulary	Meaning
Measurement model	The measurement model explicitly models the relationship between latent variables and the directly observed variables that reflect or form the underlying constructs
Structural model	The structural model explicitly models the hypothesized causal relationships among endogenous and exogenous variables
e or more formally ε or δ	"e" is used as the symbol for measurement error. Measurement error is the difference between an observed value and the true value. Latent variables measure the true concept by handling the measurement error in the observed items in the measurement model
D or more formally ζ	"D" is the symbol used for a disturbance term. A disturbance term is an unobservable (latent) variable that is the residual error from regressing an outcome on a predictor (or predictors) in a structural model

[a] Measurement error and disturbance terms are also sometimes displayed in small circles.

2.2 Latent Variables

Directly observable phenomena, such as height or weight, are routinely captured by a single measure. Measurable (directly observed) variables are also called *manifest variables*. Researchers may not have a single observed measure that adequately describes phenomena such as depression, pain behavior, happiness or anxiety. Multiple measures are often used to obtain reliable estimates, particularly for self-report or rater administered survey questionnaires. Medical researchers and practitioners alike need reliable and valid measures in order to understand symptoms, conditions and other clinically relevant measures that cannot be quantified directly. Variables that are not directly observed are considered *latent variables* and are also regularly labeled *latent traits* and/or *latent constructs*. Latent variable analyses can be useful for assessing the measurement properties of clinical screening, assessment and symptom scales.

A primary usage of latent variables is for representing a common factor reflected by multiple indicators (i.e. items). To measure a latent variable, one can use indicators on a multiple-item scale that presumably measure(s) the underlying variable. Responses to these items are directly observed and may provide a reasonable estimate of the underlying variable. *Measurement error* contained in the observed responses must also be accounted for in order to more accurately represent the relationship between the latent construct and observed responses. In this setting, measurement error is the difference between the observed value and the true value. In Figure 2.2, we illustrate that the nine items of the PHQ-9 may provide a reasonable estimate of an underlying latent variable of depression [1–4].

Since latent variables are unobserved, they do not have a natural metric or measurement scale. For this reason, this metric must be assigned to them. Assigning a metric also contributes to resolving a problem of lack of model identification. The metric can be set by

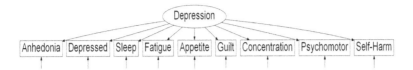

FIGURE 2.2
Latent construct of depression using the items of the patient health questionnaire (PHQ)-9.

Depression is hypothesized as the underlying cause of nine observed items describing symptoms of anhedonia, depressed mood, sleep disturbance, fatigue, appetite changes, feelings of worthlessness (guilt), concentration difficulties, psychomotor disturbances and thoughts of self-harm. Arrows pointing toward each of the nine items at the bottom of the figure represent measurement error.

assigning the latent variable a mean and variance. We introduce model identification later in this chapter and dedicate most of Chapter 5 to the topic.

Measurement error terms are also unobserved. However, measurement error terms are not a part of the causal process; thus, there are various ways to represent such error terms in a path diagram as related to continuous observed variables. We represent the measurement error terms in Figure 2.2 using arrows (edges) at the bottom of the path diagram directionally pointing toward each of the nine items. Other common representations of these error terms would be to include a freestanding symbol (not included in a circle or oval as symbolic of a latent variable), such as e or ε or δ, with a subscript unique to each item (such as subscripts 1–9), at the end of each edge. Another representation, such as in the AMOS software package, includes circles with numbered measurement error terms (i.e. $e1, e2, ..., e9$) inside. These error terms could also simply be implied in the model and left out of the path diagram.

Measurement error can be either *random* or *systematic*. Random measurement error varies from one measurement to another in an unpredictable manner. When we use the terminology "measurement error" throughout this textbook, we are referring to random measurement error unless denoted otherwise. Systematic measurement error is predictable and constant. Systematic measurement error is also known as bias and leads to incorrect model estimates. An entire group has the same error from the true value across measurements of a fixed magnitude and direction. For example, gender disparities in how a questionnaire is filled out lead to a form of systematic measurement error in scoring the questionnaire across men and women. We specifically discuss systematic measurement error and how to identify and account for it in SEM in Chapter 10.

Conventionally, latent variables in SEM analyses appear as *reflective constructs,* such as *depression* in Figure 2.2, where the latent trait influences the indicators. In *formative constructs*, indicators influence the latent trait. In health and medicine, latent variables for physical health conditions such as obesity (Chapter 1, Figure 1.4) reasonably could be considered a formative construct based on clinical characteristics, such as waist circumference, waist–hip ratio and BMI. However, including formative variables in SEMs is an application that requires special care (Chapter 7).

2.2.1 Factor Analysis

Factor analysis (FA) is a technique for investigating whether a latent variable or variables underlie a set of item responses [5–9]. If there are multiple latent variables underlying the item responses, FA is also used to evaluate the relationships among the latent variables [5–9]. *Exploratory factor analysis (EFA)* [6,10] is typically used as an investigative technique to identify the number of latent variables that underlie a set of item responses. One commonly uses EFA to describe the factor structure that is consistent with the data and leads to the most meaningful substantive interpretation of groups of questions or indicators. *Confirmatory factor analysis (CFA)* [5] is an analytic technique used to study the relationships between multiple indicators and a latent variable or variables. CFA is the most widely used technique for specifying latent variables in the measurement model within the SEM framework. Recall, the measurement model is used to evaluate the relationships between latent variables and their measurements.

The CFA model is in itself a special case of a structural equation model. Though historically EFA was not typically an SEM procedure, it can be classified as a more general latent variable procedure and is available for use in many SEM software packages. Aforementioned in Chapter 1, EFA can also be viewed as a special case of CFA and vice versa as both techniques employ the same common mathematical model under different constraints (Chapter 8).

Many health and medical researchers use both EFA and CFA in subsequent analyses (see Figure 2.3). EFA is useful for helping to determine the factor structure among multiple indicators. CFA is useful for testing and evaluating the measurement properties of a predetermined factor structure and then modifying this structure as indicated. Most often a researcher performing EFA and CFA in succession will do so using two separate samples. Otherwise, one is likely overfitting the model in confirming a factor structure that was determined by optimizing empirical criteria with the same data. A data set can be randomly split into two data sets for conducting EFA and then CFA. Alternatively, one could find two similar data sets for this purpose.

2.2.2 Principal Component Analysis

Principal component analysis (PCA) is a variable reduction technique that sometimes is mistaken for factor analysis. While FA explains the correlations (variances and covariances) among a set of variables (e.g. items), PCA explains the variance *only*. Therefore, these two techniques are different approaches and have different applications. To elaborate further, PCA does not have a causal interpretation. A principal component is a linear combination of weighted observed variables. These principal components are uncorrelated. Properly specified factors, as previously mentioned, do have a causal interpretation. Multiple latent factors in a factor analytic solution can be correlated or uncorrelated.

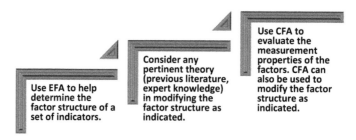

FIGURE 2.3
Step diagram for using exploratory and confirmatory factor analysis in succession for health and medical research.

A subsequent step is to evaluate for group differences (e.g. differences for males and females or across age groups) across the factor structure using multiple indicator multiple cause (MIMIC) modeling or multigroup confirmatory factor analysis. See Chapter 10 for a discussion of these techniques.

For illustration purposes of the two different methods, 15 indicators represent affective, cognitive and somatic domains of depression. In a typical application involving PCA, one would determine fewer than 15 principal components that explain a percent of the variance (say 90%) among these 15 indicators in representing depression. This is a data reduction technique.

FA, on the other hand, typically would be used for determining the factor structure of these 15 indicators and evaluating measurement properties. For example, in determining the factor structure, one may hypothesize three factors of affective, cognitive and somatic dimensions of depression rather than a single factor of depression. Then, one might evaluate how well this structure fits the data (Chapter 7 for discussion of model fit, reliability and internal validity in CFA models).

A common tactic for forming a formative latent construct in health and medicine is to use the first principal component. This approach has been applied for constructing neighborhood socioeconomic position, which some researchers have assessed using the first principal component of census tract data [11]. However, as a limitation, this first principal component alone may not explain a high enough percent of the variance in the latent construct to be useful. Multiple principal components are often necessary to explain 90% of the variance.

2.3 Path Analysis

SEM has many applications in health and medical research. SEMs are useful for understanding the measurement properties of clinical screening, assessment and symptom scales. Relationships among these scales, demographic characteristics, risk factors and health outcomes can be evaluated using SEM approaches. SEM is useful for studying latent variables and hypothesized relationships between variables.

With the preceding discussion, we have provided the reader with some background on latent variables. Now, we discuss *path analysis*. Path analysis is a technique used to examine hypothesized causal relationships between variables and is a special case of SEM with only observed variables.

In clarifying the purpose of path analysis, we discuss how it diverges from other more traditional analyses. That is, in order to apply path analysis, one needs to understand explicitly how a typical biomedical interpretation of path analysis differs from traditional regression analyses. In referencing traditional regression, we are not merely discussing a technique, but also the standard assumptions and application of the technique for evaluating an associative relationship. In these traditional applications, one hypothesizes an associative relationship and draws conclusions regarding association (or lack of). For traditional ordinary least squares linear regression, statistical assumptions include linearity, homoscedasticity, independence of errors, weak exogeneity and no or little multicollinearity in the predictors. See, for example, Neter et al. [12] or Weisberg [13] for a full review of the statistical assumptions and standard applications of traditional regression analysis.

For this introduction to path analysis, again, we are merely discussing a type of analysis as opposed to a specific statistical framework. The technique of multivariate multiple regression could be used to perform path analysis, but one makes different assumptions (i.e. causal assumptions) in path analysis than in the traditional application of multiple regression. Similarly, path analysis can be done by fitting one regression equation at a time, once the model has been established. PROCESS written by Andrew F. Hayes is a macro for SPSS and SAS that can be used to conduct path analysis using this approach [14].

Let us suppose that, from our example in Figure 2.1, we are focused on weekly exercise and BMI. We hypothesize that in our participants, BMI is inversely associated with weekly exercise. We use traditional linear regression analysis. Our hypothetical results, simulating 550 study participants, show a negative regression slope estimate with a confidence interval that does not contain zero and a statistically significant p-value (Figure 2.4).

What can we conclude? We can generally make a statement like, "in our sample, given our study assumptions, BMI is negatively associated with weekly exercise." We are assuming that we checked traditional regression assumptions and evaluated for multicollinearity, autocorrelation of residuals and high leverage values/outliers and found no substantial issues before drawing these conclusions.

We could use traditional multiple regression to evaluate other clinical risk factors (socioeconomic status, depressive symptoms, age, sex, race, etc.) that associate with BMI. Traditional multiple regression could also be used for evaluating the wellness program vs. treatment as usual for lowering BMI, while adjusting for various clinical patient characteristics, such as age, race and sex. In these examples, we have given relevant data a process for making biomedical interpretations following the left side of Figure 2.5 for traditional regression analysis. Unlike in the example corresponding to Figure 2.1, we did not make any causal assumptions in the traditional regression approach.

Path analysis is an extension of traditional regression analysis, in which a researcher estimates hypothesized causal relationships among a set of observed variables. The path analysis process flow on the right side of Figure 2.5 is importantly different from the traditional regression analysis. In path analysis, the researcher is often more interested in causal relationships rather than just associations among a set of measures. Such modeling under strong causal assumptions is more complex than traditional regression analysis.

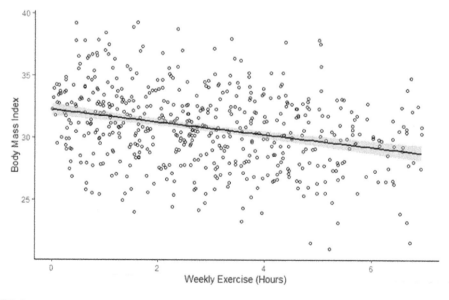

FIGURE 2.4

Scatterplot with linear regression line and 95% confidence region for regression of body mass index on weekly exercise ($N = 550$).

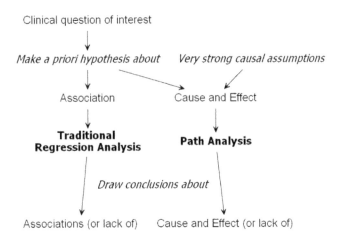

FIGURE 2.5
Process flow diagram for biomedical interpretation for traditional regression analysis vs. path analysis.

A researcher makes causal assumptions based on logic, theory and prior literature.

In a traditional univariate or multiple regression approach, only a single equation is fit at one time. Multivariate regression modeling, path modeling and SEM, in a single analysis, allow for the simultaneous estimation of multiple unknown model parameters in multi-equation models. For example, using the SEM framework, estimating the magnitude and significance of the eight causal paths in the path diagram in Figure 2.1 is done simultaneously. Likewise, estimating the parameters representing the causal paths in the four regression-type mathematical equations is done simultaneously in Figure 2.1. Recall that each regression equation in the structural model has a *disturbance term* that reflects the residual error in regressing an outcome variable on a predictor (or set of predictors).

In traditional multiple regression analysis, potential confounders are accounted for in order to decrease bias in the estimate of the main effect. The testing of any single causal path in the SEM framework can be interpreted in lieu of adjustment for potential confounders in the form of other model relationships (and covariates), since the analyses is performed at the same time. Therefore, while simultaneously estimating all paths in a structural equation model, one can focus on statistical output about a single causal path or particular relationship across causal paths (e.g. Wellness program → calorie intake → anxiety) in order to evaluate a specific research hypothesis of interest. As a result, SEM simplifies testing in complex causal models.

Hypothesized correlational relationships in addition to cause and effect relationships can still be evaluated while using path analysis or SEM. The SEM framework is sufficiently general to be used for many traditional statistical techniques. ANOVA, traditional linear regression and traditional logistic regression can also be performed in the SEM framework.

The SEM framework can handle many more specialized techniques when a researcher makes use of causal assumptions. SEM can be used to analyze feedback loops (Chapter 5), latent constructs and path analysis models. SEM can be used to conduct multiple group comparisons across the same measurement and/or structural model. The SEM framework, compared to traditional frameworks, provides more empirical and theoretical flexibility for researchers. The assumptions one makes when using a traditional linear regression approach to evaluate an associative relationship do not allow a researcher to make causal conclusions. Traditional regression analysis implies a statistical relationship based on a conditional expected value. Additionally, perfect measurement in the observed variables (i.e. no measurement error) is assumed in traditional regression analysis. Strong a priori theory is more typically used in path analysis and SEM. These approaches more typically allow a functional relationship between variables expressed via a conceptual model, path diagram and mathematical equations [15]. In this way, path analysis and other SEM approaches are a combination of data independent methods (conceptual modeling and path diagramming) and data-driven empirical analyses. The presence of latent variables and explicitly modeling measurement error is outside of the paradigm of traditional regression analysis and path analysis. The structural model in the SEM framework in which relationships between latent variables can be examined can also be thought of as the combination of CFA and path analysis.

2.4 Conducting SEM Analysis in Health and Medicine

In somewhat simplistic terms, a conventional structural equation model in health and medicine consists of a set of equations that fuse together CFA and path analysis, with a purpose in mind. That purpose is commonly to test hypotheses regarding relationships among latent and observed measures.

2.4.1 Confirmatory Data Analysis for a Single Model

Recall, exploratory data analysis is data-driven, while confirmatory data analysis is hypothesis-driven (relies on a priori hypothesis). Here we discuss a single structural equation model used for a given study. Conducting confirmatory data analysis using SEM in health and medicine may involve four basic steps (Table 2.2).

2.4.2 Model Specification

A researcher first may have a hypothesis of interest in mind and a conceptual model to represent the phenomenon being investigated. David A. Kenny has defined the process of building a structural equation model as the "translation of theory, previous research, design, and common sense into a structural model" [16]. Aforementioned in this process of model specification, a researcher translates the conceptual model into a formal structural equation model.

Model misspecification (or *specification error*) is a term to describe where the model failed to account for everything it should. For example, a model that omits important explanatory variables or a meaningful causal path or correlation between two variables is misspecified. A misspecified model leads to the possibility of coming to incorrect conclusions due to biased estimates. In practice, all models, as approximations of the truth, are somewhat

TABLE 2.2

Four Basic Steps for Conducting Confirmatory Data Analysis Using SEM

1. specify an identifiable model
2. estimate the model
3. assess model fit
4. test hypotheses of interest

misspecified. SEM researchers using a team science approach and theory, logic and prior literature in developing models are employing sensible strategies toward minimizing the amount of specification error.

2.4.3 Model Identification

Importantly, for analytical purposes, a model must meet the condition of *identifiability*. *Identifiability* is a property in which a single solution is possible for all unknown parameters. Even with "perfect" data of an infinitely large sample size one would not be able to uniquely estimate unknown parameters if a model was not identifiable. Thus, lack of identifiability is not an issue regarding data quality. We dedicate much of Chapter 5 to the topic of identifiability. In that chapter we discuss some necessary conditions for identifiability and provide some examples to help one understand the topic further.

At this point in the textbook, we broadly mention the role of model identifiability within Table 2.2. There would be no substantial statistical analysis for the model without meeting this condition. Thus, one needs to specify an identifiable model before conducting data analysis. However, keep in mind, the existence of a unique solution for unknown parameters does not ensure that estimates will be unbiased. For example, the researcher may have applied a numerical optimization procedure that did not perform well on the data at hand or there may be systematic measurement error in measurement of the variables in the sample. There are many places to go astray in the application of SEM, starting from conceptualizing a model that does not translate into an identifiable model and/or having poor quality data.

2.4.4 Model Estimation and Evaluation

An important feature of SEM analyses is that formal tests and indices are available for assessing the adequacy of the fit of a model to the observed data (Chapter 4). Much emphasis is given to model fit. The classic approaches to SEM analysis use the covariance matrix of the data to estimate the unknown parameters in a specified model. In SEM analysis, different algorithms for numerical optimization can be used to estimate parameters with the aim of closely reproducing the covariance matrix. The better the model fits the observed data, the better one reproduces the covariance matrix after plugging in the estimates of unknown parameters.

Maximum likelihood (ML) is a commonly used estimator in the SEM framework for interval data. ML is based on the assumption of multivariate normality of the endogenous variables [9]. Multivariate normality has the properties of (1) univariate normality, (2) normality of all linear combinations between variables, (3) linearity of all bivariate associations and the distribution of residuals is homoscedastic [8]. Statistical tests are available to help detect violations of univariate and multivariate normality (Chapter 3).

Continuous data in health and medical research are often not normally distributed (Chapter 3). *Robust ML* (or *ML with robust standard errors*) is a commonly used estimator in the SEM framework for interval data that violates normality assumptions [9]. Modifications of ML, *full information ML* (FIML), are useful techniques for handling missing data, under certain assumptions about the data missingness mechanism, for analysis of all available cases in a study sample. This is only a very brief sketch of model estimation and evaluation for SEM; we dedicate an entire Chapter 4 to providing details about these procedures.

2.4.5 Hypothesis Testing

Assuming the model is identifiable, we have discussed how SEM allows for the estimation of multiple equation model parameters in a single analysis for simplifying hypothesis testing in a complex causal model. One can, for example, go on to test the strength of a causal hypothesis between two variables using a corresponding point estimate and confidence interval estimate for that regression path coefficient. A plausible model with a good model fit provides evidence for internal validity and as a result has a specific set of parameters that well-defines the problem at hand. However, in conducting confirmatory data analysis, the researcher might still perform hypothesis testing even with a poor fitting model [17]. The researcher would just report all the results and note that this model should be evaluated further in future studies. An alternative, which we will discuss below briefly, is to modify the model if the fit is poor; this would then be considered more along the lines of exploratory data analysis as opposed to confirmatory data analysis. Formal hypothesis testing for a structural model in the context of mediation analysis is discussed in Chapter 9.

2.4.6 Exploratory Data Analysis, Model Re-specification and Comparison

There are many additional applications of SEM that do not involve a hypothesis of interest. One may use EFA in exploratory data analysis to help determine the factor structure of a set of questions, given no strong a priori hypothesis about the factor structure. One may also use SEM to revise an initial model for further use in reproducible research. That is, prior to any formal hypothesis testing, one may revise the model (and consider alternative models) if the model fit is not good and/or if the model is not theoretically defensible.

The analysis can be done iteratively with a single modification evaluated at each model comparison. The initial model is compared to a revised model. If the revised model has an improved model fit and is theoretically defensible, then that model may become the new standard model for the study. The new standard model may be compared to a model with another modification in a similar process until a "best" model is identified. We discuss in Chapter 6 how such an iterative procedure should be conducted prudently in which a researcher considers only a few, theoretically meaningful potential model revisions.

Model re-specification may be viewed in many applications as mostly (or entirely) exploratory data analysis. Some researchers would discourage others from using the same data for revising a model and conducting confirmatory data analysis. This may lead to overfitting the model used for confirmatory data analysis given it was revised for an improved fit based on the same data. Another view is to consider results as exploratory/preliminary when testing hypotheses about relationships between variables in the re-specified model using the same data (or holdout data). There are practical reasons a health and medical researcher may not have access to different data (other than a holdout sample). For example, the systematic collection of certain validated measures on a condition under study may only have ever been done in a single sample.

Another approach for model comparison is to begin with several plausible models for the same data and compare their fit in a more confirmatory manner [17]. Using this approach, a series of models can be compared to determine the "best" model among competing models. Plausible measurement and structural models can be determined using theory, logic and prior literature for this analysis. For example, using the PHQ-9 items one may specify and compare three measurement models: a one factor model of *depression*, two factor model of *cognitive/affective* and *somatic* and two factor model of *affective* and *somatic (and cognitive)*. Here a researcher is evaluating the dimensionality and measurement structure of a set of item responses. Hypothesis testing can be conducted using this approach (e.g. testing unidimensionality of a scale vs. plausible alternatives). We discuss model modification and comparison in Chapter 6 and measurement models and dimensionality in Chapter 7.

2.5 Longitudinal SEM

There are many researchers who view cross-sectional SEMs as inherently associational as opposed to causal because they do not allow one to identify precedents and antecedents. We discuss longitudinal SEMs in Chapters 13 and 14 and how these models may enable researchers to assess within-individual changes over time or temporality between measures, and make stronger inferences about hypothesized causality. However, more generally, one can use strong a priori theory to assume causality in both cross-sectional and longitudinal SEM analyses. Thus, we emphasize again that with strong a priori theory traditional multivariate regression analysis could be used to test a causal model with observed variables. In this context, the SEM framework (or another error-in-variables modeling approach) is extremely useful for the modeling of measurement error.

2.6 Systems-Based Models

SEM is commonly used as a tool for building and examining models in complex causal systems. In Chapter 1, Figure 1.4 depicts a graphical model of the relationships between risk for a cardiovascular event and cardiovascular event. In this example, a model of the relationships between risk factors, symptoms and cardiovascular event outcomes was developed in order to understand risk for adverse health outcomes and the interplay of intermediate outcomes (e.g. high cholesterol and blood pressure) over time in study participants.

In the context of health and medicine, *systems-based modeling* is the use of interdisciplinary, multidisciplinary or transdisciplinary approaches (see Preface for a brief overview of team science approaches) to conceptualize and construct a model of clinical systems. A researcher depicts causal dependencies between predictors, demographic information, risk factors, symptoms, outcomes and other clinical measures within these systems to help address research questions. For practical purposes, researchers should construct reasonable hypotheses that can be supported by available data for understanding relationships in systems-based models. Thus, a mental model of a systems-based model, independent of any particular hypotheses and available data may be different than the conceptual model based on study boundaries or limitations of a specific data base. SEM is a powerful technique available to researchers well-suited for analyses of casual system models.

Due to data or computing limitations, a researcher may have to parcel a system into subsystems and focus analyses on these subsystems. A drawback is that analyzing separate subsystems, one at a time, treats them independently rather than cohesively. This may lead to spurious and biased results in analyses of any subsystem. For an example of subsystem analysis, we might focus on how mental health, lipid disorders and hypertension influence the probability of a cardiovascular event as represented in Chapter 1, Figure 1.4. This is a hypothesized subsystem model to evaluate the influence of intermediate outcomes and mental health on a cardiovascular health outcome.

In actuality, the SEM strategies as discussed in this book are some of the few tools available to researchers for causal system modeling. Bayesian networks, a graphical, Bayesian approach for representing probabilistic models, could also be used for addressing causal system modeling problems.

2.7 Direct, Indirect and Total Effects

While individual causal path estimates may be of interest, researchers using SEM are often interested in *direct, indirect* and *total effects*. We illustrate these effect pathways using a conceptual causal diagram in Figure 2.6.

A direct effect is the causal effect of an independent variable on a dependent variable. Recall that an independent variable can be either strictly an independent variable (i.e. exogenous variable) or a dependent variable (i.e. endogenous variable) in another equation in a system of structural equations. An indirect effect is the causal effect of an independent variable on a dependent variable through the pathway of a third variable, an endogenous variable termed the *mediator*. The indirect effect is synonymous with the mediation effect. The mediator is both an effect with respect to the independent variable and the cause with respect to a dependent variable. In Figure 2.6, we present some of the pathways of our previous example of a wellness program (Figure 2.1) to illustrate the concepts of direct, indirect and total effects. We also introduce letters A, B, C and D in Figure 2.6 to generalize these relationships.

The effect of $A \rightarrow D$ is the sole direct effect *across the entire system*. That is, it is the only direct pathway effect (from an independent variable to a dependent variable) that is not a piece of an indirect pathway effect (from an independent variable to a dependent variable via a mediator). Other direct effects $A \rightarrow B$, $B \rightarrow D$, $A \rightarrow C$ and $C \rightarrow D$ are pieces of indirect pathway effects. The effects of $A \rightarrow B \rightarrow D$ and $A \rightarrow C \rightarrow D$ are indirect effects. From our example, these two indirect effects represent the influence of the wellness program (A) on BMI (D) through calorie intake (B) and weekly exercise (C). The total effect represents the sum of all possible pathway effects from an independent variable to a dependent variable,

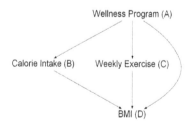

FIGURE 2.6
Conceptual causal diagram with direct and indirect pathways between wellness program, calorie intake, weekly exercise and body mass index (BMI).

including both direct and indirect effects. The total effect with respect to the dependent variable BMI (*D*) in Figure 2.5 includes the direct effect from wellness program (*A*) to BMI (*D*) and the two indirect effects. We will discuss mediation modeling for evaluating direct, indirect and total effects in Chapter 9.

One should note relationships in Figure 2.6 not indicated by an arrow are assumed to equal zero. For example, there is no effect of *B* on *C* in Figure 2.6, which implies that the value of $B \rightarrow C$ is zero. As a result, an indirect effect of $A \rightarrow B \rightarrow C$ also equals zero. Further, despite an effect of *A* on *B*, there is no effect of *B* on *A* and thus the value of $B \rightarrow A$ is zero.

2.8 Subgroup Analysis Using Latent Variable Methodology or Multigroup Analysis

Subgroup analysis is traditionally performed under the hypothesis that there will be differences in certain groups from the population that share a common characteristic (e.g. race, ethnicity, language, sex, occupation). SEM models provide in-depth and flexible analyses for performing subgroup analyses.

The condition of *measurement invariance* (*measurement equivalence*) indicates that a similar latent construct is being measured equally well across subgroups of interest. SEM allows for measurement invariance testing to evaluate if the measurement model is valid across subgroups (Chapter 10). If the measurement model is not valid across subgroups, systematic measurement error is present. In addition to merely identifying systematic measurement error, SEM approaches are available to account for this bias. Two such techniques are *multiple indicator multiple cause (MIMIC) modeling* and *multiple group analysis*. MIMIC modeling is CFA with covariates. Multiple group analysis is a stratified analysis in which each group (e.g. male and female groups) has its own model. Measurement invariance testing, especially in multigroup analysis, can be far more nuanced than traditional subgroup analyses as a researcher can evaluate multiple indices and tests to determine and describe the type of invariance.

In the SEM framework, a *moderator* is an interactive or grouping variable that affects the direction and/or strength of a hypothesized causal relationship between an independent and dependent variable. Moderation analysis is performed to test for changes in the relationship between variables across levels of a subgrouping variable (e.g. age). In an experimental study, moderation analysis can be used to help identify for whom the treatment works best. Moderation analysis can be used to test for either overall or localized (e.g. moderation of a single causal path) subgroup differences in a structural model (Chapter 9).

Subgroup techniques described above rely on the researcher defining a priori subgroups. On the other hand, there are available alternatives to *unsupervised learning* techniques with latent variable models to identify subgroups across selected indicators. *Unsupervised learning* is a type of machine learning algorithm for preprocessing and grouping input data without any corresponding output variables. These techniques with latent variable models are termed synonymously by many applied researchers as *finite mixture modeling, mixture modeling, latent variable mixture modeling* or *latent class modeling. Latent class analysis (LCA)* for categorical data (Chapter 11) and *latent profile analysis (LPA)* for continuous data (Chapter 12) are applications of such techniques. LCA and LPA are a subset of second-generation SEM, and a latent class/latent profile is represented using a categorical latent variable. Many variations and extensions of these types of techniques are available depending on the application. For example, *latent transition analysis (LTA)* is an extension of LCA for longitudinal data in which subjects can transition across classes over time.

Latent growth modeling (LGM) (Chapter 13) is used for longitudinal data analysis to estimate growth trajectories [18,19]. The LGM framework is very flexible and allows a researcher to build a statistical model corresponding precisely with a conceptual framework [19]. *Growth mixture modeling (GMM)* (Chapter 14) is an extension of LGM that can be used to identify latent subpopulations based on outcome trajectories. GMM is a case of mixture modeling using a combination of continuous and categorical latent variables.

2.9 An Introduction to MPlus

In this textbook, for particular problems and methods, we discuss the use of the software we found most well-suited for our research. Most predominately, we have used MPlus in our analyses [9]. MPlus uses a GLVM framework [20]. Examples of the diverse latent variable modeling techniques available in MPlus include full, conventional SEM with different types of variables, EFA, Bayesian analyses, LCA, GMM and item response theory. In this section we walk through some of the detailed steps necessary for implementing a path analysis model in MPlus (example diagrammed in Figure 2.7).

MPlus allows a user to perform analyses of interest either by inputting code, using a language generator or drawing a path diagram directly, with a variety of different choices

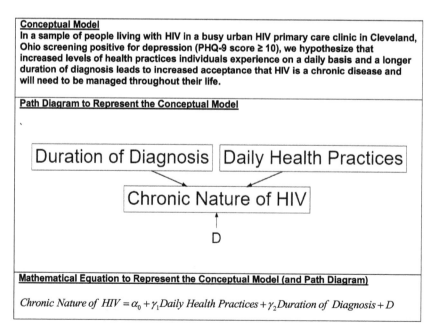

FIGURE 2.7
Path model for chronic nature of HIV self-management in people living with HIV screening positive for depressive symptoms.

for model estimators and types of models. Data for MPlus must reside in an external ASCII file (e.g. file type.dat or.txt) [21] and should not include a header for variable names.

As an example, to perform the corresponding path analysis to Figure 2.7 in a sample of 565 people living with HIV and screening positive for depressive symptoms,[1] a text file in the wide format called `Data _ HIV` is saved on a computer network drive (designated as the H drive, H:\) with the data. The data includes each subject ID, chronic nature of HIV self-management score (0–15), daily self-management health practices score (0–36) and years diagnosed with HIV from study baseline (duration of diagnosis). Here are six lines of data from the data table that forms the text file (Box 2.1)

BOX 2.1

1	−999	−999	16
2	10	36	13
3	12	31	4
4	−999	−999	23
5	4	25	11
6	5	14	18

Most analyses in software programs appropriate for SEM are performed with data in the wide format, even for longitudinal analyses, due to flexibility in specifying relationships between variables. There are exceptions for preferring to keep data in the long format, such as some multilevel modeling applications. There are also important differences in how to input the data into the software when using more complex data structures (e.g. multiple imputation). Further explanations are available in the MPlus user's guide [9].

MPlus code format for performing analyses on an existing external data set begins with a title, identifying the data sources, naming the variables and specifying which variables will be used in analyses. Other options include identifying the numeric code for missing data and specifying ordered-categorical (labeled "categorical" in Mplus), nominal or count outcomes.

While all 565 subjects in this data set had a recorded value for duration of diagnosis, a subset of 235 subjects filled out an HIV self-management scale with domains for daily self-management health practices and chronic nature of HIV self-management [22]. We have used "−999" to signify missing data in this example. In this basic illustrative example, we remove any cases with missing data and analyze the remaining data (Chapter 4 for techniques for handling missing data). In the analysis, Mplus will omit the 330 cases with a missing value on daily self-management health practices with no further coding necessary given the specification of this basic path model.[2]

All variable names must begin with a letter and must be eight characters or less. The order of variable names in the syntax must correspond to the order in the data file. MPlus is not case sensitive; for example, writing "missing" or "MISSING" are interpreted in the same manner.

---

[1] Baseline sample for a study of the collaborative care program at a public health system in Cleveland, Ohio; research funding by the Health Resources and Services Administration (H97HA27429-01-00).

[2] Note that one can also explicitly request to omit cases with any missing values in MPlus using the option LISTWISE = ON (listwise deletion; Chapter 4) in the DATA command.

Here we present an example of code for performing path analysis corresponding to Figure 2.7 using the data file `Data _ HIV` on the H drive:

BOX 2.2

```
TITLE: SEM CCM HIV PATH ANALYSIS;
DATA: FILE = "H:/Data_HIV.txt";
VARIABLE: NAMES = ID HIV_SM HLTHPRAC YRSDXHIV;
missing are all (-999);
USEVARIABLES = HIV_SM HLTHPRAC YRSDXHIV;
ANALYSIS:
ESTIMATOR = MLR;
!Regression of Chronic Nature of HIV_Self-Management (HIV_SM) on
!Daily Self-Management Health Practices (HLTHPRAC) and Duration of
!Diagnosis (YRSDXHIV)
MODEL:
HIV_SM ON HLTHPRAC YRSDXHIV;
OUTPUT: standardized;
```

As shown in Box 2.2, major headings for MPlus coding include: TITLE, DATA, VARIABLE, ANALYSIS, MODEL and OUTPUT. The user can also request various plots corresponding to the particular analysis with the PLOT heading (not used in this output). Lines of comments can be added to the code in MPlus for clarity using exclamation points.

In the ANALYSIS section, an estimator can be specified. For instance, in this example, a robust maximum likelihood (MLR option) is used (standard maximum likelihood, or ML, is often the default setting for continuous variables).

The MODEL section is where we specify both the measurement and structural models. Since we are evaluating a path model in Figure 2.7, we only specify a structural model in Box 2.2.[3] We specify the structural model for regressing chronic nature of HIV self-management (HIV _ SM) on duration of diagnosis (YRSDXHIV) and daily self-management health practices (HLTHPRAC). We used the shorter acronyms due to the variable name width limit of eight characters, and an underscore because spaces have a different syntax meaning. Coming up with suitable acronyms within the width limit sometimes becomes a task in itself. Members of a multidisciplinary team may need to see familiar variable names in order to examine how output compares to clinical expectations. OUTPUT allows the user to request more technical details in the output. For example, here standardized estimates (Chapter 4) are requested. SAVEDATA (not used in this output) allows the user to save information from a model and output datasets in a text file.

The MPLUS User's Guide (also available on the statmodel.com website) provides example programming syntax and applications for many different models within the SEM framework, and it is a great resource for learning how to program with MPlus [9]. We have provided a brief overview of MPlus coding for a basic cross-sectional path model. Depending on the model complexities, there are more MPlus coding headings. For example, coding of a multilevel latent growth model or Monte Carlo simulation would involve more MPlus coding headings.

Once code is entered, users can either choose to "Run Mplus" on the drop-down menu under the heading "Mplus" or hit Alt+R on the keyboard to run the program. Mplus will then provide technical output for the analyses. Included in the output will be a summary

---

[3] Measurement models for latent variables are specified using the BY, rather than ON, statement in the MODEL command.

of the analyses. For the example analyses, MPlus will provide the sample size, variable information and information about the estimator and convergence:

BOX 2.3

```
SUMMARY OF ANALYSIS

Number of groups                                  1
Number of observations                          235
Number of dependent variables                    1
Number of independent variables                  2
Number of continuous latent variables            0

Observed dependent variables

 Continuous

   HIV_SM

Observed independent variables

   HLTHPRAC   YRSDXHIV
Estimator                         MLR
Information matrix                OBSERVED
Maximum number of iterations           1000
Convergence criterion            0.500D-04
Maximum number of steepest descent iterations     20
Maximum number of iterations for H1         2000
   Convergence criterion for H1          0.100D-03
```

In the output, there will be a summary of any errors in the estimation. In our example, there were no errors:

```
THE MODEL ESTIMATION TERMINATED NORMALLY
```

Note that for this basic path model there is no meaningful available test of fit (Chapter 5 for discussion of a just identified or saturated model). We can evaluate the relationships between our variables from the select MPlus output (Box 2.4) to test the hypothesis in our conceptual model from Figure 2.6.

BOX 2.4

```
MODEL RESULTS

                                                Two-Tailed
                Estimate    S.E.    Est./S.E.    P-Value
SLFMGT_C ON
   HLTHPRAC      0.143     0.028     5.128        0.000
   YRSDXHIV      0.001     0.019     0.073        0.943

Intercepts
   HIV_SM        4.101     0.628     6.534        0.000
Residual Variances
   HIV_SM        5.279     0.644     8.193        0.000
```

Output for each raw path estimate is similar to output from traditional regression analysis for a regression slope, including an estimate, standard error (SE), test value (Est./SE) and p-value. The test value here is a z-test value. An important difference is that we interpret this MPlus output with respect to our causal assumptions and substantive theory for path analysis, as shown in Figure 2.4.

We find that a one unit increase in the level of daily health self-management practices leads to a statistically significant increase in the level of the chronic nature of HIV self-management ($\hat{\gamma}_1 = 0.143$, SE $= 0.028$, $p < 0.001$). Duration of diagnosis does not have a statistically significant effect on the level of chronic nature of HIV self-management.

2.10 Conclusions

Research in health and medicine may involve complex modeling of latent variables and hypothesized relationships among scales, symptoms and/or conditions. SEM is a very general, flexible multivariate technique that can be used for addressing problems involving hypothesized relationships among latent constructs and observed measures. We compared and contrasted SEM to traditional approaches throughout this chapter to give a reader a more thorough understanding of the vocabulary, concepts and uses of SEM. We also lead the reader through a basic example of path analysis using MPlus software.

References

1. Gunzler, D.D. and N. Morris, A tutorial on structural equation modeling for analysis of overlapping symptoms in co-occurring conditions using MPlus. *Statistics in Medicine*, 2015. **34**(24): pp. 3246–3280.
2. Hansson, M., et al., Comparison of two self-rating scales to detect depression: HADS and PHQ-9. *British Journal of General Practice*, 2009. **59**(566): pp. e283–e288.
3. Huang, F.Y., et al., Using the Patient Health Questionnaire-9 to measure depression among racially and ethnically diverse primary care patients. *Journal of General Internal Medicine*, 2006. **21**(6): pp. 547–552.
4. Gunzler, D., et al., Disentangling multiple sclerosis & depression: An adjusted depression screening score for patient-centered care. *Journal of Behavioral Medicine*, 2015. **38**(2): pp. 237–250.
5. Brown, T.A., *Confirmatory factor analysis for applied research*. 2012, New York: Guilford Press.
6. Tucker, L.R. and R.C. MacCallum, *Exploratory factor analysis*. 1997, Columbus: Ohio State University, Unpublished manuscript.
7. Bollen, K., *Structural equations with latent variables*. 1989, New York: Wiley.
8. Kline, R.B., *Principles and practice of structural equation modeling, fourth edition*. 2016, New York: Guilford Press.
9. Muthén, L.K. and B.O. Muthén, *Mplus: The comprehensive modelling program for applied researchers: user's guide. Eighth edition*. 1998–2017, Los Angeles, CA: Muthén & Muthén.
10. Raykov, T. and G.A. Marcoulides, *Introduction to psychometric theory*. 2010, Oxford: Taylor & Francis.
11. Dalton, J.E., et al., Accuracy of cardiovascular risk prediction varies by neighborhood socioeconomic position: A retrospective cohort study. *Annals of Internal Medicine*, 2017. **167**(7): pp. 456–464.

12. Neter, J., W. Wasserman, and M.H. Kutner, *Applied linear regression models*. 1989, Irwin: Homewood, III.
13. Weisberg, S., *Applied linear regression*. Vol. 528, 2005, Hoboken, NJ: John Wiley & Sons.
14. Hayes, A.F., *Introduction to mediation, moderation, and conditional process analysis: A regression-based approach*. 2017, New York: Guilford Publications.
15. Gunzler, D., et al., A class of distribution-free models for longitudinal mediation analysis. *Psychometrika*, 2014. **79**(4): pp. 543–568.
16. Kenny, D.A. Terminology and basics of SEM, 2011. Available from: http://davidakenny.net/cm/basics.htm.
17. Bollen, K.A. and M.D. Noble, Structural equation models and the quantification of behavior. *Proceedings of the National Academy of Sciences*, 2011. 108(Supplement 3): pp. 15639–15646.
18. Duncan, T.E., S.C. Duncan, and L.A. Strycker, *An introduction to latent variable growth curve modeling: Concepts, issues, and application*. 2013, Abingdon: Routledge Academic.
19. Preacher, K.J., et al., *Latent growth curve modeling*. 2008, Thousand Oaks, CA: Sage.
20. Muthén, B.O., Beyond SEM: General latent variable modeling. *Behaviormetrika*, 2002. 29(1; issue 51): pp. 81–118.
21. Byrne, B.M., *Structural equation modeling with AMOS: Basic concepts, applications, and programming*. 2013, Abingdon: Routledge.
22. Webel, A.R., et al., Measuring HIV self-management in women living with HIV/AIDS: A psychometric evaluation study of the HIV Self-management Scale. *Journal of Acquired Immune Deficiency Syndromes*, 2012. 60(3): p. e72.

Part II

Theory of Structural Equation Modeling

3

The Form of Structural Equation Models

3.1 Introduction to the Form of SEMs

The SEM framework is useful for evaluating hypothesized relationships among latent and observed variables [1,2]. The conceptual model involves a background presentation of these hypothesized relationships. During the model specification step, an approach is necessary for representing the conceptual model in the SEM framework. At this point, we are assuming that the conceptual model will translate into a statistical model that we can evaluate given study and data limitations. In theory, there may be a better conceptual model for a research study given no sample restrictions or data limitations. This can be an exciting and rewarding step of the research process using SEM techniques, whereby ideas about how processes drive health outcomes are reduced to visual diagrams and sets of underlying equations and mathematical relationships.

We describe the most widely used graphical and mathematical forms for representing the SEM framework. The researcher's model using these approaches is represented in a suitable form for subsequent testing of hypotheses of interest about particular relationships.

We are focused on the matrix form of conventional SEMs for continuous dependent variables in this chapter for the mathematical representation. It is worth mentioning again that the data modeled for analysis in the classic approaches to SEM are the elements of the covariance matrix. That is, one is modeling the sample covariance matrix of their data. One can also model the sample mean vector of their data in SEM. Kaplan [3] defined SEM as "a class of methodologies that seeks to represent hypotheses about the means, variances, and covariances of observed data in terms of a smaller number of 'structural' parameters defined by a hypothesized underlying conceptual or theoretical model." We will discuss the procedure for estimating the free (unknown) parameters in SEMs in Chapter 4.

In Figure 3.1, we represent a path analysis model and illustrate hypothesized causal relationships among different clinical factors influencing body mass index (BMI).

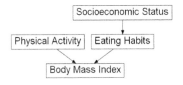

FIGURE 3.1
Path analysis model for body mass index example.

All variables in this path diagram are observed (or manifest) variables. We have not specified all potential paths of interest, including correlations (e.g. correlation between physical activity and eating habits is theoretically reasonable).

We hypothesize a higher socioeconomic status (SES) leads to better eating habits which in turn results in a lower BMI; likewise, more physical activity leads to lower BMI. An implicit assumption in Figure 3.1 is that there is no relationship between SES and physical activity or between physical activity and eating habits.

We have represented the conceptual model in a path diagram. The path diagram in Figure 3.1 makes known hypothesized relationships among SES, physical activity, eating habits and BMI. Evaluating the magnitude and significance of these particular pathways would allow us to test our hypothesis. Either implicitly or explicitly, in our representation of the SEM framework, we present the pathways in the model as a function of the free parameters. In the example in Figure 3.1, the free parameters to be estimated for the three causal paths are implied in the arrows. In more technical path diagrams and mathematical representations of the SEM framework as we will describe in this chapter, the free parameters are written explicitly.

The mathematical representation of SEM we will discuss in this chapter is generalized for a full structural equation model. SEMs that are not full (i.e. CFA models, path analysis models or structural models with both observed and latent variables) are special cases. Thus, all such SEMs (full or not full) can be represented using this mathematical approach.

3.2 Path Diagrams

As we have carefully stated in Part I of this book, causality is an assumption of the researcher and not a condition that can be scientifically proven. The conceptual model may present a carefully crafted causal theory to be tested. A path diagram is a visualization of the conceptual model. In a path diagram, latent variables are represented by a circle or ellipse. Observed variables are represented by a rectangular or square box. Error terms (measurement error or disturbance terms) are generally denoted by a letter or symbol (i.e. e or ε or δ or D or ζ) not enclosed in a shape. However, sometimes error terms are displayed in small circles, since they are unobserved random variables. In less formal path diagrams, these error terms are implied and left out of the figure. Arrows (single and double-headed) are used to represent relationships among the variables.

Path diagrams are fundamentally important for representing models aimed at testing causal theories, by displaying the temporality and causality between measures as suggested in a conceptual model. A conceptual model along with the directionality of an arrow on a path diagram makes the hypothesized causal relationship between variables explicit. One must always keep in mind that substantive and clinical theories and prior empirical evidence are necessary as study background since there is no "model magic" to make a causal path a reality. For example, clinical theory and empirical evidence dictates cigarette smoking causes lung cancer. However, we would not draw a causal path between ice cream consumption and sun poisoning despite an association (both occur more in the summer months).

The reader should be aware that a path diagram is not equivalent to a model. A path diagram is an illustration of hypothesized relationships and a representation of a model (i.e. measurement model, structural model or both). Distributional assumptions for the variables displayed in the path diagram are made separately. A model makes explicit the functional form of the relationships displayed in the path diagram and distributional assumptions.

A single straight arrow assumes a causal relation from the base of the arrow to the head of the arrow. Two straight single-headed arrows in opposing directions connecting two

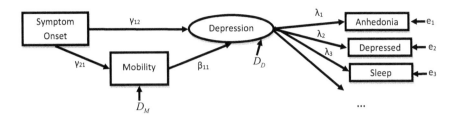

FIGURE 3.2
Path diagram representation of hypothesized multiple sclerosis-depression mediation model.

variables may be used to assume a reciprocal feedback loop. A curved two-headed arrow assumes there may be a pairwise association between two variables or error terms.

In function, any pathways left out of the path diagram (e.g. the absent pathway between SES and physical activity in Figure 3.1) are constrained to zero, unless otherwise noted. For visual ease, we most typically omit displaying such pathways constrained to zero in order to focus on the causal relations we are hypothesizing have a nonzero magnitude.

Most SEM software allows a user to interactively draw a path diagram. For example, in MPlus, AMOS and STATA, the software interface allows you to draw a path diagram and then the program will perform the analysis based on the diagram. Similarly, one can run analysis and these software programs will provide a corresponding path diagram, annotated to include estimated coefficients and results on the pathways of the model.

External to SEM analysis, one can draw a path diagram using popular software tools including Microsoft Office or Graphviz (a free graphing software). Graphviz (https://graphviz.org/) consists of a graph description language called the DOT language, and it also includes various tools that can process the DOT language [4]. DOT is highly customizable, and it allows you to control line colors, arrow shapes, node shapes and many other layout features. The DiagrammeR package in R program implements Graphviz graphs using R script [5].

Figure 3.2 is an example of a path diagram with the inclusion of parameters. We will link the parameters to the mathematical representation of the SEM framework in the second half of this chapter.

Figure 3.2 (drawn in Microsoft Office) represents the path diagram for the causal pathways in multiple sclerosis (MS) patients from time since MS symptom onset to depression. We hypothesize a longer time since symptom onset lead to higher levels of depression. We hypothesize, indirectly, a longer time since symptom onset lead to higher levels of depression through a decline in mobility function. We model *depression* as a latent variable, measured by nine observed items (via the PHQ-9 [6]) with measurement error. *Mobility* and *symptom onset* are observed (manifest) variables.

Figure 3.2 is also an example of a mediation process with a single independent variable, mediator and latent outcome. We include parameters on Figure 3.2 to represent unknown causal effects. For example, β_{11} represents the parameter for the direct effect on the causal path between *mobility* and *depression*.

Error terms are also included on the path diagram for Figure 3.2. For example D_M corresponds to the error term (disturbance term) from the regression of *mobility* on *symptom onset*, while e_1 corresponds to the unique factor variance (measurement error) for the PHQ-9 item for *anhedonia* loading on the latent variable *depression*. We did not explicitly include means and intercept parameters in the path diagram in Figure 3.2. However, we could still include these means and intercepts in analysis corresponding to the figure.

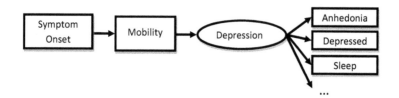

FIGURE 3.3
MS-depression mediation model modified with no path between *symptom onset* and *depression*.

Path diagrams, in general, can be understood as implying indirect and/or direct relationships between variables of interest. For example, in Figure 3.2, *symptom onset* has an indirect effect on *depression* through *mobility*. In Figure 3.2, *symptom onset* also has a direct effect on *depression* since there is a causal path from *symptom onset* to *depression*. However, in Figure 3.3, *symptom onset* has only an indirect effect via *mobility* (and no direct effect) on *depression*. We can obtain Figure 3.3 from Figure 3.2 by constraining γ_{12} to zero. Previously mentioned, in most instances, simply omitting the path from the diagram is equivalent to constraining the path to zero. In both Figures 3.2 and 3.3, *depression* and *mobility* are endogenous variables, while *symptom onset* is an exogenous variable.

3.3 Mathematical Form of the SEM Framework

In applied research, SEMs are often represented through the visual approach of a path diagram. In this section, we provide an overview of a commonly used mathematical form of the SEM framework. This mathematical approach can be used in conjunction with the conceptual model and path diagram for a comprehensive representation of the SEM framework.

A note for the reader before further discussion is this mathematical approach is presented in matrix form. In our experience, some students have struggled to understand the underlying matrix forms behind the SEM framework. However, a basic understanding of this material will support one's fluency in reading and understanding SEM-related research.

In Figure 3.2, we denoted specific parameters for pathways in the MS-depression mediation model. Presenting the parameters in Figure 3.2 in corresponding matrices for the mathematical approach will be done later in this chapter as an illustrative example.

LISREL (Linear Structural Relations) is an approach to more formally express a system of structural equations with latent variables in general matrix form [1,7]. The LISREL approach was developed by Jöreskog and Sörbom [8]. In LISREL, SEMs are divided into two parts consisting of the measurement model and the structural model (as aforementioned) [1]. The measurement model consists of regression-type equations that model the relationship between latent variables and the directly observed variables that represent the underlying constructs. There are two equations in the measurement model for the observed indicators of endogenous latent variables and the observed indicators of exogenous latent variables. The structural model consists of regression-type equations that model the hypothesized causal relationships between endogenous and exogenous variables [1,2]. The structural model relates the latent variables to each other through slopes (*structural* or *regression coefficients* or *paths*).

We present a general formulation of LISREL in the next section for examining relation-ships between latent variables for a model with a mean and covariance structure. Adding a *mean structure* in a model with a covariance structure expands the model to include means and intercepts. An intercept is a conditional mean for endogenous variables that can be interpreted at the reference level for all covariates. This intercept can be thought of similarly in concept to the intercept in a traditional multiple regression model.

Means for exogenous variables are referred to as "means." Exogenous variables are assumed to have a distribution and are treated as dependent variables in a model with a mean structure. One can also specify a structural equation model with intercepts, but treat exogenous variables as independent variables. This is the default in MPlus [9]. When an exogenous variable is treated as an independent variable, the distribution of the exogenous variable is not part of the model. In this case, the scale of an exogenous variable does not affect model estimation and analysis is conditional on the exogenous variable.

In general, the mean of a variable is assumed to be zero when a variable is excluded from the mean structure [10]. Later in this chapter, we will provide several reasons why analysis of means is often done in SEM in health and medical research.

3.3.1 LISREL Approach

A full structural equation model is presented in LISREL matrix form in Box 3.1. In greek symbols, we use lowercase bold fonts for vectors and uppercase bold fonts for full matrices.

BOX 3.1

MEASUREMENT MODEL

$$\mathbf{y} = \mathbf{v}_y + \mathbf{\Lambda}_y \mathbf{\eta} + \mathbf{\varepsilon}$$
$$\mathbf{x} = \mathbf{v}_x + \mathbf{\Lambda}_x \mathbf{\xi} + \mathbf{\delta}$$
(3.1)

$\mathbf{\eta}$ is a $m \times 1$ vector of the endogenous latent variables measured by a $p \times 1$ vector of the observed variables $\mathbf{y}$. $\mathbf{\xi}$ represents a $n \times 1$ vector of the exogenous latent variables measured by a $q \times 1$ vector of the observed variables $\mathbf{x}$. $\mathbf{\varepsilon}$ and $\mathbf{\delta}$ are vectors of error terms, of dimensions $p \times 1$ and $q \times 1$, respectively, representing measurement error. The above equations include vectors of intercepts, $\mathbf{v}_y$ and $\mathbf{v}_x$, of dimensions $p \times 1$ and $q \times 1$, respectively, and matrices of slopes (*factor loadings*), $\mathbf{\Lambda}_y$ and $\mathbf{\Lambda}_x$ of dimensions $p \times m$ and $q \times n$, respectively.

STRUCTURAL MODEL

$$\mathbf{\eta} = \mathbf{\alpha}_\eta + \mathbf{B}\mathbf{\eta} + \mathbf{\Gamma}\mathbf{\xi} + \mathbf{\zeta}$$
(3.2)

$\mathbf{\alpha}_\eta$ is a $m \times 1$ vector of intercepts for the endogenous latent variables, $\mathbf{B}$ is a $m \times m$ matrix of slopes relating the endogenous latent variables to each other and $\mathbf{\Gamma}$ is a $m \times n$ matrix of slopes relating the endogenous latent variables to the exogenous latent variables. $\mathbf{\zeta}$ is a $m \times 1$ vector of random error terms.

The relatively standard assumptions that we will review below in this section are made for every conventional structural equation model with continuous dependent variables in this textbook, unless denoting otherwise.

Each of the error terms ε, δ and ζ in (3.1) and (3.2) have an expected (mean) value of zero. The covariance matrices (or variance-covariance matrices) of ε, δ and ζ are, respectively, denoted as equal to Θ_ε, Θ_δ and Ψ_ζ. In including a mean structure in the model, ξ has an expected value of κ and covariance matrix denoted as equal to Φ.

To facilitate validation, there is a requirement of zero correlation (termed *pseudo-isolation*) between the explanatory variables and error terms in each equation in the model [1]. The researcher believes the residual terms in the model include only random errors that are not correlated with the predictors [11]. The condition of pseudo-isolation is typically explained in the context of a structural model, although it applies to a measurement model as well. It is a standard assumption in regression analysis (i.e. traditional regression analysis) [1].

For the pseudo-isolation condition, in the measurement model, ε is uncorrelated with η and δ is uncorrelated with ξ. Additionally, ε is uncorrelated with ξ and δ is uncorrelated with η. In the structural model, for the pseudo-isolation condition, the correlation between ξ and ζ is equal to zero.

The pseudo-isolation condition is particularly important for *causal inference* [12]. Causal inference is a process for determining whether a cause influences an effect. Most of the causes of the given effects should be in the model in order to justify the condition of pseudo-isolation. Otherwise, most of the causes would likely be in the error term and lead to a correlation of the error with the explanatory variables in the model [1]. In a misspecified model that omitted important explanatory variables, the causal impact of the predictors included in the model (e.g. ξ in the structural model) may be incorrectly estimated.

3.3.2 Some Extensions and Special Cases of the LISREL Model

We could use the form of either of the two equations (for **y** or **x**) in (3.1) to do CFA [13]. Thus, there is a straightforward connection between the measurement model and CFA.

We can solve for η in the equation (3.2) using some linear algebra under the assumption that $\mathbf{I} - \mathbf{B}$ is invertible (see Appendix A):

$$\eta = (\mathbf{I} - \mathbf{B})^{-1}(\alpha_\eta + \Gamma\xi + \zeta) \tag{3.3}$$

Equation (3.3) is referred to as the *reduced form* of the structural equation model. The relationships among variables in equation (3.3) are reduced to a set of equations in which the endogenous variables are functions of only the exogenous variables and error terms [14].

In the special case of no latent variables (such as the model represented in Figure 3.1), there is no explicit measurement model because all variables are measured without error (i.e. $\mathbf{y} = \eta$ and $\mathbf{x} = \xi$) [1]. The form of the structural model in equation (3.2) can be simplified to observed variables only:

$$\mathbf{y} = \alpha_y + \mathbf{B}\mathbf{y} + \Gamma\mathbf{x} + \zeta \tag{3.4}$$

Econometrics developed the idea of simultaneous equation models such as in (3.4) to relate a series of observed endogenous variables to each other as well as a series of observed exogenous variables [13].

One can extend the equations in (3.1) and (3.2) to add regressions on observed covariates (assumed to be measured without error). For example, a measurement model for the equation for **y** in (3.1) with observed covariates is part of a representation of a MIMIC model in which observed covariates influence the effect indicators of the latent variable(s) (Chapter 10).

3.3.3 Mathematical Form of the MS-Depression Mediation Model

In health and medicine, many data sets combine single item observable measures and multiple item patient-reported outcomes (PROs). We may make the assumption that the PRO is measured with imprecision, in which the observed items are composed of the true values plus some measurement error. We also might assume that an observable measure is objective and measured more precisely. For example, we consider a hemoglobin A1c test or height as observable measures. The 36-Item Short Form Health Survey (SF-36) is a set of self-report health and well-being measures, and the EQ-5D is a multiple item self-report instrument for measuring generic health status. Considering the PRO as a latent variable and the observable measure as objective are assumptions about these scales that we might make in certain cases and not others. The assumptions will depend on the particular measure, data available and the context of the study.

In the MS-depression example corresponding to Figure 3.2, we are using a single item measure, the timed 25-foot walk, for mobility function and a multiple item PRO for depression screening, the PHQ-9. Note that one may suggest that the timed 25-foot walk is an indirect measure of mobility function. Nevertheless, the timed 25-foot walk is a performance-based measure based on walking speed viewed as objectively useful in clinical settings [15]. In line with our earlier discussion, we will assume that depression is a latent variable and mobility function is an observed variable. Corresponding with these assumptions, SEMs with both observed and latent endogenous variables in health and medicine are quite common.

We present the reader with the MS-depression mediation model in a modified LISREL form for one latent and one observed endogenous variable and one observed exogenous variable. We will present a measurement model for relating the observed PHQ-9 items to *depression*, but also for *mobility* to itself.

More generally, an observed variable in a structural model that is not full (e.g. structural model with at least one latent and at least one observed variable) can be viewed as special case of a latent variable with an implicit measurement model. As such, we treat *mobility* as a special case of a latent variable in including it as part of η. *Mobility* is an observed endogenous variable that we have assumed is measured without error.

The structural model then relates the latent and observed endogenous variables to each other as well as the observed exogenous variable *symptom onset*. See Appendix B for a description of the mathematical equations.

For illustration purposes, we are assuming that each of the nine items of the PHQ-9, which can take on the discrete values of 0, 1, 2 or 3 are on an interval scale in a large sample of persons living with MS. Whether this is an acceptable assumption, as opposed to treating the items as ordered-categorical in nature, is a subject of much debate even among expert applied researchers in SEM. We return to this issue in Chapter 7.

The measurement model for the nine PHQ-9 items and *mobility* in the LISREL form (3.1) can be written as

$$
\begin{bmatrix} \text{Anhedonia} \\ \text{Depressed} \\ \text{Sleep} \\ \text{Fatigue} \\ \text{Appetite} \\ \text{Guilt} \\ \text{Psychomotor} \\ \text{Movement} \\ \text{Self-Harm} \\ \text{Mobility} \end{bmatrix} = \begin{bmatrix} v_1 \\ v_2 \\ v_3 \\ v_4 \\ v_5 \\ v_6 \\ v_7 \\ v_8 \\ v_9 \\ 0 \end{bmatrix} + \begin{bmatrix} \lambda_1 & 0 \\ \lambda_2 & 0 \\ \lambda_3 & 0 \\ \lambda_4 & 0 \\ \lambda_5 & 0 \\ \lambda_6 & 0 \\ \lambda_7 & 0 \\ \lambda_8 & 0 \\ \lambda_9 & 0 \\ 0 & 1 \end{bmatrix} \begin{bmatrix} \text{Depression} \\ \text{Mobility} \end{bmatrix} + \begin{bmatrix} e_1 \\ e_2 \\ e_3 \\ e_4 \\ e_5 \\ e_6 \\ e_7 \\ e_8 \\ e_9 \\ 0 \end{bmatrix} \quad (3.5)
$$

An additional *identifying constraint* of setting any one of the factors' loadings as a reference to one will result in eight factor loadings to estimate instead of nine. Most typically, in equation (3.5), we would set $\lambda_1 = 1$. An identifying constraint is a constraint used for model estimation purposes to decrease the number of parameters by one by fixing a particular parameter to a constant. It is necessary for the number of free parameters to be equal to or less than the amount of observed information necessary to estimate those parameters in order for the parameters of the model to have a unique solution (Chapter 5 for criteria for model identification).

There is no explicit measurement model for the observed exogenous variable *symptom onset*. Similar to *mobility* we assumed *symptom onset* is measured without error. The LISREL form, unlike the typical path diagram, makes explicit all relationships which we constrained to zero (e.g. *depression* → *mobility* is constrained to zero).

The structural model in LISREL form follows (3.2):

$$
\begin{bmatrix} \text{Depression} \\ \text{Mobility} \end{bmatrix} = \begin{bmatrix} \alpha_D \\ \alpha_M \end{bmatrix} + \begin{bmatrix} 0 & \beta_{11} \\ 0 & 0 \end{bmatrix} \begin{bmatrix} \text{Depression} \\ \text{Mobility} \end{bmatrix}
$$

$$
+ \begin{bmatrix} \gamma_{12} \\ \gamma_{21} \end{bmatrix} \begin{bmatrix} \text{Symptom Onset} \end{bmatrix} + \begin{bmatrix} D_D \\ D_M \end{bmatrix}. \quad (3.6)
$$

Means/intercepts of latent variables, such as α_D in equation (3.6) are not estimable without further constraints [10]. As previously mentioned in Chapter 2, a latent variable must be assigned a metric, including a mean. In addition, a model with a latent variable included in the mean structure necessitates additional identifying constraints [10].[1]

---

[1] Or else the model would be underidentified (Chapter 5).

In equation (3.6), we will assume that the model intercept α_D is constrained to zero. An alternative approach would be to set a reference item intercept to a constant in the measurement model (e.g. fix $v_1 = 0$ and estimate α_D). In multigroup analysis, one can constrain the mean of a latent variable in a reference group to zero and estimate the mean for the latent variable in the non-reference groups (given the model is identifiable).

In including a mean structure in the model, the exogenous variable symptom onset has mean κ_S and variance ϕ_S.

3.4 Assumptions for the Error Terms

3.4.1 Local Independence

A standard assumption of a measurement model (e.g. CFA model) is that each observed indicator is independent of every other observed indicator. This assumption is referred to as *local independence*. Local independence is a form of conditional independence. Observed indicators are independent conditional on the latent variable. Error terms for the reflective indicators of a latent variable are not correlated with each other. Importantly, this assumption leads to a useful interpretation as the latent variable alone explains why the observed indicators are related to each other [16]. We assume local independence for the measurement model of *depression* in this chapter.

Local dependence can be specified in a measurement model (Chapter 6). A *residual covariance* is a covariance between two error terms. The standardized form of the residual covariance, a *residual correlation*, is a correlation between two error terms. In a measurement model, a residual covariance represents covariance between the observed items that is not explained by the latent variable of which they are effect indicators. It may indicate that there are common causes (i.e. unmeasured confounding) that explain the relationship between two variables and are not included in the model.

3.4.2 Making Distributional Assumptions

In describing the LISREL approach, we did not assume multivariate normality for each of the error terms in equations (3.1) and (3.2). We more generally assumed a distribution with zero mean for ε, δ and ζ. Multivariate normality is not a characteristic of the model itself used in SEM, but of certain widely used estimators such as ML, which will be discussed in Chapter 4 [17].

There is a likely degree of *skewness* and *kurtosis* in variables such as the PHQ-9 items and timed 25-foot walk in a sample of persons with MS not consistent with a multivariate normal distribution. While an assumption of normality is made for the error terms, in practice a typical step toward determining whether normality is a reasonable assumption is to examine univariate and multivariate distributions of observed dependent variables and skewness and kurtosis.

3.4.3 An Introduction to Skewness and Kurtosis

The moments around the mean of a distribution can uncover departures from normality [1]. One should be aware that the first raw moment is the mean, the second central moment is the variance and the standardized third and fourth central moments are skewness and kurtosis, respectively. A well-known property of the normal distribution is that it is symmetric (i.e. centered around the mean). Skewness measures the degree of asymmetry. *Right (or positive) skewed data* has a long tail on the positive side of the peak of the distribution. *Left (or negative) skewed data* has a long tail on the negative side of the peak of the distribution.

The plot of a standard normal distribution has a bell-shaped curve with approximately 5% of the data falling in the tails. Kurtosis measures whether data are *heavy-tailed* or *light-tailed* relative to a normal distribution. A light-tailed distribution has less extreme values or outliers than the normal distribution; the tails are thinner and the distribution is shorter in a light-tailed distribution compared to the normal distribution. A heavy-tailed distribution has more extreme values or outliers than the normal distribution; the tails are fatter and the distribution is longer in a heavy-tailed distribution compared to the normal distribution.

Asymptotically, skewness can impact means while kurtosis can impact standard errors [18]. In the context of SEM, kurtosis has been found to be typically more problematic than skewness in terms of the effects on inferences [18].

The normal distribution has a skewness of 0 (for perfect symmetry) and a kurtosis of 3. Most software provide *excess kurtosis* instead of kurtosis. Excess kurtosis can be calculated by subtracting 3 from kurtosis and equals zero for the normal distribution [19]. Thus, it is a measure of "excess" kurtosis beyond the normal distribution. We use the terminology kurtosis for excess kurtosis hereafter, unless denoting otherwise.

A rule of thumb that has been used in samples larger than 300 in evaluating a univariate distribution is if the absolute value of the skewness exceeds 2 and kurtosis exceeds 4 then the distribution is non-normal [19]. However, one should also analyze graphical displays such as the histogram to help assess normality.

For samples sizes less than or equal to 300, one should evaluate the absolute z-scores rather than the raw absolute values of skewness and kurtosis. The z-score is the value divided by the standard error. For samples of size between 50 and 300, a recommended threshold is 3.29 for both skewness and kurtosis [19]. In samples smaller than 50, some researchers would opine that these statistics are far too instable to determine a trustworthy rule of thumb. Nevertheless, in these very small samples, a recommended threshold sometimes used is 1.96 for both skewness and kurtosis [19].

Extensions of univariate skewness and kurtosis are available for multivariate data [20]. Mardia's measures [21] allow one to evaluate multivariate skewness and kurtosis and test if multivariate normality is a reasonable assumption.

Consider we have p observed endogenous variables. The expected Mardia's skewness and kurtosis for a multivariate normal distribution is, respectively, 0 and $p(p+2)$. Higher values of Mardia's estimate of multivariate skewness indicate a more severe departure from normality [20]. Values lower or higher than the expected Mardia's kurtosis indicate tailedness. Tests of the departure from normality using these values can then be performed for the joint distribution of the set of p variables. A significant test statistic (i.e. p-value <0.05) for Mardia's estimate of multivariate skewness indicates significant multivariate skewness, and likewise, a significant test statistic for Mardia's estimate of multivariate kurtosis indicates significant multivariate kurtosis.

3.4.4 Distributional Assumptions in the MS-Depression Mediation Example

We used a data set of 3,507 persons living with MS extracted from an electronic health registry, Cleveland Clinic's Knowledge Program between 2008 and 2011 [22–24] (Appendix C).

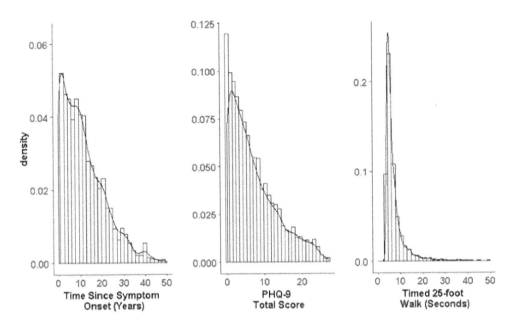

FIGURE 3.4
Density histograms in the MS-depression example (N=3,507).

We do not show time since symptom onset values above 50 years for the density histogram (some sparse values above 50 ranging until 76.5). We do not show the timed 25-foot walk scores above 50 seconds for the density histogram (very sparse values above 50 ranging all the way until 180). A PHQ-9 total score ≥10 is considered a positive screening for major depression. The PHQ-9 total score, ranging from 0 to 27, is the sum score of the nine items.

In Figure 3.4 we show density histograms of time since symptom onset (years), timed 25-foot walk (seconds) and the PHQ-9 total score (sum of the nine PHQ-9 items). The mean (standard deviation) in the data set for the PHQ-9 total score is 6.97 (6.21), timed 25-foot walk is 8.13 (9.82) and symptom onset is 11.53 (9.83). Thus, the distribution of these scores represents a wide range of self-reported depression severity, mobility impairment levels and time since symptom onset. Further, nearly 30% (n=1,005) of patients had PHQ-9≥10 (screening cutoff for depressive disorder).

The PHQ-9 total score did not show considerable skewness=1.01 or kurtosis=0.30, according to the rule of thumb guidelines. However, the density histogram in Figure 3.4 for PHQ-9 total score does not appear to be symmetric as characteristic of the normal distribution. Thus, there certainly appears to be a departure from normality for the distribution of the PHQ-9 total score. Further, when evaluating the individual nine items, the histograms (not shown) do not appear symmetric. The item for self-harm exhibits both right skewness (skewness=3.81) and heavy-tailedness (kurtosis=16.82). The timed 25-foot walk due to the spread of the data and presence of outliers (indicated in Figure 3.4) exhibits considerable right skewness (skewness=7.84) and heavy-tailedness (kurtosis=87.74). Similar to the PHQ-9 total score, time since symptom onset did not show considerable skewness (skewness=1.16) or kurtosis (kurtosis=1.58), but the density histogram did not appear symmetric.

We have data for p=11 variables to test for multivariate normality, given the model with a mean and covariance structure, including ten endogenous variables (nine PHQ-9 items and the timed 25-foot walk) and one exogenous variable treated like a dependent variable.

Mardia's estimate of multivariate kurtosis should then be approximately $11(11+2)=143$ for a multivariate normal distribution.

We used the mardia function in the psych package in R program for performing Mardia tests of multivariate skew and kurtosis. We found Mardia's estimate of multivariate skew $=99.24$ and kurtosis $=297.63$, thus indicating skewness and tailedness. Further, tests of the departure from normality indicated both significant skewness ($p<0.001$) and kurtosis ($p<0.001$) for the joint distribution of the set of 11 variables. Additional analysis to test bivariate skewness and kurtosis (between pairs of the 11 variables) revealed considerable bivariate skewness and kurtosis between many of the variables.

Aforementioned, if we did not add a mean structure in the model, the model is expressed for the endogenous variables conditional on the exogenous variable. Since the distribution of the exogenous variable is not part of the model in this case, we would examine the joint distribution of the ten endogenous variables for Mardia's test.

As a result of our analyses, we will not assume multivariate normality for the data. We assume that the error terms in the measurement model of *depression* (trivially leaving out *mobility* here) are each continuous with zero mean and positive variance.

Formally, $E(\varepsilon)=0$ and $\text{Var}(\varepsilon)=\Theta_\varepsilon$, where

$$
\varepsilon =
\begin{pmatrix}
e_1 \\
e_2 \\
e_3 \\
e_4 \\
e_5 \\
e_6 \\
e_7 \\
e_8 \\
e_9
\end{pmatrix},
\quad
\Theta_\varepsilon =
\begin{pmatrix}
\theta_{e1} & 0 & 0 & 0 & 0 & 0 & 0 & 0 & 0 \\
0 & \theta_{e2} & 0 & 0 & 0 & 0 & 0 & 0 & 0 \\
0 & 0 & \theta_{e3} & 0 & 0 & 0 & 0 & 0 & 0 \\
0 & 0 & 0 & \theta_{e4} & 0 & 0 & 0 & 0 & 0 \\
0 & 0 & 0 & 0 & \theta_{e5} & 0 & 0 & 0 & 0 \\
0 & 0 & 0 & 0 & 0 & \theta_{e6} & 0 & 0 & 0 \\
0 & 0 & 0 & 0 & 0 & 0 & \theta_{e7} & 0 & 0 \\
0 & 0 & 0 & 0 & 0 & 0 & 0 & \theta_{e8} & 0 \\
0 & 0 & 0 & 0 & 0 & 0 & 0 & 0 & \theta_{e9}
\end{pmatrix}
\tag{3.7}
$$

$\theta_{e1}, \theta_{e2}, \theta_{e3}, \theta_{e4}, \theta_{e5}, \theta_{e6}, \theta_{e7}, \theta_{e8}$ and θ_{e9} are the residual variances for the item error terms. The residual covariances in (3.7) between all pairwise item error terms under local independence are assumed to be zero. The item error terms are assumed to be uncorrelated with *depression, mobility* and *symptom onset*.

We also assume that the error terms associated with *depression* and *mobility* are both continuous with zero mean and positive variance.

Formally, $E(\zeta)=0$ and $\text{Var}(\zeta)=\Psi_\zeta$, where

$$
\zeta \sim
\begin{pmatrix}
D_D \\
D_M
\end{pmatrix},
\quad
\Psi_\zeta =
\begin{pmatrix}
\psi_D & \psi_{DM} \\
\psi_{DM} & \psi_M
\end{pmatrix}
\tag{3.8}
$$

ψ_D and ψ_M are the residual variances for the disturbance terms. We will assume the identifying constraint of $\text{Cov}(D_D, D_M) = \psi_{DM} = 0$, a typical assumption for a mediation model. In a structural model, nonzero covariance between disturbance terms represents covariance between endogenous variables that is not explained by the predictors. See Chapter 5 for discussion on model identifiability and the special care required for a model with correlated disturbance terms.

Aforementioned, we also assume the exogenous variable *symptom onset* has mean κ_S and variance ϕ_S. For the pseudo-isolation condition, *symptom onset* and the two disturbance terms are uncorrelated.

3.5 Mean Structure

Variable intercepts/means play an important role in health and medicine. Medical records, administrative, survey and longitudinal clinical trials data alike often have a lot of missing values. In models under study, there are potential sources of confounding of hypothesized relationships to account for. Health and medical researchers are commonly estimating models with multiple covariates and encountering missing data on dependent and independent variables. Researchers can include both the mean and covariance structures in such a model. Missing data can then be handled using the FIML procedure under practical assumptions about the missing data mechanism (that we shall discuss in Chapter 4) [9]. In FIML, all available information in all observations (even for cases with missing values on some of the variables) are included in the analysis. The sample means and individual-level data are required for FIML.

Means also are important for standard analysis in health and medicine involving data that violates normality assumptions. Mean-adjusted or mean- and variance- adjusted robust estimators[2] are often useful in analysis in health in medicine due to the distribution of the data (e.g. data exhibiting skewness and kurtosis).

Health or other disparities may exist across groups (e.g. race/ethnicity groups). In many studies, researchers are greatly interested to evaluate for mean differences across groups (in addition to other differences). As such researchers assess equivalence of item intercepts (i.e. equality of the levels of the underlying items) and factor means. Measurement invariance testing will be a topic of much discussion in Chapter 10. For an example, Sudano et al. [25] found unequal item intercepts (but equal factor loadings) for SF-36 version 2 scores across four tested racial/ethnic and language groups using multigroup CFA. Thus, analyses of model intercepts revealed some degree of systematic bias for Spanish-speaking Hispanics relative to the other groups [25].

Intercepts are fundamental for describing the baseline value of an outcome when performing longitudinal data analysis such as latent growth curve analysis. We discuss latent growth curve analysis in Chapter 13.

In a structural equation model with a mean structure, the means of the endogenous variables are a function of intercepts, regression slopes and the means of the exogenous variables. The interested reader should refer to Bentler and Yuan [26] for more technical details on adding a mean structure to a covariance structure model.

To illustrate the makeup of the mean structure in a basic manner [27,28], consider a simple model with a regression of a single dependent variable Y on a single independent variable X, such that

$$Y = \alpha_0 + \gamma_1 X + D \tag{3.9}$$

---

[2] For example, MLM and MLR options for continuous data and the WLSMV option for ordered-categorical data in MPlus.

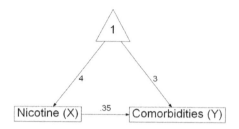

FIGURE 3.5
Regression of the number of comorbid illnesses on the level of nicotine dependence.

We assume that the expected value of the error term D is equal to zero. We can decompose the raw mean of Y, into a function of its intercept, a regression coefficient and the raw mean of X. Taking the expectation of both sides of equation (3.9) [18]:

$$\mu_y = \alpha_0 + \gamma_1 \mu_x \tag{3.10}$$

where μ_x is the mean of X and μ_y is the mean of Y. We include in (3.10) parameters for the intercept of Y, α_0 and a regression coefficient, γ_1, for the direct effect of X on Y.

Means are included in SEM by regressing exogenous and/or endogenous variables on a constant that equals one [10]. In a path diagram, these means can either be implied (left out of the path diagram) or explicitly drawn. Generally, in this book, we will not show, but rather imply means/intercepts in path diagrams. The triangle in a path diagram explicitly presents the mean structure.

In the example in Figure 3.5, we explicitly show the mean structure for the regression of a single dependent variable representing the number of comorbid illnesses (Y) on a single independent variable representing the level of nicotine dependence (X).

The mean of *nicotine* is equal to four from the regression of *nicotine* on a constant that equals one. The mean of *comorbidities* follows from formula (3.10): $3.00 + 0.35(4.00) = 4.40$.

3.5.1 Free Parameters in the MS-Depression Mediation Model

In nearly all models, there are multiple possible ways to relate a set of variables to each other. For example, in the MS-depression example, one could have alternatively hypothesized, rather unreasonably, that *depression* and *mobility* both influence *symptom onset*. The two hypothesized models for MS-depression represented in Figures 3.2 and 3.3 are both plausible.

When specifying a structural equation model, one is hypothesizing using logic, theory and prior evidence how a set of variables are related to each other. These relationships can be illustrated in a path diagram or represented using the LISREL approach as discussed in this chapter. In the model specification, pathways in the model are a function of the parameters. In a system of equations to describe relationships for a given model specification, the parameters are embedded in the equations (e.g. intercepts and slopes). These parameters can be estimated using observed information, such as observed means, variances and covariances (Chapter 4). In this section, we are merely explaining how to determine the free parameters in a structural equation model. In the simple path model in Chapter 2 regressing Chronic Nature of HIV on Daily Health Services and Duration of Diagnosis, the unknown parameters included an intercept, two slopes and a residual variance (Chapter 2, Figure 2.7) to relate the dependent variable to the two independent

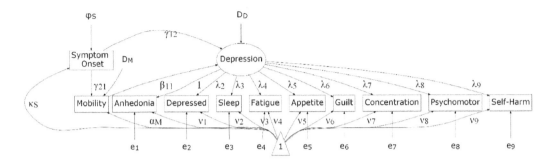

FIGURE 3.6
MS-depression mediation model with a mean structure and explicitly indicating all unknown parameters.

We include three identifying constraints (among other assumptions) that the first factor loading λ_1 for anhedonia is fixed to one, the intercept for depression α_D is fixed to zero and the covariance for the two residual errors D_D and D_M is fixed to zero. Note that for the error terms $e_1, e_2, e_3, e_4, e_5, e_6, e_7, e_8$ and e_9 and D_D and D_M the unknown parameters are the residual variances $\theta_{e1}, \theta_{e2}, \theta_{e3}, \theta_{e4}, \theta_{e5}, \theta_{e6}, \theta_{e7}, \theta_{e8}$ and θ_{e9} and ψ_D and ψ_M, respectively.

TABLE 3.1

The Breakdown of the 34 Free Parameters for the MS-Depression Mediation Model Corresponding to the Symbols in Figure 3.6

Parameters	Symbols
Nine factor intercepts	$\nu_1, \nu_2, \nu_3, \nu_4, \nu_5, \nu_6, \nu_7, \nu_8, \nu_9$
Eight factor loadings	$\lambda_2, \lambda_3, \lambda_4, \lambda_5, \lambda_6, \lambda_7, \lambda_8, \lambda_9$
Nine factor residual variances	$\theta_{e1}, \theta_{e2}, \theta_{e3}, \theta_{e4}, \theta_{e5}, \theta_{e6}, \theta_{e7}, \theta_{e8}, \theta_{e9}$
One structural regression intercept	α_M
Three structural regression slopes	$\beta_{11}, \gamma_{12}, \gamma_{21}$
Two error residuals variances	ψ_D, ψ_M
One estimated mean for symptom onset	κ_S
One estimated variance for symptom onset	ϕ_S

Note that omitting a parameter (e.g. path or covariance) in the model represented in Figure 3.6 is equivalent to constraining that parameter to zero.

variables in the model under the model specification. Multi-equation models with latent variables involve many more parameters.

In Figure 3.6, we revisit the example from Figure 3.2 for the MS-depression mediation model explicitly indicating all free parameters under the model specification. The free parameters for the equations for the measurement and structural model for this specification were also previously indicated using a modified LISREL approach. Here we should formally distinguish that one may have t^* total parameters and t free parameters to estimate, where $t < t^*$. The other $t^* - t$ parameters are known and fixed to a value given a prior assumption. A free parameter is one that can be adjusted by the optimization routine to make the model fit the data. After making three previously mentioned identifying constraints (summarized in Figure 3.6) and several other assumptions (e.g. local independence), we have 34 free parameters [28]. The breakdown of these 34 free parameters is listed in Table 3.1.

In traditional simple linear regression utilizing ordinary least squares, we estimate a typical set of parameters such as the intercept and slope. In SEM, depending on the specification of the model, we may get a different number of parameters; there is no typical set of parameters. In the SEM framework a model is specified (and dependent upon) one's conceptual model and hypotheses of interest.

Analysis of the total effect from *symptom onset* to *depression* corresponding to Figures 3.2 and 3.6 would include consideration of the three structural regression slopes in the structural model $(\beta_{11}, \gamma_{12}, \gamma_{21})$ that make up the direct and indirect effects. In Figure 3.3, under a different specification of the same variables considered in Figure 3.2, there are only two structural regression slopes in the structural model to consider in the indirect pathway between *symptom onset* and *depression* (i.e. *symptom onset* → *mobility*, *mobility* → *depression*).

There are also assumptions regarding the mean structure that influence the number of parameters in the model. For example, alternatively, we might include 32 parameters in our model and exclude the estimated mean and variance for the exogenous variable *symptom onset*. In this case, one would view *symptom onset* strictly as a fixed measure to be conditioned on during model estimation similar to how one typically treats covariates in traditional multiple regression analysis. The model with no mean structure (i.e. no means/intercepts) includes 22 parameters. When z-scores as standardized scores are used in place of the raw scores for variables prior to analysis the means are close to zero [10].

3.6 Conclusions

This chapter provided an overview of path diagrams and the LISREL model. These approaches allow a researcher to represent a conceptual model in the SEM framework. We used an example from a study evaluating depression-related issues in persons with MS to illustrate these approaches. When using PRO data and other health-related outcomes, one should consider that an assumption of multivariate normality is likely not valid.

Appendix

A. Solving the Structural Equations for η

Using straightforward algebra under the assumption that $\mathbf{I} - \mathbf{B}$ is invertible (which is in general a rather mild assumption, and one that's satisfied in all models used in this book).

$$\eta = \alpha_\eta + \mathbf{B}\eta + \mathbf{\Gamma}\xi + \zeta$$

$$\eta - \mathbf{B}\eta = \alpha_\eta + \mathbf{\Gamma}\xi + \zeta$$

$$(\mathbf{I} - \mathbf{B})\eta = \alpha_\eta + \mathbf{\Gamma}\xi + \zeta \qquad (3.11)$$

$$\eta = (\mathbf{I} - \mathbf{B})^{-1}(\alpha_\eta + \mathbf{\Gamma}\xi + \zeta)$$

B. Mathematical Equations Corresponding to the MS-Depression Mediation Model in Figure 3.2

Equations that provide a measurement model of the latent variable *depression*:

$$\text{Anhedonia} = v_1 + \lambda_1 \text{Depression} + e_1,$$

$$\text{Depressed} = v_2 + \lambda_2 \text{Depression} + e_2,$$

$$\text{Sleep} = v_3 + \lambda_3 \text{Depression} + e_3,$$

$$\text{Fatigue} = v_4 + \lambda_4 \text{Depression} + e_4,$$

$$\text{Appetite} = v_5 + \lambda_5 \text{Depression} + e_5, \tag{3.12}$$

$$\text{Guilt} = v_6 + \lambda_6 \text{Depression} + e_6,$$

$$\text{Concentration} = v_7 + \lambda_7 \text{Depression} + e_7,$$

$$\text{Psychomotor} = v_8 + \lambda_8 \text{Depression} + e_8,$$

$$\text{Self-Harm} = v_9 + \lambda_9 \text{Depression} + e_9$$

Equations that provide a structural model:

$$\text{Depression} = \alpha_D + \beta_{11}\text{Mobility} + \gamma_{12}\text{Symptom Onset} + D_D,$$

$$\text{Mobility} = \alpha_M + \gamma_{21}\text{Symptom Onset} + D_M \tag{3.13}$$

Each equation above is both linear in the variables and parameters [1]. Equations in SEMs (e.g. models with interaction terms or quadratic relationships) can be nonlinear in the variables.

C. Observational Data of Persons Living with MS (N = 3,507)

Information about Cleveland Clinic's Neurological Institute and The Knowledge Program can be found at http://my.clevelandclinic.org/neurological_institute/about/default.aspx. The Mellen Center (https://my.clevelandclinic.org/departments/neurological/depts/multiple-sclerosis) manages more than 21,000 visits and 8,000 patients every year for MS treatment. The Knowledge Program tracked illness severity and treatment efficacy over time across the Mellen Center population (2008–2016).

We used a retrospective cohort study design with data collected between 2008 and 2011. Inclusion criteria included individuals making at least one visit to the Mellen Center with measurements of PHQ-9 score and a timed 25-foot walk available. In the sample, typical of the United States' MS population, the majority were female (73%) and Caucasian (83%). MS is typically diagnosed in individuals in their early 30s. In our sample, the average age was 46 (SD=12). Also, in our sample, the average time since symptom onset was 10 (SD=9) years ago with 81% relapsing and 16% progressive with the remaining patients falling into other categories, or under evaluation for a potential MS diagnosis. See Gunzler et al. [22] and Gunzler and Morris [23] for further description of the cross-sectional data and scales for this sample of persons living with MS which is used throughout this textbook.

References

1. Bollen, K., *Structural equations with latent variables.* 1989, New York: Wiley.
2. Kline, R.B., *Principles and practice of structural equation modeling, fourth edition.* 2016, New York: Guilford Press.
3. Kaplan, D., *Structural equation modeling.* 2001, Thousand Oaks, CA: Sage.
4. Ellson, J., et al., *Graphviz: Open Source Graph Drawing Tools.* 2002, Berlin, Heidelberg: Springer.
5. Iannone, R., DiagrammeR: Graph/network visualization. *R Package Version,* 2018. **1**.
6. Kroenke, K., R.L. Spitzer, and J.B. Williams, The Phq-9. *Journal of General Internal Medicine,* 2001. **16**(9): pp. 606–613.
7. Joreskog, K. and D. Sorbom, *LISREL 8 user's reference guide.* 1996, Chicago, IL: Scientific Software.
8. Jöreskog, K.G. and M. Thiilo, Lisrel A general computer program for estimating a linear structural equation system involving multiple indicators of unmeasured variables. *ETS Research Report Series,* 1972. **1972**(2): pp. 171.
9. Muthén, L.K. and B.O. Muthén, *Mplus: The comprehensive modelling program for applied researchers: user's guide.* Eighth edition. 1998–2017, Los Angeles, CA: Muthén & Muthén.
10. Kline, R.B., Supplemental Chapter B: Introduction to Mean Structures, in *Principles and practice of structural equation modeling.* 2000, New York: Guilford Press.
11. Tarka, P., An overview of structural equation modeling: its beginnings, historical development, usefulness and controversies in the social sciences. *Quality and Quantity,* 2018. **52**(1): pp. 313–354.
12. Gunzler, D., et al., A class of distribution-free models for longitudinal mediation analysis. *Psychometrika,* 2014. **79**(4): pp. 543–568.
13. Bollen, K.A. and M.D. Noble, Structural equation models and the quantification of behavior. *Proceedings of the National Academy of Sciences,* 2011. 108(Supplement 3): pp. 15639–15646.
14. Long, J., *Covariance structure models: An introduction to LISREL.* 1983, Thousand Oaks, CA: Sage.
15. Kieseier, B.C. and C. Pozzilli, Assessing walking disability in multiple sclerosis. *Multiple Sclerosis Journal,* 2012. **18**(7): pp. 914–924.
16. Lazarsfeld, P.F. and N.W. Henry, *Latent structure analysis.* 1968, New York: Houghton, Mifflin.
17. Posted in CBA Help Desk, News and Updates, Statistics & Research Methods, Structural Equation Modeling. Can I estimate an SEM if the sample data are not normally distributed? Curran-Bauer Analytics 2019 January 23 [cited 2020 August 28].
18. Byrne, B.M., *Structural equation modeling with Mplus: Basic concepts, applications, and programming.* 2013, Abingdon: Routledge.
19. Kim, H.-Y., Statistical notes for clinical researchers: assessing normal distribution (2) using skewness and kurtosis. *Restorative Dentistry and Endodontics,* 2013. **38**(1): pp. 52–54.
20. Cain, M.K., Z. Zhang, and K.-H. Yuan, Univariate and multivariate skewness and kurtosis for measuring nonnormality: Prevalence, influence and estimation. *Behavior Research Methods,* 2017. **49**(5): pp. 1716–1735.
21. Mardia, K.V., Measures of multivariate skewness and kurtosis with applications. *Biometrika,* 1970. **57**(3): pp. 519–530.
22. Gunzler, D., et al., Disentangling multiple sclerosis & depression: An adjusted depression screening score for patient-centered care. *Journal of Behavioral Medicine,* 2015. **38**(2): pp. 237–250.
23. Gunzler, D.D. and N. Morris, A tutorial on structural equation modeling for analysis of overlapping symptoms in co-occurring conditions using MPlus. *Statistics in Medicine,* 2015. **34**(24): pp. 3246–3280.
24. Katzan, I., et al., The Knowledge Program: An innovative, comprehensive electronic data capture system and warehouse. *AMIA Annual Symposium Proceedings,* 2011. 2011: pp. 683–692.
25. Sudano, J.J., et al., Measuring disparities: Bias in the SF-36v2 among Spanish-speaking medical patients. *Medical Care,* 2011. **49**(5): pp. 480–488.

26. Bentler, P.M. and K.-H. Yuan, On adding a mean structure to a covariance structure model. *Educational and Psychological Measurement*, 2000. **60**(3): pp. 326–339.
27. Bentler, P.M. and E.J. Wu, *EQS 6.1 for Windows*. 2005, Encino, CA: Multivariate Software INC.
28. Byrne, B.M., Structural equation modeling with Mplus: Basic concepts, applications, and programming. 2013, Abingdon: Routledge.

4

Model Estimation and Evaluation

4.1 Introduction to Model Estimation in SEM

In Chapter 3, we discussed frameworks for representing a structural equation model as a function of its free (unknown) parameters. Here we describe a procedure that can be used for estimating these parameters using sample data. Models are specified, combined with data, and structures of equations are implemented to calculate results and thereby inform theoretical interpretations.

A novice SEM researcher might initially assume that only a mystical, wildly confusing process could simultaneously combine multi-equation models and handle measurement error. Instead, a clever aspect of the procedure that we will outline in this chapter is that it is grounded in sound multivariate statistical theory. The reader should always keep in mind that SEM researchers make strong assumptions, multiplied by the number of hypothesized causal paths, to infer causal relations [1]. In other words, one should never believe that SEM can magically produce sensible results from a baseless conceptual model!

For clarity for the novice SEM researcher, we illustrate this type of procedure with a simple example in a traditional setting. We hypothesize that infant fat mass is associated with maternal adiposity. How do we estimate this association and test this hypothesis? We could proceed by regressing infant fat mass on maternal adiposity using the ordinary least squares (OLS) estimation method in the traditional regression framework. Then, we could test our hypothesis through evaluation of the OLS regression slope estimate and standard error for maternal adiposity.

Model estimation in linear SEMs can be seen as a multifaceted extension of traditional linear regression model estimation. In the SEM framework, we estimate free parameters from observed variables. Estimation in a typical structural equation model involves many free parameters in order to evaluate complex relationships among latent and observed variables. As a consequence, an estimation procedure in SEM typically requires a larger sample size (e.g. at least 200 observations for meaningful results) and much more observed information, including observed variances and covariances, than a traditional regression model.

Conducting SEM analysis using small samples may lead to convergence problems (iterative optimization algorithm was unable to find a suitable solution), improper solutions and inaccurate parameter estimates, especially standard errors. In analyses using a very large sample, the evaluation of model fit is done with special considerations. For example, the chi-square test (to be discussed in this chapter) can be sensitive to even small specification errors in the model and therefore impractical for studies with very large sample sizes or many parameters to be estimated.

One can perform SEM analysis based on summary statistics such as observed variances and covariances. However, as we will discuss within this chapter, individual level data allows for far more flexibility and complexity in the statistical analysis. A researcher makes strong causal assumptions in addition to other standard statistical assumptions (e.g. when appropriate, linearity and multivariate normality) in using SEM.

4.2 Estimating Model Parameters from Sample Data and Statistics

In an OLS traditional linear regression, the conditional mean is modeled as a linear predictor function of model parameters (i.e. intercept and slopes). Then, the key idea is to minimize the sum of the squared residuals in order to choose the model parameters.

In the classic covariance-based approaches to SEM, relationships are modeled among observed and latent variables in a system of equations. The covariance matrix of the observed variables in these equations can then be represented as a function of the model parameters [2,3].

The key idea used in covariance-based SEM estimation methods is to choose the model parameters θ, which minimize the distance between the observed covariance matrix and a covariance matrix "implied" or reproduced by the parameters in the model. The model-implied covariance matrix is meant to represent the population covariance matrix. Aforementioned, one can (and typically does) fit a structural equation model to the raw data using software such as MPlus in a manner similar to traditional regression analysis.

Diagonal elements in the sample (empirical) covariance matrix are the sample estimates of the variances of the observed variables, while the off-diagonal elements are the sample estimates of the covariances between the observed variables [4]. The implication in this approach is that if the model is correct then the model-implied covariance matrix and the observed covariance matrix should be an exact match [5]. Thus the covariance matrix is "implied" or reproduced in the sense of looking to reproduce the observed covariance matrix for a given model and estimated parameters values [6]. For more technical details regarding the form of the model-implied covariance matrix in SEMs, the interested reader should refer to the classic textbook by Bollen [2].

Formally, suppose one aims to estimate t unknown model parameters from a total of k observed and w^* unobserved (latent) variables. In classic covariance-based approaches to SEM, the null hypothesis is $\Sigma = \Sigma(\theta)$ [2]. θ is a vector of unknown parameters of dimension $t \times 1$. The population covariance matrix Σ and model-implied covariance matrix $\Sigma(\theta)$ are both of dimension $k \times k$. The sample covariance matrix is used as an approximate of Σ in practice to estimate the unknown parameters.

We may perform both mean *and* covariance structure analysis. In addition to the covariance matrix, the mean vector of the observed variables can be represented as a function of the model parameters. Thus, one can additionally choose the model parameters θ to minimize the distance between the observed and model-implied mean vector. That is, one can test the null hypotheses that $\mu = \mu(\theta)$ *and* $\Sigma = \Sigma(\theta)$. The population mean vector μ and model-implied mean vector $\mu(\theta)$ are both of dimension $k \times 1$. The sample mean vector is used as an approximate of μ in practice to estimate unknown parameters.

Formally the distance between the vector of sample means and sample covariance matrix on the one hand, and the model-implied mean vector and covariance matrix on the other, must be given by some non-negative discrepancy function $F(\mu(\theta), \Sigma(\theta), \bar{z}, S)$ [5,7–9]. Here, $\bar{z}$ is the vector of the sample means $\bar{y}$ and $\bar{x}$ for all the observed endogenous and exogenous variables, and $\mu(\theta)$ is the model-implied mean vector (as notated previously). S is the sample covariance matrix, and $\Sigma(\theta)$ is the model-implied covariance matrix (as notated previously).

Numerical optimization is used to find the (values of) θ, which best fits the observed data in the sense of minimizing this discrepancy function [10,11]. That is, parameters are estimated by defining a discrepancy function in line with the variable distribution assumptions and then using an iterative method for minimization of this discrepancy function. For an example, for performing estimation using *maximum likelihood (ML)*, the negative of the log-likelihood may also be considered as a discrepancy function, because minimizing the negative of the log-likelihood is the same as maximizing the log-likelihood.

The discrepancy function to be minimized for performing estimation using ML can be defined as [5]:

$$F_{ML} = \log(|\Sigma(\theta)|) + \mathrm{tr}(S\Sigma(\theta)^{-1}) - \log(|S|) - k + (\bar{z} - \mu(\theta))^T \Sigma(\theta)^{-1}(\bar{z} - \mu(\theta)). \qquad (4.1)$$

Here, $|.|$ is the determinant, $\mathrm{tr}(.)$ is the trace function and $\log(.)$ is the logarithmic function. The number of observed variables is k.

The ML estimator assumes that the joint distribution of the observed variables in the model is a multivariate normal distribution. Then, ML searches for the set of parameter estimates $\hat{\theta}$ that minimizes discrepancy function in (4.1).

Although less commonly used than ML-based methods for SEM research in health and medicine, other discrepancy functions such as generalized least squares (GLS) or unweighted least squares (ULS) can be used under the assumption of multivariate normality [2]. In terms of traditional regression, ULS is analogous to OLS and GLS is analogous to weighted least squares [12]. Likewise, both ULS and GLS are less restrictive in terms of assumptions than ML-based methods. Asymptotically, ML and GLS are the same and will yield similar results if the data is approximately normally distributed. However, ML-based methods are more computationally efficient than both ULS and GLS.

The ML approach has been shown to still perform well in estimating parameter values compared to the true parameter values in many cases when multivariate normality does not hold [13]. For example, ML usually performs quite well in estimating the parameters with slightly skewed data. However, the ML approach may not perform as well in calculating model standard error values under these same violations of parametric assumptions.

4.3 Robust Estimation

Robust approaches are insensitive to departures from certain assumptions of the model (i.e. no clustering effect) and about the data (i.e. normality). *ML with robust standard errors* (or *robust ML*) is a commonly used estimator that provides robust estimation where parametric assumptions may be violated [14]. In practice, as previously mentioned, many health-related outcomes within health and medicine exhibit skewness and kurtosis. We have also noted how problematic multivariate kurtosis can be in impacting standard errors [15]. The ML approach with robust standard errors uses ML to estimate the parameters but uses a robust sandwich type estimator (Huber-White sandwich estimator) to calculate standard errors as well as to correct the overall model fit indices [16]. This approach can be carried out with standard errors computed using different sandwich estimator methods within MPlus for the MLM option (for complete data) or the MLR option (for complete or incomplete data) [14]. Similar options are available in most other SEM software (e.g. AMOS).

Bootstrapping the ML estimator is a more computationally intensive approach to calculating robust standard errors and confidence intervals [17]. Different versions of the bootstrap, such as a percentile, bias-corrected and bias-corrected and accelerated bootstrap [14,18,19], may be available depending on the SEM software.

We provide a sketch of the bootstrap procedure for calculating the 95% confidence interval around ML estimates for model parameters using the percentile method.

1. The original data set is sampled with replacement R times. Each bootstrapped data set will have the same number of observations as the original sample. By sampling with replacement, some of the original data points in each bootstrapped subsample will contain repeat values.

2. The model is fit using ML on the series of R bootstrap datasets.

3. From this procedure the average across the bootstrap samples can be obtained for each of the model parameters.

4. Out of our R bootstrapped estimates of a parameter find the 2.5th percentile estimate and the 97.5th percentile estimate (values that put 2.5% and 97.5% of the results to the left), which leaves 95% of the estimates in the middle.

At minimum, users should set $R = 1,000$, and many users will set $R = 10,000$. In mediation analysis, Preacher and Hayes [20] recommended using at least 5,000 samples for final reporting, even if one uses 1,000 for preliminary research.

The confidence interval can then be asymmetrical since it is based on an empirical estimation of the sampling distribution of each parameter estimate, rather than on an assumption that the sampling distribution is normal [20]. The *bias-corrected (BC) bootstrap* corrects further for bias in the distribution of the bootstrap estimates. The point estimate for a parameter via bootstrapping will not necessarily equal the original estimate. For example, a bootstrapped estimate of the median may be different from the original sample median. The BC bootstrap includes a bias correction parameter obtained from the proportion of bootstrap samples below the original estimate in the total number of bootstrap samples taken [19]. This bias correction parameter is then used to adjust the bootstrapped CI based on the percentile method to correct for bias.

In addition to model parameters, bootstrapping can be used to calculate model fit indices. Bootstrapping can be used for the purpose of validation to understand if there is any bias and sampling variation in the model parameters due to overfitting. The bootstrap may still be unreliable on smaller samples and works best on a moderately large sample size [20].

4.4 Non-normal Data

Numerous approaches exist for using SEM when dealing with non-normal endogenous variables. For analysis with non-normal continuous endogenous variables, techniques that may be useful include robust approaches such as ML with robust standard errors and bootstrapping and applying a data transformation (e.g. log transformation for right skewed or heavy-tailed data). One requires potentially a very large sample for these types of analyses using transformations. In practice, it may be difficult to interpret model estimates from some transformed variables compared to non-transformed variables.

A transformation is also performed on univariate data. The ML estimator does assume multivariate normality. Multivariate normality implies marginal normality. However, marginal normality does not imply multivariate normality. That is, a multivariate distribution may have standard normal margins but is not multivariate normal. Non-normality influences the estimation undesirably irrespective of where the non-normality may be. A transformation alone may not be adequate enough in some cases.

The *weighted least squares (WLS)* estimator uses a weight matrix constructed from direct estimation of the fourth-order moments of the residuals in an asymptotically distribution free (ADF) discrepancy function [10]. ADF estimators do not require multivariate normality [10]. The WLS estimator is robust to parametric assumptions and the type of data (ordered-categorical or continuous). The WLS estimator is also an example of an approach to SEM in which information is used outside of the covariance matrix (i.e. the fourth-order moment) [9].

Modifications to WLS to accommodate small samples are commonly used for performing CFA for a scale with dichotomous or ordinal items or for analysis of structural models with dichotomous or ordinal endogenous variables. These approaches are also typically paired with a robust sandwich type estimator to calculate standard errors as well as to correct the overall fit indices. Thus, these approaches are sometimes referred to as robust WLS.

Requesting WLS and modifications to WLS in most SEM software is accomplished within a line of code. For example, in MPLUS, one would request the WLSMV option (a robust WLS estimator) in the ANALYSIS section: ESTIMATOR = WLSMV. Another line of code under the VARIABLES section is available for treating outcome variables as ordered-categorical. For example, if items Y1, Y2, Y3 and Y4 are ordered-categorical variables used in a measurement model, one could input code under the VARIABLES section in MPlus: CATEGORICAL ARE Y1 Y2 Y3 Y4.

In a commonly used latent variable model for ordered-categorical data, a normally distributed latent variable (referred to as the *latent response variate*) exists which leads to the different levels of the ordered-categorical outcome if the latent variable exceeds some threshold level. The interpretation follows from probit analyses. Parameter estimates of the probit model are interpreted in terms of a one-unit increase in the z-score for the probability of being in a particular category vs. the reference category. We will discuss more technical details about this latent variable model for ordered-categorical data in Chapter 7.

Likelihood approaches are often used in the estimation of this latent variable model for ordered-categorical data. A three-stage procedure described by Muthén [7] can be used for estimating a CFA or structural equation model incorporating latent response variates using ML and WLS estimation.

MULTISTAGE WEIGHTED LEAST SQUARES (WLS) APPROACHES

For observed ordinal data, the WLS approach can be part of a three-stage procedure involving *polychoric correlations* [7]. Polychoric correlations estimate the linear relationship between two unobserved continuous variables given only observed ordered-categorical data [21]. The thresholds and polychoric correlations are estimated using two-stage ML estimation [22,23]. The third stage consists of estimating unknown model parameters using the discrepancy function for WLS:

$$F_{\text{WLS}} = \left[\mathbf{s} - \sigma(\theta) \right]^{T} \mathbf{W}^{-1} \left[\mathbf{s} - \sigma(\theta) \right] \qquad (4.2)$$

where $\mathbf{s}$ is a vector of polychoric correlations, $\sigma(\theta)$ is a vector of elements of the model-implied covariance matrix and $\mathbf{W}$ is the positive-definite weight matrix. $\mathbf{W}$ must be a consistent estimator of the asymptotic covariance matrix of $\mathbf{s}$. Different choices of $\mathbf{W}$ will lead to different versions of WLS. A simulation study by Flora and Curran [21] exhibited that CFA models using polychoric correlations were robust to the moderate levels of non-normality in the latent response variates under consideration.

The multistage procedure described above could be applied to different types of observed variables. A *polyserial correlation* is a linear relationship between two unobserved continuous variables when one of the observed distributions is ordered-categorical and one is continuous [21]. A *tetrachoric correlation* is a special case of the polychoric correlation when both observed variables are dichotomous. A *biserial correlation* is a special case of the polyserial correlation when the ordered-categorical observed variable is dichotomous.

We can generalize the multistage procedure to estimate (1) the correlation (e.g. polychoric, polyserial) depending on the distributions of the observed variables and (2) the unknown parameters of a model by WLS using a weight matrix which must be a consistent estimate of the asymptotic covariance matrix of the estimated correlations [24].

Diagonal weighted least squares (DWLS) [7,25] is a modification of WLS. The DWLS approach is computationally more practical as it uses the diagonal of the weight matrix whereas WLS uses the full weight matrix in the estimation procedure. Since the weight matrix is inverted in WLS estimation as in equation (4.2), this can be computationally problematic with the full weight matrix with a large number of variables. DWLS has been shown to perform better than WLS for small samples [26]. The WLSMV option in MPlus [14] is a commonly used variation of DWLS, using a different weight matrix, with adjusted mean and variance. One can additionally use bootstrap techniques with WLS or modifications of WLS estimators.

Binary, ordinal or nominal categorical outcomes can also be handled using ML-based approaches (e.g. ML or MLR option in MPlus) with numerical approximations, such as Monte Carlo integration [27]. Individual-level data is necessary for such analyses. This procedure can lead to familiar interpretations of the model parameter estimates. For example, analysis with a binary outcome may have a logit interpretation. ML-based approaches with numerical approximations are also available for count outcomes with a log interpretation [14].

In small data sets, Bayesian approaches to SEM analysis have been shown to perform well [28]. Bayesian SEM approaches can also be used for handling of non-normal parameters as they can deal with asymmetric distributions [29]. Many latent variable software program, such as MPlus and AMOS, allow for Bayesian estimation using powerful computational algorithms referred to as *Markov Chain Monte Carlo (MCMC)* methods. See Chapter 15 for a basic overview of Bayesian SEM.

4.4.1 Outliers

Many datasets used in health and medicine (e.g. real-world datasets) contain some invalid, unusual (or outlying) values that necessitate correction or removal before any analyses. However, some outlying values are assumed to be valid and not the result of typos or bad data entry. Outliers can be the cause of non-normality. We discuss briefly how to detect and handle such outliers here.

A univariate outlier is an outlying score on a single variable. In SEM, one conducts multivariate analysis. Multivariate outliers are a pattern of outlying scores across two or more variables. Outliers can affect estimates if they are also influential observations. Sample means, variances and covariances as used in SEM estimation procedures can all be sensitive to influential observations.

Univariate outliers can be detected by examination of a frequency distribution or a box plot. One also should review the summary statistics (e.g. mean, median, standard deviation, interquartile range, minimum, maximum, skewness and kurtosis) of a set of variables as well as correlations between variables as descriptive analysis before performing SEM. Outliers may have a large effect on the degree of skewness and kurtosis. Kurtosis in itself is a measure of outliers present in the distribution (Chapter 3).

Variables showing a high degree of skewness and kurtosis can be transformed, given previously mentioned limitations to using transformations. Robust estimators such as robust ML are constructed to perform reasonably well in the presence of outliers as long as the number of outliers is not too large [30].

Another possible recommendation for dealing with outliers is to trim/remove or modify cases that can be flagged as outliers. An approach sometimes used to identify multivariate outliers is based on exceeding the critical value threshold on a multivariate distance metric. For example, one can calculate the *Mahalanobis distance* (MD)[1] for each vector of responses on all the observed endogenous and exogenous variables z_i for individual i, where:

$$MD = \sqrt{(z_i - \bar{z})^T S^{-1} (z_i - \bar{z})} \qquad (4.3)$$

Again, $\bar{z}$ is the mean vector and S is the covariance matrix as previously notated. Mahalanobis distance is based on a chi-square distribution. A Mahalanobis distance value larger than the critical chi-square value for degrees of freedom = k (for the number of observed variables in the model) at a value of alpha equal to 0.001 indicates the presence of a multivariate outlier. One can trim those cases with a Mahalanobis distance value exceeding the critical value threshold prior to conducting analysis.

---

[1] Can use the Mahalanobis function in *R* program for this purpose.

This approach, however, may suffer from masking [31]. That is if some outliers are present in the data, the largest distances may not be associated with the outlying observations because the mean and covariance used in the calculation of Mahalanobis distance will have been shifted by the outliers. In general, detection of multidimensional outliers may still be a work in development [2]. See Bollen [2] for a more thorough discussion about univariate and multivariate outliers in SEM.

In practice, in health and medicine, outliers may contain important information about the distribution of the data in a study sample. For example, in a study of joint conditions, very high blood pressure levels may be found in some individuals as a side effect to localized steroid treatment. Assessment of outliers/influential observations should be done using empirical criteria as well as consideration of theory, logic and prior literature before deciding how to proceed (e.g. eliminate or modify none, some or all of the outliers).

4.4.2 Floor and Ceiling Effects

Ordered-categorical variables in research samples may show a *floor effect* or *ceiling effect*. A floor effect occurs when a high proportion of individuals endorse the minimum score on the observed variable. In contrast, a ceiling effect occurs when a high proportion of individuals endorse the maximum score on the observed variable. For an example, the frequency counts in the first category (endorsing the category for "not at all") were high relative to the other categories in each of the nine items for the PHQ-9 in a sample of 644 hemodialysis patients, thus exhibiting a floor effect. As a consequence, the presence of floor and ceiling effects reduce variability in the reported data with most of the values at an extreme value. Robust WLS or ML with numerical integration can be used to analyze ordered-categorical data with a floor or ceiling effect.

Another approach is to collapse categories that more evenly distribute the data to reduce the floor or ceiling effect. However, this approach may be done at a loss of information and power that may alter the meaning for many health-related outcomes that consist of a well-defined range of possible responses.

4.5 Unstandardized and Standardized Estimates

Unstandardized (or "raw" estimates) and *standardized estimates* may be presented in SEM output. Determining which one (or both) to evaluate depends on the particular analysis. Standardized estimates recast SEM model regression coefficients and covariance estimates on a scale similar to a correlation coefficient. A standardized estimate can be thought of as the z-score version of the unstandardized estimate. Therefore, using standardized estimates may be preferable when trying to compare the effect sizes of different causal paths within a model. Different scales could lead to vastly different raw estimates. We can represent in most health and medical research null (0.0), small (0.1), moderate (0.3), large (0.5) and very large (0.8) effects on a standardized coefficient scale.

In the HIV path analysis example in MPlus in Chapter 2, the raw estimate (0.143) for the regression of chronic nature of HIV on daily health practices did not necessarily provide contextual information for the size of the effect. However, we can describe the size of the effect as moderate due to the standardization of estimates (standardized estimate = 0.368).

In MPlus, standardized estimates can be requested in the OUTPUT option with the STANDARDIZED command.[2]

There are limitations to standardized estimates. Using standardized estimates removes the original unit of measure from the value. One typically prefers the original unit of measure for comparing across groups and describing baseline means/intercept values. Also, standardized estimates can be biased. The mean and standard deviation used for standardization could be biased for a small sample size or if distributional assumptions are violated.

4.6 Missing Data

Research studies reliant on a lot of recorded information about subjects will often have missing observations on one or more variables across subjects. Additionally, studies reliant on having subjects show up to visits and appointments in a timely manner will often have missing observations on one or more variables across time. Parameter estimates may be biased if missing observations are not handled in an appropriate manner during the estimation process. In order to appropriately handle these missing observations, it is necessary to make assumptions about the mechanism of missingness (Table 4.1).

The *missing at random (MAR)* assumption is an assumption that the missingness is dependent on the data at hand such as outcome values from prior time points, treatment assignment and/or observed covariates. The MAR assumption should not be confused with the *missing completely at random (MCAR)* assumption. The MCAR assumption is a stronger assumption and implies truly random missingness. In the MCAR assumption, there is no association between whether a data value is missing and any other values in the data set.

TABLE 4.1

Missing Data Assumptions

Can Be Addressed with Observed Variables		Cannot Be Addressed with Observed Variables Alone
Missing Completely at Random (MCAR)	**Missing at Random (MAR)**	**Missing Not at Random (MNAR)**
Missingness mechanism is what we think of as "random"; missing observations are a random subset of all observations	Systematic differences between the missing and observed values, but these differences can be explained by observed variables in the data set	Systematic differences between the missing and observed values and these differences *cannot* be explained by observed variables in the data set

Definitions for MCAR and MAR referenced from Bhaskaran, K. and L. Smeeth, What is the difference between missing completely at random and missing at random? *International Journal of Epidemiology*, 2014. 43(4): pp. 1336–1339.

---

[2] There are different standardized solutions included in the STANDARDIZED command. STDYX option standardizes all latent variables and observed endogenous and exogenous variable. The STDYX option is preferable for standardization of causal path estimates with continuous covariates. STDY option standardizes all latent variables and observed endogenous variables. For binary covariates, standardization has no meaning and the STDY option is preferable.

To illustrate the MAR assumption, we are evaluating a weight loss program for subjects interested in losing weight. Subjects have multiple follow-up visits to track their weight loss progression. In this study, older subjects have more missing values than younger subjects. We have an observed variable for age that explains the systematic differences between the observed and missing values. In a second example, subjects with weight gain in the first follow-up visit do not show up for the next visit.

Missing values may be assumed to be missing based on information not captured in the data. This assumption for the missing data mechanism is referred to as *missing not at random (MNAR)*.

The MAR assumption is the most typically used missing data assumption in health and medical research. It provides some flexibility in that the missingness is not completely random and is associated with other factors, which is likely for most studies in health and medicine. For example, clinic appointment nonadherence for subjects with serious mental illness and type 2 diabetes was found to be associated with demographic and mental health characteristics [32].

Now that we have differentiated the terminology for describing the missingness mechanism, we can discuss approaches for handling missing data. In *listwise deletion*, cases with any missing values on any of the variables are deleted from the sample. In other words, listwise deletion uses only the subset of cases with complete data in the analysis. Given a large enough sample, under the MCAR assumption, removing some cases is not expected to produce biased results since the missing values are a random subset of all observations.

Pairwise deletion uses all available data when calculating a statistic; data on variables with missing values for an individual are not included in the estimate. For illustration, we are calculating correlations between height, weight and systolic blood pressure. Consider a case with values on height and weight but a missing value on systolic blood pressure. In pairwise deletion, this case would be included in the calculation of the correlation between height and weight, but not in the calculation of the correlation between systolic blood pressure and either height or weight. Generally, both listwise deletion and pairwise deletion are well-suited to handle missing data under the MCAR assumption but not under the MAR assumption or MNAR assumption.

Modifications of ML techniques within SEM provide methods for dealing with missing data under the MAR or MCAR assumption [33]. In the *full information ML (FIML) approach* [14], the likelihood function is adjusted so that each individual contributes information only on the variables that are observed for that particular individual. The FIML uses individual level raw data. In general, the raw data always contain more information than the sample covariance matrix since the same sample covariance matrix can be reproduced by different raw data sets, but a raw data set only has one sample covariance [34]. Individual level data is also fundamental for multilevel modeling of longitudinal data in accounting for individual-level variability. No observations are thrown away in using FIML, as all available information is used to estimate model parameters. FIML is the default missing data technique in MPlus [14]. The *expectation-maximization (EM) algorithm* can be used with FIML for numerical optimization of parameter estimates.

The EM algorithm is an iterative method that consists of alternating between two steps, performing an expectation step (E-step) and a maximization step (M-step). An initial estimate is first made for the parameter values. The E-step consists of finding the expected value of the log-likelihood function using the current estimates for the parameter values. The expectation is also taken over the possible replacement values of the missing data. The M-step consists of maximizing the expected log-likelihood to derive new estimates for the parameters values. The iteration between the E-step and M-step stops when there is no longer any change in the parameter estimates from one iteration to the next [35]. In general, the EM algorithm is commonly used for parameter estimation with more complex models including models with missing data, mixture models (Chapters 11, 12 and 14) and nonlinear SEMs.

Multiple imputation approaches are available within most software used for SEM such as MPlus [14]. For example, there are multiple imputation approaches based on MCMC algorithms or bootstrapping-based algorithms (e.g. AMELIA II) [36]. In theory, results should be equivalent to FIML given similar assumptions under MAR or MCAR. However, two advantages of FIML over multiple imputation are (1) a separate missing data model does not need to be specified and (2) repeated runs of the same model should produce similar results.

WLSMV estimates with missing data uses a technique for handling missing data under MCAR along with a weaker missing data assumption in which covariates can also influence the missingness [37]. This technique does not handle missingness under the full MAR assumption, in which other dependent variables can influence the missingness. Note that in a model with only outcome variables and no covariates, such as a CFA model, this technique is similar to pairwise deletion. See Asparouhov and Muthén [37] for details regarding this approach for WLSMV estimates with missing data.

Further methods for handling data under the MNAR assumption are beyond the scope of this book. The SEM framework can be used to model this type of missingness under strong assumptions regarding the missing data pattern. The MNAR assumption can be seen as an extension of the MAR assumption in which missingness may also depend on latent variables [38].

4.7 Covariates

A *confounder* is an extraneous variable whose presence affects the relationship between variables being studied [39]. A confounder is associated with both an independent variable and an outcome being examined. The results may not reflect the actual relationship between variables being studied if confounders of that relationship are not controlled for in the statistical model. For example, consider a study of the relationship between alcohol consumption and lung cancer. Smoking is a confounder of this relationship since smoking is associated with alcohol consumption and a cause of lung cancer. After accounting for smoking, there is no significant association between alcohol consumption and lung cancer [40].

A *covariate* is a variable that is controlled for in the statistical model that may or may not be related to the outcome. A covariate is included in the model because the researcher deemed it is a potential confounder. If the covariate does affect the relationships between variables being studied, then it is indeed a confounder.

Similar to traditional multiple regression, inclusion of potential confounders of particular hypothesized relationships in SEM is done with the intent of reducing bias. In SEM analysis, the list of potential confounders may be different for each dependent variable within the same model. In a mediation study, different covariates may be potential confounders of the independent variable-mediator, mediator-outcome and independent variable-outcome relationships.

Conceptually, covariates are different than exogenous variables which are of interest to evaluate within a causal network. For example, time since symptom onset is an exogenous variable within the causal network in the MS-depression example. However, model estimation in SEM analysis proceeds in a similar manner for all exogenous variables. In a model in which covariates that are exogenous variables are included in a mean structure, means, variances and covariances are estimated for the covariates. The scales of exogenous variables do not affect model estimation when the respective variables are not included in a mean structure. In this case, analysis is conditional on the exogenous variables. One may not explicitly show potential confounders in the causal structure in a path diagram, but instead note in a table legend or in text the list of covariates controlled for in the model. Alternatively, one could explicitly show them in a path diagram.

4.8 MPlus Output for the MS-Depression Example with Covariates

We now present an example analysis to illustrate concepts discussed in this chapter. We again used data from an EHR registry of 3,507 persons with multiple sclerosis [41]. Analysis in this example using the model represented in Chapter 3, Figure 3.3 was focused on cross-sectional study data for each subject. Recall too for illustration purposes we are assuming that each of the nine items of the PHQ-9 is on an interval scale (Chapter 7 for a discussion of this assumption). If we did not consider that this is a reasonable assumption we could, for example, treat these nine items, each of a 0–3 range, as ordered-categorical items and use the WLSMV option in MPlus.

All but two patients had both a PHQ-9 self-reported depression screening score [42] and a timed 25-foot walk (mobility function variable). Approximately 90% of patients had no missing data on any of the variables assessed in this example. In Box 4.1, we print out selected portions of MPlus code with comments to perform this analysis.

BOX 4.1

```
Analysis: Estimator=MLR;

Model:
!Latent Variable of Depression (D) Using Nine PHQ-9 Items
!Measurement Model
D BY PHQ9_A1 PHQ9_A2 PHQ9_A3 PHQ9_A4 PHQ9_A5
   PHQ9_A6 PHQ9_A7 PHQ9_A8 PHQ9_A9;

!Model for Pathways Between Symptom Onset (Onset), Mobility
!and Depression (D) While Controlling for Race, Age and MS Type (Type)
!Structural Model
D ON Mobility Sex Race Age Type;
Mobility ON Onset Sex Race Age Type;

!Means, Variances and Covariances for Exogenous Variables Will be
!Estimated from a Line of Code Explicitly Requesting Variances
```

```
Onset Sex Race Age Type;

!Request Standardized Estimates
Output: Standardized;
```

In this example, we extend the model corresponding to Chapter 3, Figure 3.3 to include potential confounders of the hypothesized causal relationships between *symptom onset* and *mobility* and *mobility* and *depression*. We control for sex (male or female), race (Caucasian or other), age and MS type (relapsing or progressive) in both of the equations in the structural model in Box 4.1. In this model, we have 63 free parameters.[3]

We hypothesized that a longer time since symptom onset would lead to a longer timed 25-foot walk (decreased mobility function) which would lead to a higher level of depression. We used a ML estimator with robust standard errors (MLR option in MPlus) to account for the skewness and kurtosis of the measures as previously discussed. Alternatively, we could have used a bootstrap procedure for the ML estimator for this purpose.

Despite cross-sectional data, we assume a temporality and causality of measures in the path diagram. We make the MAR assumption for missingness. We assume that values that are missing are dependent on subject demographic information, disease characteristics and progression as recorded in the data at hand and captured in the variables used for analysis. In order to perform the FIML procedure to include cases with missing data on some but not all variables, we include the means, variances and covariances of the exogenous variables as parameters in the model. Alternatively, we could have used multiple imputation to handle missing data for the purpose of including all cases in the analyses.

In Figure 4.1, we report all standardized estimates for the model for ease of interpretation of the magnitude of the regression path, factor loading and error variance estimates. We also include the standard errors in parenthesis for the three regression path estimates. Since we have not yet discussed the analysis of measurement model output (Chapter 7), we will refrain from any substantial comment on the factor loadings.[4]

The causal paths between (1) *symptom onset* and *mobility* and (2) *mobility* and *depression* are statistically significant. In line with our hypothesis, there is a positive relationship between longer time since symptom onset and less mobility function (i.e. higher values for timed 25-foot walk) and less mobility function and higher depression. These relationships, however, are of a smaller effect size. Due to the very small effect size (standardized estimate less than 0.10), the causal effect between *symptom onset* and *depression* may not be considered clinically that meaningful.

We note that when encountering data patterns that include more than one issue (e.g. missing data *and* nonnormality), such as in this example, then researchers should select estimation approaches and make interpretations with care. There are many approaches available to consider.

In the model used in this example, as opposed to the mediation model represented in Chapter 3, Figure 3.2, we omitted the regression path for the relationship between *symptom onset* and *depression*. Whether this model specification is theoretically plausible is

---

[3] Parameters include nine factor intercepts, eight factor loadings, nine factor residuals, one structural regression intercept, two structural regression slopes, eight regression paths with the covariates, two error residuals, five means, five variances and ten covariances. Not shown in code are four residual correlations (anhedonia and depressed, depressed and guilt, sleep and fatigue, concentration and psychomotor).

[4] The estimates of the factor loadings are all reasonably high, ranging between 0.50 and 0.78. There is a moderate to high proportion of variance in each of the PHQ-9 items explained by the latent variable *depression*.

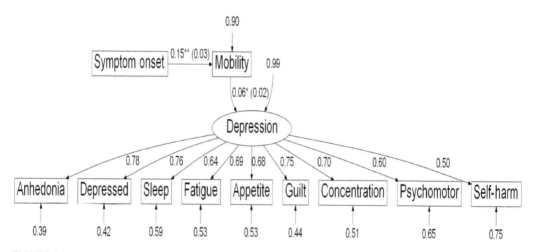

FIGURE 4.1

MS-depression model with no regression path between *symptom onset* and *depression*.

*p = 0.001; **p < 0.001. Standardized estimates reported on the figure using MPlus. In the structural model, we also include standardized estimates of the standard errors in parenthesis. We used the MLR option and the FIML procedure to handle missing data and the STDYX option for all reported standardized estimates. We controlled for sex, race, age and MS type in the structural model. We included four residual correlations (anhedonia and depressed, depressed and guilt, sleep and fatigue, concentration and psychomotor) in this analysis that all are theoretically sensible. However, we do not include these residual correlations in the diagram or discussion since we have not yet sufficiently discussed measurement models, residual correlations or modification indices.

dependent on clinical theory, logic and prior literature. In actuality, both model specifications are theoretically reasonable. We discuss how to choose between competing models in Chapter 6. In this particular illustrative analysis, we utilized theory that omitting this path may be in line with the nature of MS [43,44] since depression occurs early in and throughout the condition.

Formal testing of an indirect (mediation) effect in a mediation model, such as the MS-depression mediation model represented in Chapter 3, Figure 3.2, is discussed in Chapter 9. Mediation analysis will help us explain structural model output in terms of direct, indirect and total effects. We will build up to performing mediation analysis for a more complex systems-based model for the MS-depression study in Chapter 9.

4.9 Introduction to Model Fit

There is no single "gold standard" measure of model fit in SEM. For illustration, we contrast model fit in SEM with traditional linear regression modeling. Given some assumptions and limitations, a single measure R^2 (or adjusted R^2) can provide a reasonable evaluation of model fit in the context of a traditional linear regression model. In this context if you output an $R^2 = 0.90$, after some considerations, you reasonably could conclude a strong model fit: 90% of the model variance is explained by the predictors. In SEM, a researcher typically reports instead multiple model fit statistics and indices, interpreted collectively to evaluate model fit.

A reasonable expectation of model fit in SEM is that a researcher will not be able to prove a model, but will be able to show that the discrepancy between model and data does not surpass the limits of chance. Different fit statistics and indices are often reported in different clinical journals or articles. Some of the general limitations of fit statistics and indices in SEM are: some parts of the model may fit poorly even if the model fit overall is good, a single statistic or index only reflects a particular aspect of model fit or a model can accurately reflect a relative lack of predictive validity [45].

Even when the model is a good fit, the model path coefficients may still not make sense. This situation would be straightforward to assess if an evident positive path coefficient is negative or vice versa. However, some counterintuitive results should not be dismissed as false findings. Thus, we encourage strong collaboration and team science, for the appropriate development of conceptual models to the interpretation of output, when using SEM in health and medicine.

In spite of these limitations, interpreted collectively and with caution, evaluation measures in SEM help one choose a model and plausibly assess model performance for the observed data. Most modeling approaches do not have the availability of such criteria and thus cannot put so much emphasis on model evaluation.

The measures discussed in this chapter assess global model fit, in which we seek to understand in its entirety how well the model fits the observed data. These model fit statistics and indices can be categorized into *absolute fit, incremental fit*, and *noncentrality-based indices*. Local measures of how particular parameters influence the model fit, such as the *modification index*, are more useful for model modification and will be discussed in Chapter 6.

Absolute fit statistics and indices measure overall fit for a substantive model. Incremental fit indices compare the substantive model to the *null model* for relative improvement. The null model is made up of the unconstrained estimate of the mean and variance based on the observed values [46]. The null model is also commonly referred to as the *baseline model* or *independence model*. Different software may assume slightly different constraints for the null model for the same data. For example, in EQS all of the covariances between observed values are assumed to be zero, while in MPlus only the covariances among endogenous observed variables are assumed to be zero.

Noncentrality-based measures do not approximate a central distribution and are adjusted for model complexity by the model degrees of freedom. Typically, these indices are also sample size-adjusted.

Model selection criteria such as *Akaike information criteria (AIC), Bayesian information criteria (BIC)* and *Browne-Cudeck criterion (BCC)* [45] are also commonly provided in SEM output. However, we defer discussion of these measures which hold the most value when comparing between a series of competing models for the chapter about model specification (Chapter 6).

4.10 Chi-squared Test Statistic

We now begin our discussion of particular model fit statistics and indices for a substantive model of interest M. Recall that estimates of the free parameters, $\hat{\theta}$, were derived to minimize the discrepancy between the observed mean vector and covariance matrix, on the one hand, and the model-implied mean vector and covariance matrix, on the other. Under certain regularity conditions, plugging $\hat{\theta}$ in a discrepancy function we obtain a minimized discrepancy function. If the model is correct and fitted to the observed mean vector and covariance matrix, under the assumption of asymptotic normality, the minimized discrepancy function will yield a test statistic with an asymptotic chi-squared distribution. For example, if we chose the estimator $\hat{\theta}$ that minimized the ML fit function in (4.1), we obtain the minimized discrepancy function $\hat{F}_{ML}$. Then we can use the test statistic

$$\chi^2_M = (N-1)\hat{F}_{ML} \qquad (4.4)$$

where N is the sample size.

The distribution of χ^2_M is the central chi-squared distribution. The number of degrees of freedom for χ^2_M (which we will refer to as df_M) will depend on the number of freely estimated parameters t in our vector of parameters θ and the number of observed variables k in our model [47]. More formally, in our model with a mean structure let

$$k^* = \frac{k(k+3)}{2} \qquad (4.5)$$

Then, $df_M = k^* - t$.

In the formula (4.5), k^* is equal to the total number of variances, unique covariance terms and means of all the model observed variables [48].[5] As a result, k^* gives the total number of pieces of information necessary to estimate the model parameters [48]. In the MS-depression mediation model example in Chapter 3, we have 11 observed variables (*symptom onset*, *mobility*, nine PHQ-9 items). Thus, using formula (4.5):

$$k^* = \frac{11(11+3)}{2} = 77$$

Also, recall from Chapter 3 as we provided a breakdown of the free parameters from this model that $t = 34$ free parameters. In this model, the degrees of freedom $df_M = 77 - 34 = 43$.

The chi-square test statistic in (4.4) can similarly be obtained using likelihood ratio theory in comparing the substantive model to a *saturated model*. The saturated model perfectly reproduces all of the means, variances and covariances of the observed variables. Thus, it has the best fit possible of all potential models for the data making it a standard for comparison with the substantive model.

The chi-square test statistic will provide a basis for assessing model fit in other evaluation criteria discussed below. In itself, the chi-square test statistic is used to test absolute model fit. The null hypothesis of equal fit is that there is no difference between the proposed model and the data. The alternative hypothesis is that there is a difference between the proposed model and the data. A large chi-square test statistic with a corresponding small p-value indicates that the model does *not* fit the data well. A chi-square test statistic of zero indicates the best fit. The saturated model has a chi-square test statistic of zero with zero degrees of freedom.

There is a correction to the statistic χ^2_M for ML with robust standard errors [14,49]. To calculate the *Satorra-Bentler scaled chi-square value*, χ^2_M in equation (4.4) is adjusted to $\dfrac{\chi^2_M}{c}$

---

[5] With no mean structure, we would just modify the formula by subtracting k (number of observed means for k observed variables) from (4.5) for $k^* = \dfrac{k(k+1)}{2}$

for an estimated scaling factor c based on the robust asymptotic covariance matrix [49,50]. If data are truly multivariate normally distributed, then the estimated scaling factor $c = 1$ and the estimator will lead to the same solution as ML. The scaling factor c is corrected for multivariate kurtosis for too-thin distribution tails (< 1) or too-fat distribution tails (> 1). The Bollen-Stine bootstrapping method [51] also provides a robust method for bootstrapping the chi-square test statistic from the sample observations [52]. There are modifications to the chi-square test statistic under different estimators available in SEM software. For example, a chi-square test statistic for the WLSMV option is available in MPlus [14].

Do not be dismayed by a small p-value for the chi-square test statistic given indication of acceptable model fit by other evaluation measures. The chi-square statistic has noted limitations in SEM research that often lead to rejection of the null hypothesis. The chi-square statistic is affected by non-normality, correlation size, low power and sample size (both too small or too large). As mentioned, to help account for non-normality, alternative scale corrected statistics are commonly used [14,49–51]. However, these adjustments do not protect the model from being rejected because there is some seemingly small misspecification in it. Since model misspecification has such a strong bearing on the chi-square test statistic, it becomes a very useful statistic in specification searches (Chapter 6).

Variations of the chi-square statistic, such as $\frac{\chi^2_M}{df_M}$, have been proposed to potentially scale down the power of the usual test with larger sample sizes [2]. Bollen [2] reasons that such variations still have a similar relationship with sample size (no N in the formula) and thus do not correct the excessive power problem.

4.11 Descriptive and Alternative Fit Indices

A model fit index is a continuous measure of model fit. Each model fit index is a measure of *goodness-of-fit* or *badness-of-fit* [45]. The higher the magnitude of the measure the better the model fit in goodness-of-fit measures; the lower the magnitude of the measure, the better the model fit in badness-of-fit measures.

Currently, the most commonly used noncentrality-based index is the Root Mean Square Error of Approximation (RMSEA) [53]. RMSEA is a badness-of-fit point estimate that builds on the chi-square statistic, but also penalizes for model complexity and is sample size corrected. RMSEA is scaled to range between zero and one, where zero indicates the best fit. As a rule of thumb, a RMSEA ≤ 0.08 is considered an acceptable fit, while a RMSEA ≤ 0.05 is considered an excellent fit [53,54].

Under ML, if $\chi^2_M \geq df_M$:

$$RMSEA = \sqrt{\frac{\chi^2_M - df_M}{df_M(N-1)}} \tag{4.6}$$

RMSEA is set to zero if $\chi^2_M < df_M$.

Part of the versatility of RMSEA is that confidence intervals and hypothesis tests can also be derived for the point estimate in (4.6). Confidence intervals can be constructed around the point estimate RMSEA because the index asymptotically follows a rescaled noncentral chi-square distribution with noncentrality parameter $\lambda = \chi^2_M - df_M$. The estimated noncentrality parameter reflects the degree of misfit in the proposed model; thus, the smaller the estimated noncentrality parameter, the better the fit in the proposed model [55]. The confidence interval can be used to evaluate the precision of the RMSEA point estimate where the width of the interval should be relatively tight. In MPlus software, a 90% confidence interval is constructed for the RMSEA point estimate [14].

A close fit hypothesis test can be performed for the model using RMSEA. That is, the null hypothesis is that RMSEA ≤ 0.05 for a close fit (excellent fit) while the alternative hypothesis is that RMSEA > 0.05. Rejecting the null hypothesis means that the model fit is worse than close fitting. There are several noted limitations to RMSEA. The fit index may not exactly follow a noncentral chi-square distribution, may be sensitive to non-normality and may favor larger models.

Another commonly reported fit index for researchers, the comparative fit index (CFI) [56], is an incremental fit goodness-of-fit measure. Let I be the null (independence) model. Given normal asymptotic theory holds, CFI can be derived using the ML estimator to quantify the incremental improvement in fit of our substantive model M in comparison to the independence model I. Here χ_I^2 is the fitting function value for the independence model which is approximately central chi-square distributed with degrees of freedom df_I.

$$CFI = 1 - \frac{\chi_M^2 - df_M}{\chi_I^2 - df_I} \tag{4.7}$$

If the CFI index is greater than one, it is set at one and if less than zero, it is set to zero. The closer the CFI index is to one, the better the model fit. As a rule of thumb, a CFI ≥ 0.90 is considered an acceptable fit, while a CFI ≥ 0.95 is considered an excellent fit [54].

The Tucker-Lewis index (TLI) [57] is another commonly reported incremental fit measure with a higher penalty for adding parameters than CFI. TLI also does not have the zero to one range restriction. As a rule of thumb, similar to CFI, a TFI ≥ 0.90 is considered an acceptable fit, while a TFI ≥ 0.95 is considered an excellent fit [54]. Under the same assumptions as we used to derive CFI,

$$TLI = \frac{\dfrac{\chi_I^2}{df_I} - \dfrac{\chi_M^2}{df_M}}{\dfrac{\chi_I^2}{df_I} - 1} \tag{4.8}$$

The formulas given in (4.6), (4.7) and (4.8) can also be corrected for ML with robust standard errors based on using the corrected chi-square statistic values divided by estimated scaling factors.

Aforementioned, programs for the analysis of SEMs may assume slightly different constraints for the null models for the same data. Different software may yield different CFI and TLI for the same model.

A commonly used absolute fit index, based on the average difference between the observed and model-implied correlation matrix, is the *standardized root mean square residual (SRMR)* [58]. As a rule of thumb, a SRMR ≤ 0.08 is considered an acceptable fit, while a SRMR ≤ 0.05 is considered an excellent fit [54]. TLI and CFI are relatively stable across sample sizes. RMSEA and SRMR are larger with smaller sample sizes.

The *weighted root mean square residual (WRMR)* is an available absolute fit index for models with ordered-categorical outcome variables [59]. A rule of thumb is that a WRMR of

TABLE 4.2

General "Rule of Thumb" Guidelines in SEM Literature for Select Model Fit Statistics and Indices

Model Fit Value	"Rule of Thumb" Guidelines	
	Excellent	Acceptable
Chi-Square Test[a]	$p \geq 0.05$	Smaller values of test statistic
RMSEA[b]	≤ 0.05	≤ 0.08
CFI	≥ 0.95	≥ 0.90
TLI	≥ 0.95	≥ 0.90
SRMR	≤ 0.05	≤ 0.08

RMSEA, CFI, TLI and SRMR should all reach acceptable (preferably excellent) levels before designating a model as good fitting. [a]In analyses with small and very large sample sizes, the chi-square test typically rejects models and is sensitive to even small model misspecifications. [b]The confidence interval for RMSEA should be reasonably tight given the confidence threshold (e.g. 90%), and the upper limit should be reasonably close to acceptable (preferably within excellent) levels.

less than 1.0 indicates good fit [59]. WRMR is size-dependent and can be unreliable with large sample sizes [60].

Many other fit measures have been proposed for SEM, such as the *Bentler-Bonett normed fit index (NFI)* [61], an incremental fit index and the first model fit measure proposed in the SEM literature [62]. NFI does not penalize for adding parameters whereas TLI is an incremental fit index with this added penalty [62].

The *Jöreskog-Sörbom goodness-of-fit index (GFI)* [63] is also an early absolute fit index in SEM [62,64]. Jöreskog and Sörbom also proposed an adjusted GFI that adjusts for the degrees of freedom of a model relative to the number of observed variables [2]. GFI and adjusted GFI are both affected by sample size and not used as often in modern SEM analyses [2,62,64].

We recommend, when available, to at minimum report the values of the model fit statistics and indices in Table 4.2. These criteria will allow a researcher to reasonably evaluate model fit for a given substantive structural equation model of interest.

4.12 MPlus Output for Model Evaluation for the MS-Depression Example

We include abridged MPlus model fit output information for the MS-depression example (corresponding to Figure 4.1) in Box 4.2. We find an acceptable to excellent fitting model according to rule of thumb criteria in Table 4.2. RMSEA, CFI, and SRMR all meet the excellent fitting model criteria. TLI is just below excellent fitting model criteria. This example then illustrates the challenge of strict decision rules based on rules of thumb. The TLI seems too high to be considered merely acceptable. The chi-square test does not meet excellent fitting model criteria according to Table 4.2. We have noted the potential sensitivity of this test to even a small misspecification and with a very large sample size ($N = 3,507$ in this example).

BOX 4.2   MODEL FIT INFORMATION

```
Number of Free Parameters              63

Chi-Square Test of Model Fit

    Value                         530.283
    Degrees of Freedom                 72
    P-Value                        0.0000
    Scaling Correction Factor      1.1621
      for MLR


RMSEA (Root Mean Square Error Of Approximation)

    Estimate                        0.043
    90 Percent C.I.         0.039  0.046
    Probability RMSEA <= .05        1.000


CFI/TLI

    CFI                             0.960
    TLI                             0.947


SRMR (Standardized Root Mean Square Residual)

    Value                           0.026
```

Note that MPlus provided the scaling correction factor for the MLR option in the output. The scaling factor is greater than one; thus the distribution of the data is heavy-tailed. The chi-square test has been corrected for this scaling factor in the output.

Some SEM researchers would be critical of any published analysis as not trustworthy that does not at least reach acceptable model fit levels for all statistics and indices using guidelines in Table 4.2. Imposing constraints and making modifications to a model that does not meet these criteria may lead to these acceptable levels. For example, adding an additional regression path, constraining a certain regression path to zero or adding residual correlations between items of a scale if theoretically warranted can all at times meaningfully improve model fit. Modification indices (Chapter 6) can be helpful for these approaches but special care must be taken not to "fish" for good model fit in revising a model without strong theoretical justification.

In health and medicine, depending on the context and setting, a researcher may not stringently follow guidelines suggested in Table 4.2 given available resources and data. The model in the current form may not have reached acceptable model fit levels, but may be precisely constructed in line with theory for intended purposes. The researcher may consider further revisions or re-specifications to the model theoretically unwarranted. Under such circumstances, a researcher might decide to present model results with less than acceptable model fit levels. The researcher should openly acknowledge limitations of the available data and study and discuss future directions.

4.13 Sample Size and Power

Power analysis helps determine the minimum sample size required to observe statistically significant results, if a researcher should reject the null hypothesis. SEM analysis often involves estimating many free parameters in a covariance matrix of large dimensions. As a result a large sample size is typically required for achieving adequate power in studies involving SEM. This may mean that a researcher conducting a proposed study with a limited number of participants will have to simplify or even abandon a proposed SEM analysis.

In some large observational studies within health and medicine, there are anywhere from tens of thousands to even millions of records in a registry. In this case, a sample size calculation will often be used to confirm that the study is more than adequately powered.

When performing power analysis within the context of SEM in health and medicine, there are four main approaches we will outline in this section:

- Rule of thumb guidelines
- Monte Carlo simulations
- Calculations based on model fit and modification measures and tests
- Calculations based on limited available information and the structure of the proposed structural equation model

Various rule of thumb guidelines have been derived for sample size for SEM. Given no other information, such as preliminary analysis or literature, to inform a researcher about expected parameter estimates, the most basic rule of thumb for conducting SEM analysis is to use a sample size of at least 200. This rule of thumb should, of course, be used within reason. A researcher cannot reasonably conduct SEM analysis for a complex systems-based model containing many dozens of variables with a sample size of around 200! Given that a model is not overly complex, a sample size of 200 could be acceptable for a study and is often referred to as the "typical" SEM sample size [45]. Factoring in model complexity, ratio of sample size to free parameter rule of thumbs, ideally 20:1, with 10:1 acceptable but less than ideal, have been discussed by Kline [45] referencing Jackson [65]. For example, given Chapter 3, Figure 3.1 with four observed variables and three causal paths, we regress eating habits on SES and body mass index on physical activity and eating habits. In the model with a mean structure (with the covariance between exogenous variables constrained to zero), we estimate eleven parameters. That is, for the endogenous variables we estimate two intercepts, three regression paths and two residual variances and for the exogenous variables two means and two variances. Thus, given a sample size of 220, we would have adequate power according to any of these above rules of thumb, since the ratio of our sample size to free parameters is 20:1 given no other preliminary estimates.

Monte Carlo simulations have been used for power analysis in the context of SEM [66]. These simulations are often done for the purpose of calculating the power to detect the estimated value of a model parameter of interest is non-zero (as opposed to zero). They rely on having suitable preliminary estimates for model parameters. For an example, we can use Monte Carlo simulations to calculate power for performing CFA on the SF-36 Health

Survey. We can use estimates from analysis with a prior sample to evaluate how large a sample would be necessary to detect two factors of physical and mental health of a particular non-zero correlation such as 0.25 (as opposed to zero correlation). The focus of this power simulation for CFA is on the correlation between the two constructs since it is a measure not attenuated by measurement error [66]. Simulations can be used to determine the sample size necessary to detect at least two unobserved subgroups in a mixture model (e.g. growth mixture model), rather than a single group.

Monte Carlo simulation could also be used to calculate power for testing a hypothesis in a structural model. Using the MS-depression mediation example corresponding to Chapter 3, Figure 3.2, a researcher could use a Monte Carlo simulation approach to estimate power as the proportion of tests that reject the null hypothesis in which the indirect (mediated) effect from *symptom onset* to *depression* through *mobility* is equal to zero vs. a suitable alternative effect size. However, in order to perform this simulation, the user would need to provide preliminary estimates of the 34 parameters in the model. Just imagine the task of coming up with appropriate preliminary estimates for all 34 parameters before undertaking the study!

A third approach to calculate power in the SEM framework is based on model fit and modification measures and tests. Preacher and Coffman have a web page (http://quantpsy.org/rmsea/rmsea.htm) that generates *R* code that can perform power analysis using RMSEA [67]. This power analysis is based in part on work by MacCallum [68]. Satorra [69] introduced a method for power analysis based on the likelihood ratio test. Methods for power analysis using modification indices were developed by Satorra [70] and in tandem with expected parameter changes by Saris et al. [71] and Kaplan [72]. Multivariate methods of model modification for two or more parameters, simultaneously using a multivariate Wald test, have been proposed for power analysis in SEM [73]. Multivariate methods, compared to univariate methods, minimize Type I or Type II errors incurred by model modification. However, multivariate methods might detract from the interpretation of the model since it becomes difficult to monitor individual changes. The Wald test has also been used to evaluate power in the multigroup CFA setting [74].

A fourth approach is to calculate power based on preliminary estimates or prior literature from a less complex model while incorporating structural features of the proposed structural equation model. A single effect size may be the only quantitative information available a priori. However, a researcher has a proposed model and knows the number of latent variables, observed variables and hypothesized causal paths. For such a study, the researcher can calculate a reasonable lower bound on the sample size using methods developed by Westland [75]. For example, a researcher might have a preliminary estimate of 0.2 for the correlation between loss of appetite and symptom severity in adults with influenza from a pilot study. The researcher is proposing a model with a latent variable and ten observed variables. A sample size calculation to achieve 90% power at a probability level of 0.05 given the number of observed and latent variables in the model and the anticipated effect size of 0.2 is 1600 [75,76].[6]

---

[6] This calculation done using an online calculator provided by Soper (2018) for a priori sample size for SEMs, which reference the work of Westland (2010). Soper, D.S., A-priori sample size calculator for structural equation models [software]. (2018); Available from http://www.danielsoper.com/statcalc. Westland, J.C., Lower bounds on sample size in structural equation modeling. *Electronic Commerce Research and Applications*, (2010). 9(6): pp. 476–487.

4.14 Conclusions

This chapter presented the procedure for estimating parameters and standard errors in a structural equation model. Methods were discussed for different types of data (e.g. non-normal, missing) commonly encountered in research studies in health and medicine.

We provided an overview of model fit in this chapter. Multiple statistics and indices, all with noted strengths and limitations, are useful for evaluating how well a substantive model of interest fits the data beyond the limits of chance.

A nuanced presentation in this chapter of standardized and unstandardized estimates, covariates and how to use model fit guidelines may prove fruitful to the reader. Finally, we ended the chapter with an overview of power analysis for SEM studies in health and medicine.

References

1. Gelman, A. and J. Hill, *Data analysis using regression and multilevel/hierarchical models.* 2006, New York: Cambridge University Press.
2. Bollen, K., *Structural equations with latent variables.* 1989, New York, NY: Wiley.
3. Hildreth, L., Residual analysis for structural equation modeling. 2013.
4. Long, J., *Covariance structure models: An introduction to LISREL.* 1983, Thousand Oaks, CA: SAGE Publications, Inc.
5. Bollen, K.A. and M.D. Noble, Structural equation models and the quantification of behavior. *Proceedings of the National Academy of Sciences*, 2011. 108(Supplement 3): pp. 15639–15646.
6. Steiger, J., Measures of fit in structural equation modeling: An introduction. 2009; Available from: Statpower.com.
7. Muthén, B., A general structural equation model with dichotomous, ordered categorical, and continuous latent variable indicators. *Psychometrika*, 1984. **49**(1): pp. 115–132.
8. Morris, N.J., R.C. Elston, and C.M. Stein, A framework for structural equation models in general pedigrees. *Human Heredity*, 2009. **70**(4): pp. 278–286.
9. Gunzler, D.D. and N. Morris, A tutorial on structural equation modeling for analysis of overlapping symptoms in co-occurring conditions using MPlus. *Statistics in Medicine*, 2015. **34**(24): pp. 3246–3280.
10. Browne, M.W., Asymptotically distribution-free methods for the analysis of covariance structures. *British Journal of Mathematical and Statistical Psychology*, 1984. **37**(1): pp. 62–83.
11. Browne, M.W., Covariance structures, in *Topics in applied multivariate analysis*, D.M. Hawkins, Editor. 1982, Cambridge: Cambridge University. pp. 72–141.
12. Blunch, N., *Introduction to structural equation modeling using IBM SPSS statistics and AMOS.* 2012, Thousand Oaks, CA: SAGE Publications, Inc.
13. Olsson, U.H., et al., The performance of ML, GLS, and WLS estimation in structural equation modeling under conditions of misspecification and nonnormality. *Structural Equation Modeling*, 2000. 7(4): pp. 557–595.
14. Muthén, L.K. and B.O. Muthén, *Mplus: The comprehensive modeling program for applied researchers: User's guide. Eighth edition.* 1998–2017, Los Angeles, CA: Muthén & Muthén.
15. Byrne, B.M., *Structural equation modeling with Mplus: Basic concepts, applications, and programming.* 2013, New York and London: Routledge.
16. Huber, P.J. The behavior of maximum likelihood estimates under nonstandard conditions, in *Proceedings of the fifth Berkeley symposium on mathematical statistics and probability.* 1967, Berkeley, CA: University of California Press.

17. Nevitt, J. and G.R. Hancock, Performance of bootstrapping approaches to model test statistics and parameter standard error estimation in structural equation modeling. *Structural Equation Modeling*, 2001. **8**(3): pp. 353–377.

18. Efron, B., Better bootstrap confidence intervals. *Journal of the American Statistical Association*, 1987. **82**(397): pp. 171–185.

19. MacKinnon, D.P., C.M. Lockwood, and J. Williams, Confidence limits for the indirect effect: Distribution of the product and resampling methods. *Multivariate Behavioral Research*, 2004. **39**(1): pp. 99–128.

20. Preacher, K.J. and A.F. Hayes, Asymptotic and resampling strategies for assessing and comparing indirect effects in multiple mediator models. *Behavior Research Methods*, 2008. **40**(3): pp. 879–891.

21. Flora, D.B. and P.J. Curran, An empirical evaluation of alternative methods of estimation for confirmatory factor analysis with ordinal data. *Psychological Methods*, 2004. **9**(4): p. 466.

22. Olsson, U., Maximum likelihood estimation of the polychoric correlation coefficient. *Psychometrika*, 1979. **44**(4): pp. 443–460.

23. Li, C.-H., The performance of MLR, USLMV, and WLSMV estimation in structural regression models with ordinal variables. 2014, Michigan State University.

24. Jöreskog, K.G., Structural equation modeling with ordinal variables. *Lecture Notes-Monograph Series*, 1994. 24: pp. 297–310.

25. Muthén, B.O., Goodness of fit with categorical and other nonnormal variables. *SAGE Focus Editions*, 1993. **154**: pp. 205–205.

26. Rhemtulla, M., P.É. Brosseau-Liard, and V. Savalei, When can categorical variables be treated as continuous? A comparison of robust continuous and categorical SEM estimation methods under suboptimal conditions. *Psychological Methods*, 2012. **17**(3): p. 354.

27. Skrondal, A. and S. Rabe-Hesketh, Structural equation modeling: Categorical variables. 2005, Wiley Online Library.

28. Lee, S.-Y. and X.-Y. Song, *Basic and advanced Bayesian structural equation modeling: With applications in the medical and behavioral sciences*. 2012, John Wiley & Sons.

29. van de Schoot, R., et al., A gentle introduction to Bayesian analysis: Applications to developmental research. *Child Development*, 2014. **85**(3): pp. 842–860.

30. David, H.A., Robust estimation in the presence of outliers, in *Robustness in Statistics*, R.L. Launer and G.N. Wilkinson, Editors. 1979, New York: Academic Press. pp. 61–74.

31. Cerioli, A., A.C. Atkinson, and M. Riani, Some perspectives on multivariate outlier detection, in *New perspectives in statistical modeling and data analysis. Studies in Classification, Data Analysis, and Knowledge Organization*, Ingrassia S., Rocci R., Vichi M. Editors. 2011, Berlin, Heidelberg: Springer. pp. 231–238. doi:10.1007/978-3-642-11363-5_26.

32. Gunzler, D.D., et al., Clinic appointment attendance in adults with serious mental illness and diabetes. *American Journal of Health Behavior*, 2017. **41**(6): pp. 810–821.

33. Little, R.J. and D.B. Rubin, *Statistical analysis with missing data*. 2014, New York: John Wiley & Sons.

34. Heck, R.H. and S.L. Thomas, *An introduction to multilevel modeling techniques: MLM and SEM approaches using Mplus*. 2015, New York, NY: Routledge.

35. Allison, P.D., Missing data techniques for structural equation modeling. *Journal of Abnormal Psychology*, 2003. **112**(4): p. 545.

36. Honaker, J., G. King, and M. Blackwell, Amelia II: A program for missing data. *Journal of Statistical Software*, 2011. **45**(7): pp. 1–47.

37. Asparouhov, T. and B. Muthén, Weighted least squares estimation with missing data. *Mplus Technical Appendix*, 2010. **2010**: pp. 1–10.

38. Muthén, B., et al., Growth modeling with non-ignorable dropout: Alternative analyses of the STAR*D antidepressant trial. *Psychological Methods*, 2011. **16**(1): pp. 17–33.

39. Pourhoseingholi, M.A., A.R. Baghestani, and M. Vahedi, How to control confounding effects by statistical analysis. *Gastroenterology and Hepatology from Bed to Bench*, 2012. **5**(2): p. 79.

40. Larsson, S.C., et al., Smoking, alcohol consumption, and cancer: A mendelian randomisation study in UK Biobank and international genetic consortia participants. *PLOS Medicine*, 2020. **17**(7): p. e1003178.

41. Gunzler, D., et al., Disentangling multiple sclerosis & depression: An adjusted depression screening score for patient-centered care. *Journal of Behavioral Medicine*, 2015. **38**(2): pp. 237–250.

42. Blacker, D., Psychiatric rating scales, in *Kaplan and Sadock's Comprehensive Textbook of Psychiatry*, Eighth Edition, B.J. Sadock and V.A. Sadock, Editors. 2005, Philadelphia, PA: Lippincott Williams & Wilkins. pp. 929–955.

43. Bermel, R.A., et al. Impact of comorbid depression on patient-reported physical disability measures in multiple sclerosis. *Neurotherapeutics*. 2013. **10**(3): p. 539.

44. Gunzler, D., N. Morris, A. Perznski, D. Miller, S. Lewis, and R.A. Bermel, Mediation analysis of co-occurring conditions for complex longitudinal clinical data. *SM Journal of Biometrics & Biostatistics* 2017. **1**(1): p. 1004.

45. Kline, R.B., *Principles and practice of structural equation modeling*, fourth edition. 2016, New York: Guilford Press.

46. Widaman, K.F. and J.S. Thompson, On specifying the null model for incremental fit indices in structural equation modeling. *Psychological Methods*, 2003. **8**(1): p. 16.

47. Bollen, K.A. and A. Maydeu-Olivares, A polychoric instrumental variable (PIV) estimator for structural equation models with categorical variables. *Psychometrika*, 2007. **72**(3): pp. 309–326.

48. Kline, R.B., Supplemental Chapter B: Introduction to mean structures, *Principles and Practice of Structural Equation Modeling* (1998), 2000. New York: Guilford Press.

49. Yuan, K.H. and P.M. Bentler, Three likelihood-based methods for mean and covariance structure analysis with nonnormal missing data. *Sociological Methodology*, 2000. **30**(1): pp. 165–200.

50. Satorra, A. and P.M. Bentler, Corrections to test statistics and standard errors in covariance structure analysis, in *Latent variables analysis: Applications for developmental research*, A. von Eye and C.C. Clogg, Editors. 1994, Thousand Oaks, CA: Sage Publications, Inc., pp. 399–419.

51. Bollen, K.A. and R.A. Stine, Bootstrapping goodness-of-fit measures in structural equation models. *Sociological Methods & Research*, 1992. **21**(2): pp. 205–229.

52. Kim, H. and R. Millsap, Using the Bollen-Stine bootstrapping method for evaluating approximate fit indices. *Multivariate Behavioral Research*, 2014. **49**(6): pp. 581–596.

53. Browne, M.W., et al., Alternative ways of assessing model fit. *Sage Focus Editions*, 1993. **154**: pp. 136–136.

54. Hu, L.t. and P.M. Bentler, Cutoff criteria for fit indexes in covariance structure analysis: Conventional criteria versus new alternatives. *Structural Equation Modeling: A Multidisciplinary Journal*, 1999. **6**(1): pp. 1–55.

55. Chen, F., et al., An empirical evaluation of the use of fixed cutoff points in RMSEA test statistic in structural equation models. *Sociological Methods & Research*, 2008. **36**(4): pp. 462–494.

56. Bentler, P.M., Comparative fit indexes in structural models. *Psychological Bulletin*, 1990. **107**(2): p. 238.

57. Tucker, L.R. and C. Lewis, A reliability coefficient for maximum likelihood factor analysis. *Psychometrika*, 1973. **38**(1): pp. 1–10.

58. Hu, L.-t. and P.M. Bentler, Fit indices in covariance structure modeling: Sensitivity to underparameterized model misspecification. *Psychological Methods*, 1998. **3**(4): p. 424.

59. Yu, C. and B. Muthén, *Evaluation of model fit indices for latent variable models with categorical and continuous outcomes. 2002.* 2005, Los Angeles: University of California.

60. Ayuso-Mateos, J.L., et al., Multi-country evaluation of affective experience: Validation of an abbreviated version of the day reconstruction method in seven countries. *PloS One*, 2013. 8(4): p. e61534.

61. Bentler, P.M. and D.G. Bonett, Significance tests and goodness of fit in the analysis of covariance structures. *Psychological Bulletin*, 1980. **88**(3): p. 588.

62. Kenny, D.A. *Measuring model fit*. 2015; Available from: http://davidakenny.net/cm/fit.htm.

63. Joreskog, K.G. and D. Sorbom, *Lisrel VI: Analysis of linear structural relationships by maximum likelihood, instrumentals variables and least squares methods: User's guide.* 1985, Mooresville: Scientific Software.

64. Sharma, S., et al., A simulation study to investigate the use of cutoff values for assessing model fit in covariance structure models. *Journal of Business Research*, 2005. **58**(7): pp. 935–943.

65. Jackson, D.L., Revisiting sample size and number of parameter estimates: Some support for the N: Q hypothesis. *Structural Equation Modeling*, 2003. **10**(1): pp. 128–141.

66. Muthén, L.K. and B.O. Muthén, How to use a Monte Carlo study to decide on sample size and determine power. *Structural Equation Modeling*, 2002. **9**(4): pp. 599–620.

67. Preacher, K.J. and D.L. Coffman, *Computing power and minimum sample size for RMSEA [Computer software].* 2006; Available from: http://quantpsy.org/.

68. MacCallum, R.C., M.W. Browne, and H.M. Sugawara, Power analysis and determination of sample size for covariance structure modeling. *Psychological Methods*, 1996. **1**(2): p. 130.

69. Satorra, A. and W.E. Saris, Power of the likelihood ratio test in covariance structure analysis. Psychometrika, 1985. **50**(1): pp. 83–90.

70. Satorra, A., Alternative test criteria in covariance structure analysis: A unified approach. *Psychometrika*, 1989. **54**(1): pp. 131–151.

71. Saris, W.E., A. Satorra, and D. Sörbom, The detection and correction of specification errors in structural equation models. *Sociological Methodology*, 1987. **17**: pp. 105–129.

72. Kaplan, D., Model modification in covariance structure analysis: Application of the expected parameter change statistic. *Multivariate Behavioral Research*, 1989. **24**(3): pp. 285–305.

73. Kaplan, D. and R.N. Wenger, Asymptomatic independence and separability in covariance structure models: Implications for specification error, power, and model modification. *Multivariate Behavioral Research*, 1993. **28**(4): pp. 467–482.

74. Kaplan, D. and R. George, A study of the power associated with testing factor mean differences under violations of factorial invariance. *Structural Equation Modeling: A Multidisciplinary Journal*, 1995. **2**(2): pp. 101–118.

75. Westland, J.C., Lower bounds on sample size in structural equation modeling. *Electronic Commerce Research and Applications*, 2010. **9**(6): pp. 476–487.

76. Soper, D.S., A-priori Sample Size Calculator for Structural Equation Models [Software]. Available from https://www.danielsoper.com/statcalc.

5

Model Identifiability and Equivalence

5.1 Introduction to Model Identifiability

In traditional regression analysis, there is a dependable model structure. We can specify a traditional OLS multiple regression model using statistical software by selecting an outcome and covariates in embedded code. Once we run this code, we typically assume we have converged upon a unique solution for the given model and data. We may instead agonize about a host of other modeling issues, including, for example, violations of traditional regression assumptions or a low R^2 value and, in the process, change our model specification.

A novice SEM researcher may be anticipating a solution after developing a sound conceptual model and inputting some carefully crafted MPlus code using a large dataset. However, the said researcher may receive the following confusing message:

THE DEGREES OF FREEDOM FOR THIS MODEL ARE NEGATIVE. THE MODEL IS NOT IDENTIFIED. NO CHI-SQUARE TEST IS AVAILABLE. CHECK YOUR MODEL.

We will decode this error message as we elaborate on the condition of model *identifiability* and some tips on how handle it.

Identifiability is a condition under which it is possible to determine unique estimates of the unknown parameters which best fit the observed data for a given model. A non-identifiable model fails on the condition of identifiability. Formally, *non-identifiability* is a condition where multiple possible values of the unknown parameters lead to the exact same probability distribution of observed variables.

An identifiable model requires that the number of unknown parameters is less than or equal to the total number of pieces of information available for model estimation. This is a necessary (but not yet sufficient) condition for identifiability. That is a model must, at minimum, meet this requirement to be identifiable, but a model can meet this requirement and still be non-identifiable.

Consider two examples. First, to illustrate the necessary condition above, if one is presented with two equations, X + Y + Z = 9 and X − Y − Z = 16, one cannot solve for X, Y and Z using these two equations. There are more unknowns (the variables) than available information (the values 16 and 9). One would need a third equation that did not introduce any new variables to solve for X, Y and Z. Second, to illustrate why this necessary condition may not yet be sufficient, consider a traditional OLS multiple regression model. In order to be identified, the sample size must be greater than the number of predictors (similar to the necessary condition we just mentioned for an identifiable structural equation model) *and* the covariance matrix of predictors must be nonsingular.

Recall that the total number of pieces of information, the number of means, variances and covariances of the observed variables can be derived using the formula for $k*$ in

TABLE 5.1

Summary of Input Pieces of Observed Information Used to Output Estimated Parameters

Information from Observed Variables as Input	Estimated Parameters to Output
Mean for endogenous variable	Intercept
Mean for exogenous variable	Mean
Variance for endogenous variable	Residual (error) variance
Variance for exogenous variable	Variance
Covariance between variables	Causal path or covariance

For k observed variables, the total number of observed means and variances is each k and the total number of observed covariances is $\dfrac{k(k-1)}{2}$.

equation (4.5) in Chapter 4. We summarize the observed information that is used to estimate unknown parameters in Table 5.1. This basic table should be interpreted with flexibility as depending on the model and restrictions input information may be used to estimate different unknown parameters.

In classic SEM approaches, one looks to reproduce the population covariance matrix (approximated in practice using the sample covariance matrix) by the model-implied covariance matrix under a model specification. Each model-implied variance and covariance is a function of one or more unknown parameters. That is, under a model specification, some or all of the model-implied variances and covariances are represented by the addition and/or multiplication of multiple unknown parameters, rather than just a single unknown parameter. Once again we refer the interested reader for more technical details regarding the form of the model-implied covariance matrix in SEMs to the classic textbook by Bollen [1].

Formally, we can notate the necessary condition for identifiability (total number of pieces of information available for model estimation is greater than or equal to the number of unknown parameters) as $k^* - t \geq 0$, given t unknown parameters in the model. Recall from Chapter 4, that the model degrees of freedom $df_M = k^* - t$. Thus, the necessary condition for identification is also analogous to stating that a model has non-negative degrees of freedom. Our MPlus error message for a hypothetical non-identifiable model warned us that our degrees of freedom were negative.

Previously alluded to, another necessary condition for identifiability is that all latent variables, including residual terms, in a model must be assigned a metric [2]. For example, in performing CFA for a latent factor and a single group, a metric is assigned by either fixing:

1. The latent factor on a metric with mean zero and variance one.
2. One of the factor loadings as a reference loading to one.

In fixing a factor loading to one, the latent factor is measured on the same metric as the reference variable. MPlus by default will set the factor loading to one for the first item of the scale [3].

In a single factor model with three effect indicators of the latent variable and uncorrelated errors, fixing the metric makes the model identifiable. We will discuss later in this chapter why it is preferable to have at least four effect indicators of the latent variable in a single factor model (given no additional variables). We will also illustrate how a latent variable that is part of a model incorporating other variables can "borrow" information from other observed variables that are not indicators of the latent variable.

A single factor model with two effect indicators and uncorrelated errors can be identified given additional restrictions such as the two factor loadings are constrained to be equal to each other and variance of the factor is one. As part of a measurement model with more than one latent variable, the restriction of equal factor loadings becomes unnecessary. In the chapter Appendix, we discuss identification of a measurement model of a latent variable with a single effect indicator. See Bollen [1] for more detailed rules for determining identifiability of CFA models, including multiple factor models.

Most typically, in a non-identifiable structural equation model, the matrix of second derivatives of the log-likelihood with respect to the model parameters is numerically not of full rank. An interested reader should refer to the SEM textbooks by Bollen or Kline [1,2] for a description of the rank and order conditions for diagnosing identifiability problems.

5.2 Underidentified, Just-Identified and Overidentified Models

A model is *underidentified* if the model degrees of freedom is less than zero. As a result, the model has infinite solutions for the unknown parameters and is not identifiable. Underidentification is not an issue about data quality and quantity or measurement precision; underidentification is a problem of model specification [4]. In other words, one can have an infinitely large sample and such a model is still nonidentifiable.

An identifiable model with zero degrees of freedom is called *just identified*. The just identified model is the same as the saturated model as discussed in Chapter 4. Recall that the saturated model fits the data exactly and model fit measures yield ideal results. There is no formal assessment of model fit in just identified models.

The preference in SEM is, in general, for an *overidentified* model with positive degrees of freedom. Overidentified models provide some meaning to evaluation criteria such as the chi-square test, RMSEA, CFI, TLI and SRMR in order to determine if the model fits the observed data well.

5.2.1 Assessing Identifiability in Illustrative Examples

We next provide the reader with some examples of underidentified, just identified and overidentified models. All observed variables are continuous in these examples. We will discuss any nonstandard assumptions for these models below. In the figures provided for each example, we list the number of observed means, variances and covariances as input observed information to output estimated parameters. The reader can review Table 5.1 as a reference. The difference in the number of input pieces of information and the number of output estimated parameters is the model degrees of freedom.

Consider the models corresponding to Figure 5.1.[1] *Physical activity* and *BMI* have a positive *feedback loop* in Figure 5.1a. In a feedback loop, some or all of the output of a system returns as input in a circular fashion [5]. A feedback loop between two variables is a reciprocal relationship. We have assumed that *BMI* affects *physical activity*, but *physical activity* also affects *BMI* in Figure 5.1a. Thus, there are two structural regressions, the regression of *physical activity* on *BMI* and the regression of *BMI* on *physical activity*. Unknown parameters in each regression equation include an intercept, slope and residual variance.

---

[1] The formula for k^* in equation (4.4) in Chapter 4 will correspond to our count of the number of means, variance and covariances of the observed variables in our figures. In 5.1a $k^* = \dfrac{2(5)}{2} = 5$ and in 5.1b $k^* = \dfrac{3(6)}{2} = 9$.

(a)

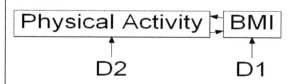

Path Model

$$BMI = \alpha_1 + \beta_1 Physical\ Activity + D1,$$
$$Physical\ Activity = \alpha_2 + \beta_2 BMI + D2$$

α_1 and α_2 are intercepts and β_1 and β_2 are regression paths. $D1$ and $D2$ are error terms assumed to be both continuous with mean zero and positive variance. The unknown parameters for the error terms are the residual variances ψ_1 for $D1$ and ψ_2 for $D2$.

Input: 1 Mean for *BMI*, 1 Mean for *Physical Activity*, 1 Variance for *BMI*, 1 Variance for *Physical Activity*, 1 Covariance Between *BMI* and *Physical Activity*
Output: 2 Intercepts, 2 Residual Variances, 2 Regression Paths
Model degrees of freedom = -1

(b)

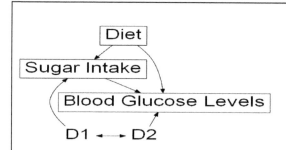

Path Model

$$Sugar\ Intake = \alpha_1 + \gamma_1 Diet + D1,$$
$$Blood\ Glucose\ Levels = \alpha_2 + \beta_1 Sugar\ Intake + \gamma_2 Diet + D2$$

α_1 and α_2 are intercepts and γ_1, γ_2 and β_1 are regression paths. $D1$ and $D2$ are correlated error terms assumed to be both continuous with mean zero. The unknown parameters for the error terms are the residual variances ψ_1 for $D1$ and ψ_2 for $D2$ which are assumed be positive and $Cov(D1, D2) = \psi_{12} \neq 0$. There is also a mean and variance for *Diet* with the mean structure.

Input: 2 Means for Endogenous Variables (*Blood Glucose Levels* and *Sugar Intake*), 1 Mean for *Diet*, 2 Variances for Endogenous Variables, 1 Variance for *Diet*, 3 Covariances Between *Blood Glucose Levels* and *Sugar Intake*, *Blood Glucose Levels* and *Diet*, *Sugar Intake* and *Diet*
Output: 2 Intercepts, 1 Mean, 2 Residual Variances, 1 Variance, 3 Regression Paths, 1 Residual Covariance
Model degrees of freedom = -1

FIGURE 5.1

Examples of underidentified nonrecursive models: (a) Feedback loop; (b) Correlated disturbance terms.

Figure 5.1b is in the form of a basic mediation model between three observed variables. However, instead of assuming the error terms for *sugar intake* and *blood glucose levels* are uncorrelated, we have incorporated a nonzero residual correlation in Figure 5.1b.

Both path models represented in these Figures in 5.1a and 5.1b are underidentified. In model 5.1a, the feedback loop has two structural regression slopes β_1 and β_2. We only have one piece of information (observed covariance between *physical activity* and *BMI*) to estimate these two parameters. This is not possible and leads to a negative degree of freedom. Figure 5.1b has three regression paths $(\gamma_1, \gamma_2, \beta_1)$ and one residual covariance ψ_{12}. We have three observed covariances to estimate these four parameters. This again results in a negative degree of freedom.

The underidentified models corresponding to Figure 5.1 are examples of *nonrecursive* models. Nonrecursive models contain at least one feedback loop or correlated disturbance terms. *Recursive* models, on the other hand, do not have these features. That is, in a recursive model [4]:

1. Causation among the variables is strictly unidirectional
2. Disturbance terms in the model are uncorrelated with each other

Therefore, nonrecursive models violate at least one of these two conditions.

Recursive models are not always appropriate given theory. There are available approaches to making nonrecursive models identifiable. Similar approaches can be used to make a just identified model into an overidentified model, since these approaches add degrees of freedom.

One approach would be to use *instrumental variables*, as discussed in the econometrics literature [6]. In the SEM context, an instrumental variable is a predictor that has a direct path to one endogenous variable but no direct path to the other endogenous variable in a nonrecursive relationship [7]. In a feedback loop with two endogenous variables Y1 and Y2, instrumental variables IV1 and IV2 can be used such that we assume IV1→Y1 and IV2→Y2 and no path from IV1 to Y2 and IV2 to Y1.

We now reassess the feedback loop in the physical activity-BMI example using an instrumental variable approach (see Figure 5.2a). We can define an instrument as a *dietary supplement* that we assume only directly effects *BMI*, but not *physical activity*. Also, the instrument *fitness tracker* we assume only directly effects *physical activity*, but not *BMI*. Indirectly, use of the *fitness tracker* influences *BMI* through *physical activity* and the *dietary supplement* influences *physical activity* through *BMI*. We also assume that use of the *fitness tracker* and *dietary supplement* are correlated. This model is overidentified with one degree of freedom.

Another approach is to constrain particular parameters in a model increasing model degrees of freedom [4]. For example, constraining the direct path *BMI*→ *physical activity* in the feedback loop to zero makes *physical activity* solely an exogenous variable (see Figure 5.2b). The model is a regression of *BMI* on *physical activity* which is just identified. In more complex models, parameters can be constrained to be equal across different equations, groups or repeated measures. Importantly, these types of constraints, as well as the use of instruments, should be theoretically reasonable and not simply done to achieve identification. A feedback loop can also be analyzed using autoregressive longitudinal modeling (Chapter 13) given the availability of time varying measures of the endogenous variables in the nonrecursive relationship.

Figure 5.3 is an example of a just identified mediation model. This path model includes an assumption of no residual correlation between the two endogenous variables, *self-efficacy*

(a)

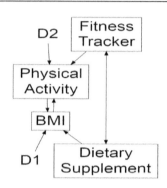

Path Model

$BMI = \alpha_1 + \beta_1 Physical\ Activity + \gamma_1 Dietary\ Supplement + D1,$

$Physical\ Activity = \alpha_2 + \beta_2 BMI + \gamma_2 Fitness\ Tracker + D2$

α_1 and α_2 are intercepts and $\beta_1, \gamma_1, \beta_2$ and γ_2 are regression paths. $D1$ and $D2$ are error terms assumed to be both continuous with mean zero and positive variance. The unknown parameters for the error terms are the residual variances ψ_1 for $D1$ and ψ_2 for $D2$. There are also two means, two variances and a covariance between *Fitness Tracker* and *Dietary Supplement* with the mean structure.

Input: 2 Means for Endogenous Variables (*Physical Activity* and *BMI*), 2 Means for Instrumental Variables (*Fitness Tracker* and *Dietary Supplement*), 2 Variances for Endogenous Variables, 2 Variances for Instrumental Variables, 6 Covariances (Pairwise Between *Physical Activity, BMI, Fitness Tracker* and *Dietary Supplement*)

Output: 2 Intercepts, 2 Means, 2 Residual Variances, 2 Variances, 4 Regression Paths, 1 Covariance

Model degrees of freedom = 1

(b)

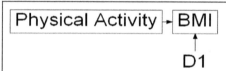

Path Model

$BMI = \alpha_1 + \gamma_1 Physical\ Activity + D1$

α_1 is an intercept and γ_1 is a regression path. $D1$ is an error term assumed to be continuous with mean zero and positive variance ψ_1. There is also a mean and variance for *Physical Activity* with the mean structure.

Input: 1 Mean for *BMI*, 1 Mean for *Physical Activity*, 1 Variance for *BMI*, 1 Variance for *Physical Activity*, 1 Covariance Between *BMI* and *Physical Activity*

Output: 1 Intercept, 1 Mean, 1 Residual Variance, 1 Variance, 1 Regression Path

Model degrees of freedom = 0

FIGURE 5.2

Approaches for identifying the nonrecursive *physical activity-BMI* model: (a) Instrumental variables; (b) Constraining a regression path to zero.

and *glucose control*. We can follow this template and constrain the residual correlation between *sugar intake* and *blood glucose levels* to zero (i.e. $\psi_{12} = 0$) in Figure 5.1b for a just identified model. That is, assuming this constraint is theoretically warranted.

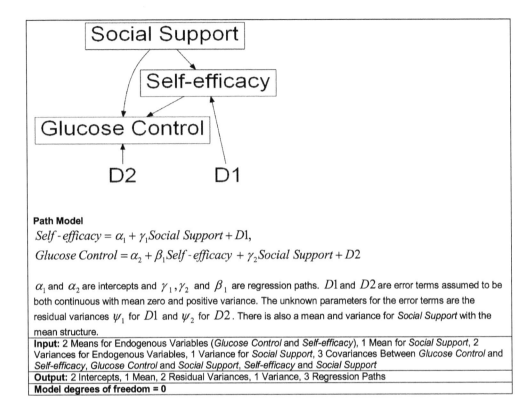

Path Model

$Self\text{-}efficacy = \alpha_1 + \gamma_1 Social\ Support + D1,$

$Glucose\ Control = \alpha_2 + \beta_1 Self\text{-}efficacy + \gamma_2 Social\ Support + D2$

α_1 and α_2 are intercepts and γ_1, γ_2 and β_1 are regression paths. $D1$ and $D2$ are error terms assumed to be both continuous with mean zero and positive variance. The unknown parameters for the error terms are the residual variances ψ_1 for $D1$ and ψ_2 for $D2$. There is also a mean and variance for *Social Support* with the mean structure.

Input: 2 Means for Endogenous Variables (*Glucose Control* and *Self-efficacy*), 1 Mean for *Social Support*, 2 Variances for Endogenous Variables, 1 Variance for *Social Support*, 3 Covariances Between *Glucose Control* and *Self-efficacy*, *Glucose Control* and *Social Support*, *Self-efficacy* and *Social Support*

Output: 2 Intercepts, 1 Mean, 2 Residual Variances, 1 Variance, 3 Regression Paths

Model degrees of freedom = 0

FIGURE 5.3
Just identified mediation model example.

Consider the MIMIC model corresponding to Figure 5.4.

We have constrained the intercept for the structural model for the latent variable to zero as an identifying constraint. We also fixed the factor loading for emotional well-being to one to assign the metric for *mental health*. This model is overidentified with two degrees of freedom.

A single factor model with three indicators and uncorrelated errors (and an assigned metric) will be just identified. A single factor model requires at least four indicators (given other identifying constraints) to be overidentified. The latent variable of *mental health* in Figure 5.4 has three observed indicators. In the model represented in Figure 5.4, we "borrowed" information from the observed variable *medical comorbidities* to make the model overidentified. *Medical comorbidities* has an observed mean and variance and observed covariances with *emotional, psychological* and *social*.

We want to emphasize here that a model with positive degrees of freedom may still not be identifiable. Lack of identification is not simply due to negative degrees of freedom. For example, if we do not assign a metric to the latent variable in the model represented in Figure 5.4 (i.e. remove the constraint that the factor loading for emotional well-being is one), the model still has a positive degree of freedom, but is no longer identifiable. More generally mistakes could be made in the specification that mean that even with positive degrees of freedom a model is not identifiable. Further, in a complex model, even for a seasoned SEM researcher, it can be difficult to determine the exact issue that leads to a non-identified model. Thus, when having problems with identification in a complex model,

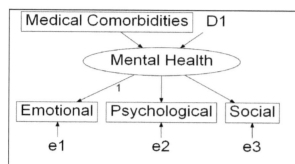

Measurement Model

$Emotional = v_1 + \lambda_1 Mental\ Health + e1$

$Psychological = v_2 + \lambda_2 Mental\ Health + e2$

$Social = v_3 + \lambda_3 Mental\ Health + e3$

v_1, v_2 and v_3 are the factor intercepts, λ_1, λ_2 and λ_3 are the factor loadings. We assign the metric of *Mental Health* by fixing $\lambda_1 = 1$. $e1, e2$ and $e3$ are measurement error terms assumed to each be continuous with mean zero and positive variance. The unknown parameters for the error terms are the factor residual variances θ_{e1}, θ_{e2} and θ_{e3} for $e1, e2$ and $e3$, respectively.

Structural Model

$Mental\ Health = \alpha_1 + \gamma_1 Medical\ Comorbidities + D1$

α_1 is an intercept and γ_1 is a regression path. $D1$ is an error term assumed to be continuous with mean zero and positive variance ψ_1. There is also a mean and variance for *Medical Comorbidities* with the mean structure. We have constrained $\alpha_1 = 0$ as an identifying constraint.

Input: 3 Means for Observed Indicators (*Emotional, Psychological* and *Social*), 1 Mean for *Medical Comorbidities*, 3 Variances for Observed Indicators, 1 Variance for *Medical Comorbidities*, 6 Covariances (Pairwise Between *Emotional, Psychological, Social* and *Medical Comorbidities*)
Output: 3 Factor Intercepts, 1 Mean, 3 Factor Residual Variances, 1 Variance, 2 Factor Loadings, 1 Regression Path, 1 Error Residual Variance
Model degrees of freedom = 2

FIGURE 5.4
Overidentified MIMIC model example.

we recommend that one start with a simpler model that can be run successfully in software for the analysis of SEMs and build up to the more complex model. This will also help one decode the problematic parameters and decipher occasionally cryptic error messages produced by software in the presence of model identification problems.

5.3 Equivalent Models

The issue with a nonidentifiable model, as aforementioned, is that there are numerous possible solutions for the unknown parameters. Another not uncommon problem in SEM (and, incidentally, in all of statistics/model building) is the result of multiple models leading to the same numerical output. We use the term in this book *equivalent models* when multiple models yield the same sample and model-implied covariance matrices.

Equivalent models yield identical model fit statistics and indices [2]. However, each model in a series of equivalent models leads to a different interpretation of the data. A series of equivalent models do have the same observed variables and number of unknown parameters. Two equivalent models may have the same probability distribution of data (termed *observationally equivalent models*) or merely have the same covariance matrices (termed *covariance equivalent models*). Observational equivalence is thus a broader form of equivalence that requires the identity of individual level data whereas covariance equivalence requires the identity of summary statistics [8].

For a basic (and somewhat trivial) example, consider the path model regressing *BMI* on *physical activity* in Figure 5.2b. A path model changing the directionality of the relationship in regressing *physical activity* on *BMI* is equivalent. In these two models we have the exact same input values (same 2 observed means, 2 variances and 1 covariance). We also have the same parameters to estimate (2 means/intercepts, 2 variances/residual variances, 1 regression path) (see Figure 5.2b). The model fit values would be the same perfect fit for these two just identified models. The actual path model estimates for the same observed data, such as the intercept and slope coefficients, will be different. These values depend on the direction of the relationship such as which variable is defined as the dependent variable and which variable is defined as the independent variable.

We can consider an extension of this path model above, adding in a single exogenous latent variable (e.g. attitude towards health and fitness) with four, uncorrelated indicators that is hypothesized to influence both *physical activity* and *BMI*. This extended model is overidentified. We will obtain the same non-trivial model fit whether *physical activity→BMI* or *BMI→physical activity* for the same observed data as discussed above.

Quantitative analysis cannot be used to distinguish which model fits the data best in a series of equivalent models. Logic, theory and prior evidence must be used to make a decision about the model or models to consider for a study. For example, it is not possible to distinguish using data alone whether cigarette smoking causes lung cancer or lung cancer causes cigarette smoking in a model. The decision to choose one causal ordering above the other is based on theoretical reasoning regarding the subject matter. The results of past scientific studies and sound scientific knowledge have dictated that cigarette smoking causes lung cancer.

5.3.1 Examples of Equivalent Models

We now present two relevant examples of equivalent models for health and medicine. The first example in Figure 5.5 uses the observational data on persons living with multiple sclerosis ($N = 3507$). Figure 5.5 visualizes equivalent one and two factor models.

In these measurement models, we used the PHQ-9 items as indicators of depression. The first two items of the PHQ-9 describe symptoms of anhedonia and depressed mood. These two items summed together termed the PHQ-2 have been commonly used as a first screening tool for depression in clinic. An application is if an individual has a total score greater than or equal to three on the PHQ-2, they will be asked to fill out the rest of the PHQ-9 to screen for depressive symptoms. An approach to distinguishing the PHQ-2 items from the other seven items in the PHQ-9 in a one factor model is to specify a residual correlation between the first two items. Alternatively, we could model the PHQ-2 items as a single factor in a two factor model. These two models represented in Figure 5.5 include the same nine observed items and the same number of parameters (28). The model fit for these two models is identical and relatively good (see Figure 5.5).

Choosing between equivalent models may depend on the context of a particular study. For example, corresponding to the mediation model in Figure 5.6a, we hypothesize

(a)

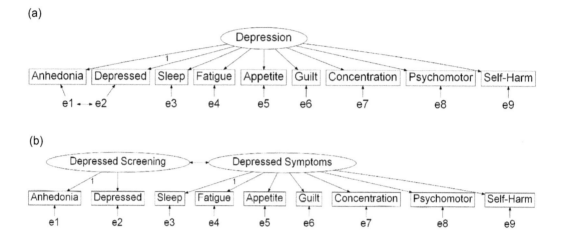

(b)

FIGURE 5.5
Equivalent CFA models for the PHQ-9 items in persons living with multiple sclerosis ($N = 3,507$): (a) One factor with residual correlation; (b) Two factors.

For both models: $\chi^2 (26) = 674.43, p = \leq.001$; CFI = .930; TLI = .903; RMSEA = .057. (90% CI 0.044, 0.070); SRMR = 0.040. We used the MLR option in MPlus to conduct analysis with these CFA models. In the single factor model reference factor loading for Anhedonia is constrained to one. In the two factor model reference factor loadings for the items for Anhedonia and Sleep are constrained to one.

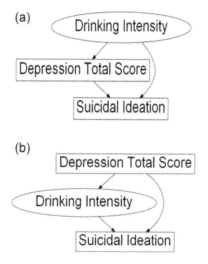

FIGURE 5.6
Equivalent mediation models of drinking and suicidal risk ($N = 1,726$): (a) Depression is a mediator; (b) Drinking intensity is a mediator.

For both models: $\chi^2 (59) = 218.288, p = <.001$; CFI = .947; TLI = .933; RMSEA = .042. Drinking intensity is a latent variable constructed from 3 months of observed data on drinking intensity. Depression total score is an observed sum score. Suicidal Ideation is a binary measure of suicidal thoughts. In analyses of these models, we assumed longitudinal invariance over 15 months (constrained model estimates across four repeated measures to be equal). Example using the first specification, with depression as the mediator, is adapted from Conner, K.R., Gunzler, D., et al., Test of a clinical model of drinking and suicidal risk. *Alcoholism: Clinical and Experimental Research*, 2011. 35(1): pp. 60–68.

drinking intensity causes depression. Prior research in a sample of alcohol dependent individuals lead us to hypothesize that depression is a potential mediator of the relationship between drinking intensity and suicidal ideation [9].

A researcher in a different setting may reasonably hypothesize that intense drinking is a potential mediator of the relationship between depression and suicidal ideation (Figure 5.6b). In the model represented in Figure 5.6b, we have simply reversed the directionality of the causal path between drinking intensity and depression from the model represented in Figure 5.6a. Thus the two models are equivalent.

5.3.2 Generating Equivalent Models

In this section thus far we have described model equivalence as a problematic issue in SEM research. However, it can also play a role in helping a researcher identify the optimal model for a study. Identifying equivalent models can provide support for a substantive model of interest if the equivalent models can be ruled out or can reveal previously unrecognized plausible alternative models [10]. Rules have been developed for many types of widely used SEMs for obtaining an equivalent model from a substantive model of interest through what may appear to be a minor model modification. The interested reader should refer to Lee and Hershberger [10], Stetzl [11] and Bentler and Satorra [12] for more on this topic.

5.4 Conclusions

We discussed model identifiability in this chapter. The necessary but not sufficient conditions we illustrated for identifiability are nonnegative degrees of freedom and assignment of a metric for all latent variables, including residual terms [2]. In very complex system-based models, assessing model identifiability may be challenging and is beyond the scope of this book. We once again refer the interested reader to Bollen or Kline [1,2] for a description of the rank and order conditions for diagnosing identifiability problems. Models with positive degrees of freedom (overidentified models) allow a researcher to meaningfully assess model fit. Equivalent models, multiple models that yield identical model fit statistics and indices, but a different interpretation of the data, were also discussed in this chapter.

The authors of this book recommend a team science strategy to specify a model in order to minimize potential issues of nonidentifiability, model equivalence and other commonly encountered challenges. In team science, an expert panel of multidisciplinary researchers use theory, logic and a prior literature review to make informed decisions for model specification. In practice, any nonidentifiable model must be revised.

Team members may see the optimal model specification differently. Therefore, an organized structure for evaluating input fairly from different members of the expert panel is necessary.

We briefly provide a recommendation on this structure. The principal investigator of a study can set guidelines before presenting the task at hand to the expert panel of developing a substantive model (or series of models). These guidelines can include a definitive list of variables for the model and some hypothesized known paths (Chapter 6 on model specification). Each member of the expert panel may independently use these guidelines along with theory, logic and prior literature to complete the task. The principal investigator may then use commonalities in the results for helping to make model development decisions.

5.4.1 Appendix: Single Indicator Latent Variable

Consider the following measurement model for a study sample of size N (for simplicity we omit an individual level subscript):

$$y_1 = \lambda_1 \eta_1 + e_1 \tag{5.1}$$

where y_1 is an observed variable, η_1 is a latent variable, λ_1 is a factor loading and e_1 is the measurement error term. A single systolic blood pressure (SBP), temperature or nonfasting blood sugar reading are some examples of tests that can be highly variable in individuals depending on the time of day, method and/or setting of administration. Thus, such a model as in (5.1) may be appropriate for such tests in order to account for measurement error associated with the observed reading.

We set the factor loading λ_1 as a reference loading to one as an identifying constraint. We also assume the expected value of the error term is zero and the covariance between the latent variable and error term is zero. Under these restrictions, we still have just one piece of information (variance of the observed indicator) to estimate two parameters (residual variance and variance of the latent variable). The model is underidentified.

A typical approach to identifying such a measurement model as above is to assume an implicit measurement model in which the residual variance is fixed to zero (i.e. $y_1 = \eta_1$). This may be a limitation with some measures, such as SBP, but is still the common approach. The observed variable then can be used as is in a structural model.

One can also instead fix the error variance to a nonzero quantity in assuming some level of uncertainty. The interested reader can refer to Brown [13] for an overview of an approach to estimating the proportion of measurement error for a single indicator factor on the basis of the observed indicator's variance and assumed reliability (consistency of measurement).

We considered here only a single observed measurement for each individual (e.g. single SBP reading). We can use the average of two or more measurements, if available in the data, as an observed variable instead for a potentially more accurate measure. Multiple measurements can also be used as indicators of a latent variable.

References

1. Bollen, K., *Structural equations with latent variables*. 1989, New York: Wiley.
2. Kline, R.B., *Principles and practice of structural equation modeling*, fourth edition. 2016, New York: Guilford Press.
3. Muthén, L.K. and B.O. Muthén, *Mplus: The comprehensive modelling program for applied researchers: user's guide*. Eighth edition, 1998–2017, Los Angeles, CA: Muthén & Muthén.
4. Berry, W.D., *Nonrecursive causal models*. Vol. 37. 1984, Beverly Hills, CA: Sage.
5. Ford, A. and F.A. Ford, *Modeling the environment: An introduction to system dynamics models of environmental systems*. 1999, Washington, DC: Island Press.
6. Heckman, J.J., Econometric causality. *International Statistical Review*, 2008. **76**(1): pp. 1–27.
7. Martens, M.P. and R.F. Haase, Advanced applications of structural equation modeling in counseling psychology research. *The Counseling Psychologist*, 2006. **34**(6): pp. 878–911.
8. Hancock, G.R. and R.O. Mueller, *Structural equation modeling: A second course*. 2013, Charlotte, NC: IAP.

9. Conner, K.R., et al., Test of a clinical model of drinking and suicidal risk. *Alcoholism: Clinical and Experimental Research*, 2011. **35**(1): pp. 60–68.

10. Lee, S. and S. Hershberger, A simple rule for generating equivalent models in covariance structure modeling. *Multivariate Behavioral Research*, 1990. **25**(3): pp. 313–334.

11. Stetzl, I., Changing causal relationships without changing the fit: Some rules for generating equivalent LISREL models. *Multivariate Behavior Research*, 1986. **21**: pp. 309–331.

12. Bentler, P.M. and A. Satorra, Testing model nesting and equivalence. *Psychological Methods*, 2010. **15**(2): pp. 111–123.

13. Brown, T.A., *Confirmatory factor analysis for applied research*. 2014, New York: Guilford Publications.

Part III

Applications and Examples of Structural Equation Modeling for Health and Medical Research

6

Choosing among Competing Specifications

6.1 Introduction to Model Specification and Re-specification

Model specification in the context of SEM is the translation of a conceptual model into a formal structural equation model. In model specification, a researcher selects which variables to include in the model as well as the functional form of the model. Further, a researcher indicates causal paths and directionality between latent and observed variables under study.

The initial model specification should be in line with theory, logic and prior studies. Although in many studies the researcher has no intention of revising a model, even the most carefully specified models sometimes require re-specification. In the HIV example with MPlus in Chapter 2, the path model evaluated if increased levels of health practices and a longer duration of diagnosis had led to increased acceptance that HIV is a chronic disease. This straightforward model was specified precisely to address a particular research hypothesis; re-specification was neither planned nor implemented.

The model for our HIV example was also just identified. In general, just identified models provide less flexibility for re-specification according to empirical fit criteria. In an overidentified initial model, a wider array of nontrivial model fit indices are available, and model fit could be less than desirable, prompting consideration of a revised, but still plausible model. In health and medical studies, even in a good fitting model, relationships between measures are often uncertain, especially as model complexity arises and when the possible regression paths and directionality may be numerous.

A revised model can be viewed as an alternative model to the initial model. Thus, a study looking to potentially respecify a model is a type of study involving model comparison between competing models. A researcher either retains the initial model or chooses an alternative, modified model as the "best" model. There is another type of study involving model comparison. The researcher can begin with multiple plausible models in pursuit of the "best" model among the competing models. In this chapter, both these approaches will be applied and sometimes even in succession. For example, one may begin by comparing between multiple plausible models and then, after choosing a single model, revise it further.

We focus primarily on competing structural models in this chapter for a given data set and set of variables. We do present some competing measurement models.

There is an important place for both subjective and quantitative analysis in making model modifications and comparisons. We recommend that researchers use a three-step procedure:

Three-step procedure for selecting a "best" model among competing models

1. Logic, theory and prior empirical evidence to specify the initial, plausible model (or models)
2. Quantitative analyses to make model revisions as indicated or model comparisons
3. Interpret subjective and quantitative evidence to choose the model most appropriate for a given study

Note that steps (2) and (3) can be iterative, in that one may consider one revision (or comparison) at a time, and then determine the "better" model before evaluating the next competing model. An overview of empirical criteria for making model comparisons is particularly important, since there is as yet no gold standard. Applying and interpreting the results of several measures, which in the ideal scenario all indicate the same model preference, can help balance the strengths and weaknesses of each individual measure. In turn, a revised model can still be modified further before denoting it as the "best" model. For example, the revised model may still have a poor overall model fit and require further modification. Note that the authors of this book have chosen our nomenclature carefully using the "best" model instead of "best-fitting" model since this model will not be chosen using quantitative methods alone.

While in practice many model possibilities may fit a given data set well, for research purposes, valuable information can be gained by assigning a single "best" model or identifying a subset of candidate models that are preferred over other models. A "best" model explicitly denotes the nature of the relationships among measures for research hypothesis testing and future studies. An important potential drawback is that in the absence of a gold standard, even the "best" model may be misspecified or non-parsimonious and ill-fitting.

The three-step procedure for "best" model selection is useful for researchers looking to provide both clinically meaningful and generalizable results. In this procedure there is a strong theoretical basis for both the initial model and competing models (or multiple models from the outset). Data-driven approaches then allow a researcher to more objectively make model comparisons. In this chapter, we discuss *specification searches* which are algorithms for modification of an initial model with the goal of finding the "best" model for the given data. Due to the computation time and labor involved in making a series of model comparisons, specification searches built into software can be invaluable for researchers looking to simultaneously consider different criterion and different models in search of a "best" model.

MacCallum [1,2] has demonstrated that specification of models can be influenced by characteristics of the data, especially in small to moderate sized samples. Researchers have incorrectly used specification searches to modify an initial model, regardless of interpretability. In this chapter, an application to a real-world, practical example using health self-ratings and physical performance measures illustrates how we can use theory and empirical criteria together to avoid these shortcomings. Researchers contemplating possible mechanisms for understanding relationships between measures in very large health data sets may find these approaches particularly useful.

6.2 Path Diagrams for Making Model Comparisons

Figure 6.1 represents the path diagram for the health self-ratings and physical performance measures applied example to be described later in this chapter.

In path diagrams for making model comparisons between competing models for a given study, "known" paths are depicted by solid lines. These "known" paths are not optional for testing of the model; all versions of the model include these paths as specified. The presence of such paths is determined according to previous theory or prior evidence. "Unknown" paths to be evaluated for inclusion or exclusion in the model are depicted by broken lines. Typically, these "unknown" paths are theoretically defensible. It is just not clear if they should be incorporated within the model under study.

Keep in mind, that one may find models that are equivalent and/or non-identifiable among competing models. Thus, one must pay attention to such potential problems from the outset when deciding on what models to consider in a study.

In a theoretically sound model in health and medicine, certain paths will be known. As a result, changing the direction of the relationship between certain measures within an "unknown" path may not be a possibility. We may be able to rule out some or all equivalent models. For example, from Figure 6.1, we specify as a "known" path that *Education* influences *Physical Performance*. We use an assumption of temporal causality to specify that *Education* influences *Physical Performance* and not vice versa. It may be "unknown" whether *Social Support* influences *Physical Performance* or *Physical Performance* influences *Social Support* (i.e. equivalence). We might further hypothesize that, like *Education*, *Social Support* has a causal effect on *Physical Performance*. In this sample of adults as discussed later in this chapter, educational attainment occurred many decades before the physical performance measure was collected. Thus, using knowledge about the system as a whole we are able to eliminate an equivalent model. In this chapter, the competing models we will consider for the health self-ratings and physical performance measures applied example are all identifiable and none are equivalent.

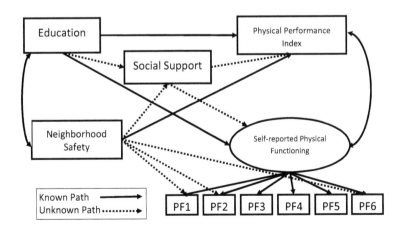

FIGURE 6.1
Path diagram for health self-ratings and physical performance measures example.

PF1–PF6 are six indicators of self-reported physical functioning.

6.3 Nested vs. Non-nested Models

In Figure 6.1, let model M1 include both "known" and "unknown" paths, and model M2 only includes the "known" paths. Then, M1 and M2 are *nested models*, in that M2 can be derived from putting parameter restrictions (constraining regression paths to zero) on M1. The fixed parameters in M2 are a subset of the fixed parameters in M1. The reduced model (M2) is nested within the larger model (M1).

We can derive many other nested models from both M1 and M2. For example, constraining the regression path for *Education* to *Social Support* to zero in M1 results in a model such that M2 is nested within this model which is nested within M1.

In a measurement model for the same data, a two factor model with a fixed zero correlation between the factors is nested within a two factor model with a non-zero correlation between the factors. Alternately, a one factor model can be perceived as a reduced version of a two factor model with a perfect correlation between the factors [3].

Non-nested models are not hierarchically related. In a series of non-nested models, none of the individual models can be obtained from each other by restricting parameters through a limiting process. For example, in non-nested path models among the same set of variables, regression paths will both need to be removed *and* added. Figure 6.2a displays a path diagram for a mediation process. A nested model can be derived from constraining c' to zero.[1] Figure 6.2b is a non-nested model under a different specification which cannot be derived from putting parameter restrictions on Figure 6.2a.

While in simpler cases, determining if models are equivalent, nested or non-nested may be straightforward, as model complexity grows, this may be increasingly harder to determine. Bentler and Satorra [4] developed the Nesting and Equivalence Test (NET)[2] to help make these distinctions.

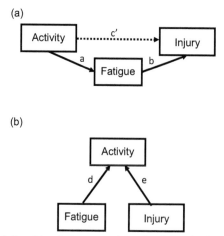

(a)

(b)

FIGURE 6.2 Hypothesized relationships between activity level, level of fatigue and number of physical injuries.

---

[1] See Chapter 9 for a description of full mediation.
[2] Function *net1.R* is available for NET Computations in *R* and EQS.

6.4 Chi-square Test of Difference

Let us now consider two SEMs, such that model B is nested within model A. Let us assume we used ML to estimate unknown parameters in these models and can use the chi-square test statistic as discussed in Chapter 4. In order to evaluate if the additional parameters in model A, as compared to model B, contribute to a good fit between the proposed model and the data, we can perform the *chi-square test of difference*.

Formally, let the model chi-square test statistic be χ_A^2 for model A and χ_B^2 for model B and the respective associated degrees of freedom df_A and df_B. Then we can derive the chi-square test of difference statistic χ_{Diff}^2 with associated degrees of freedom df_{Diff}:

$$\chi_{\text{Diff}}^2 = \chi_B^2 - \chi_A^2 \tag{6.1}$$

where $df_{\text{Diff}} = df_B - df_A$

Since model B is nested in model A, model A contains more parameters than model B. Therefore, model A has less degrees of freedom than model B and $df_{\text{Diff}} > 0$. If the test statistic in (6.1) is sufficiently large, which can be arbitrarily assessed by a p-value for a given level of α such as 0.05, then the fit of model A is better than that of model B (not equal fit). We might then conclude that the additional parameters in model A improve the fit of the model for a given data set. If we do not reject the null hypothesis of equal model fit, then including the parameters in model A that are not in model B will not provide a better fitting model. This does not necessarily mean model A is a worse fitting model, but at minimum less parsimonious.

Performing the chi-square test of difference using a more robust estimator such as ML with robust standard errors requires additional steps. These additional steps involve adjustment for the correction factors in using the robust estimator [5–7].

Satorra-Bentler scaled chi-square difference test can be used for both the MLM and MLR options in MPlus [5,8,9]. As before, model B is nested within model A. To perform the test using the MLM or MLR option in MPlus, let c_A be the scaling correction factor for model A and c_B be the scaling correction factor for model B. The Satorra-Bentler scaled chi-square value is SB_A for model A and SB_B for model B, and the respective associated degrees of freedom are df_A^{SB} and df_B^{SB}. The test statistic can be calculated as

$$T_{\text{Diff}} = \frac{\left(SB_B c_B - SB_A c_A\right)}{c_{\text{Diff}}} \tag{6.2}$$

where

$$c_{\text{Diff}} = \frac{\left(df_B^{SB} c_B - df_A^{SB} c_A\right)}{df_B^{SB} - df_A^{SB}} \tag{6.3}$$

Then, T_{Diff} is distributed chi-square with associated degrees of freedom df_{Diff}^{SB} where

$$df_{\text{Diff}}^{SB} = df_B^{SB} - df_A^{SB} \tag{6.4}$$

There are modified tests for difference for ordered-categorical data. For example, under the WLSMV option[3] in MPlus for ordered-categorical data, there is a modified chi-square test for difference [5]. Degree of freedom for this modified chi-square test is itself mean- and variance- adjusted.

6.5 Modification Indices

A fundamental assessment for model modification in SEM is through the evaluation of *modification indices (MIs)*. MIs are calculated individually for every parameter that is fixed to zero (or a constant), through estimate of a chi-square test statistic with one degree of freedom. Recall that fixing parameters to zero is not always explicitly done, but may be implicitly done in what is not included in a path diagram. For example, in Figure 6.1, all pairwise residual correlations between the six indicators of self-reported physical functioning PF1, PF2, ..., PF6 (i.e. 15 residual correlations total) have been constrained to zero. A theoretically warranted residual correlation may lead to improvements in the overall model fit.

The higher the value of the MI, the better the predicted improvement in model fit if that parameter were included to the model. Here we discuss guidelines on how to use MIs for continuous outcomes with maximum likelihood estimators. Jöreskog [10] suggested that a MI should be at least five before the researcher considers freeing that restricted parameter. In MPlus, when requested and applicable, the MIs for all restricted parameters in the model will be output. Further, a researcher can request to only print out the MIs that reach a certain threshold.[4]

MIs can be evaluated using a *p*-value approach. However, if the sample size is not large or the magnitude of the estimate is small, using such criterion may automatically include or exclude a path. Similarly, if the sample size is very large, we might mistakenly conclude that all of the changes are important, since there could be incremental benefits in trivial changes. This may not be consistent with the conceptual and theoretical grounds in the study. Therefore, it is preferred to examine the actual estimates in relation to other such estimates in the model instead [11].

A researcher must be very careful to use MIs "responsibly." What do we mean by "responsibly"? We encourage manual use of a limited number of MIs under strong theoretical underpinnings.

For starters, there should be a substantive reason for looking at MIs for revising a model beyond just using them to analytically improve model fit. For example, there may be a priori theory for evaluating MIs for residual correlations between certain items in a measurement model.

An example of theoretically warranted residual correlations can be demonstrated using the items of the Center for Epidemiologic Studies Depression (CESD)-20 depression symptom inventory [12]. In the CESD-20 scale, there are particular items addressing feeling good, hope about the future, happiness and enjoying life that are positively worded in contrast to other scale items that are negatively worded. In a single factor model of this

---

[3] There is a procedure DIFFTEST available in MPlus for performing the modified chi-square test for difference under the WLSMV option for comparing nested SEMs.

[4] To request only MIs greater than or equal to five in MPlus use the option in OUTPUT: modindices(5).

scale, residual correlations could be specified between such positively worded items. These residual correlations then account for the associations between items of a similar affirmative language when evaluating the underlying level of depression of the person taking the questionnaire.

One should "trust" MIs when the actual estimates are large enough (i.e. above a threshold such as five) and they represent meaningful parameters. Further, one should not use more than a few MIs for model modification. Some researchers will only use MIs to modify a model in a replication study and not for initial model building.

In practice, MIs can be used for applications involving both adding parameters to a model of interest and removing parameters from a model of interest. That is, one can test the value of adding a parameter to the model that was not a part of the hypothesized model, such as a residual correlation in Figure 6.1 for re-specification of the measurement model. One can also test the value of constraining a parameter to zero and removing it from the model. For example, in the model M1, we discussed earlier for Figure 6.1 with all "known" and "unknown" paths, and we can test the value of removing the regression path for *Education* to *Social Support*.

Changes in models based on MIs should be very carefully assessed for their impact on the overall model. As an example, the removal of a regression path according to a low MI value may not be theoretically appropriate. It may be more appropriate to leave the path in the model to maintain the conceptual meaning of the model. Also, when adding a parameter based on a MI consider whether the direction and magnitude of the actual parameter estimate is consistent with theory.

We recommend in practice researchers should add or remove parameters in a revised model based on MIs *one at a time* in an iterative process. Each parameter tested should be of theoretical relevance. Commonly, when adding a parameter, the corresponding MI value is above a threshold (such as five) and is the largest out of all the MIs in the model output. If the largest MI value corresponds with a parameter that is nonsensical for the model, then one should not consider adding it. When removing a parameter, the corresponding MI is typically below such a threshold. If the parameter must be included in the model for conceptual reasons, then one should not consider removing it. After each revision, one should re-evaluate whether to leave the updated model alone or to make a further modification. We will provide an illustrative example of this iterative process in the next section. A researcher may make no further additions to a model if

- there are no more parameters of theoretical relevance to consider adding into the model
- no remaining MI values higher than a threshold
- there have already been a few modifications made and any further changes may lead to overfitting the model.

Saris et al. [13] proposed using both the MI and the *expected parameter change (EPC)* simultaneously for performing model modifications. EPC represents how much the given parameter would be expected to change if it were freely estimated [5,14]. Standardized EPCs allow the researcher to make relative comparisons across parameters. Parameters with large MIs and large EPCs should be freed first for model modification provided it makes theoretical sense. Many software packages for SEM (e.g. MPlus, *Lavaan*) allow a user to view MI and EPC values close to each other in the output for concurrent evaluation.

6.5.1 Categorical Outcomes and Modification Indices

MIs are based on the first order derivatives for categorical outcomes with robust WLS estimators (e.g. WLSMV option in MPlus). These derivatives are rescaled by a correction factor for the estimator so that they are on the chi-square scale [5]. Due to the approach, these MIs are interpreted in rank ordering and absolute size, but there are no established rules of thumb as to how high a value to consider before freeing a restricted parameter. A researcher should only consider MIs that make substantive sense [5].

6.6 Manual Approaches for Model Re-specification

A simplified approach to model modification could involve dropping parameters in which estimates were not statistically significant and then re-running the model. However, this simplistic approach leads to a potential bias in fitting the data alone. The researcher is testing parameters and then discarding them, then calculating new estimates and performing hypothesis testing without any regard to the original model.

Another manual approach to specification would involve constraining each parameter for an "unknown" path one at a time and checking the value of the MI. If the value is high (e.g. above five), then one can free the parameter. One can also perform model modification through analyzing the MIs in tandem with EPCs as suggested by Saris et al. [13].

As an example of using MIs and EPCs in tandem for model modification, we revisit observational data of persons with multiple sclerosis ($N = 3,507$). We considered one and two factor measurement models for the nine PHQ-9 items for self-reported depression [15–17]. The two factor model is represented in Figure 6.3a. The two factors can be interpreted as a variation of affective and somatic underlying dimensions for the PHQ-9.

The model fit criteria discussed in Chapter 4 (e.g. chi-square, CFI, TLI, RMSEA and SRMR) can also be used for model comparison across competing models. In a series of competing models, the model with the highest CFI and TLI and lowest chi-square value, RMSEA and SRMR is the better-fitting model. The criteria can also be used to evaluate if the model has an acceptable fit as well. In the MS-depression example, the two factor model has a better fit according to each of these criterion compared to the one factor model (see Table 6.1). The two factor model also has a relatively acceptable fit, with a slightly high RMSEA value. The TLI and RMSEA values for the one factor model are both less than desirable according to guidelines for acceptable thresholds (Chapter 4).

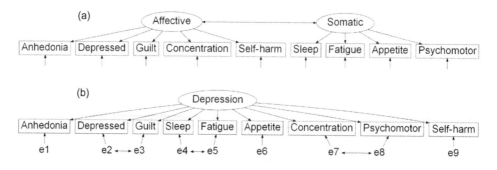

FIGURE 6.3
Measurement models of the PHQ-9 items in persons with multiple sclerosis: (a) Two factor model; (b) One factor model with residual correlations.

TABLE 6.1

Model Fit Evaluation for the Multiple Sclerosis-Depression Measurement Model Example

	One Factor	Two Factor	One Factor with Residual Correlations[a]
χ^2 (df)	754.344 (27) $p < 0.001$	401.83 (26) $p < 0.001$	416.63 (24) $p < 0.001$
CFI	0.922	0.960	0.958
TLI	0.896	0.944	0.937
RMSEA (90% CI)	0.088 (0.082, 0.093)	0.064 (0.059, 0.070)	0.068 (0.063, 0.074)
SRMR	0.042	0.031	0.033

[a]Residual correlations are shown in Figure 8.3B between depressed and guilt, sleep and fatigue and concentration and psychomotor. The estimated values of these residual correlations in the model were depressed and guilt = 0.237, sleep and fatigue = 0.297 and concentration and psychomotor = 0.195.

We evaluated the correlation between the *affective* and *somatic* factors in the CFA model corresponding to Figure 6.3a. The correlation was large at 0.86, which could imply poor *discriminant validity*. In a multidimensional model with correlated factors, discriminant validity is the degree to which measures of different constructs are unrelated. A high correlation between factors of greater than or equal to 0.85 has been used as a cutoff that implies poor discriminant validity [18,19]. Poor discriminant validity suggests that a more parsimonious factor solution is preferred [14]. In this case, it suggested the two factors could be combined into a single factor.

Note that a large factor intercorrelation could also signal unmodeled *cross-loadings* (Chapter 7) [19]. A cross-loading occurs when a single item influences (or loads onto) multiple factors in a measurement model. As a result, the cross-loaded item measures more than one dimension or domain.

In lieu of these results, we determined that a compromise solution would be a single factor model with residual correlations (see Figure 6.3b). An analysis of the MIs and EPCs between the covariance of the error terms for each pair of PHQ-9 items was used to help determine residual correlations of interest. A cutoff for adding a residual correlation to the measurement model was a MI above five and a standardized EPC in absolute value ≥ 0.10, implying at least a small effect size [20]. We used an iterative process (Box 6.1):

BOX 6.1

1. An initial model was specified as a single factor model with no residual correlations (Model P1)

2. We evaluated for the residual correlation parameter with the largest MI and EPC.

3. If the residual correlation exceeded the cutoff values (MI above five, standardized EPC in absolute value ≥ 0.10), it was included in a revised model (Model P2). If not, then we would proceed no further.

4. We then evaluated for the largest MI and EPC in Model P2.

5. Again, if the residual correlation exceeded the cutoff values, it was included in a new model (Model P3). If not, then we would proceed no further.

6. We continued with a similar iterative process, until we could proceed no further as criteria were not met.

Any residual correlation under consideration had to have a strong theoretical basis. In the interest of parsimony, we did not consider the same item for use in more than one residual correlation.

Using these criteria (Box 6.1), correlations between items for *sleep* and *fatigue* (MI = 207.323, standardized EPC = 0.331), *depressed* and *guilt* (MI = 100.541, standardized EPC = 0.291) and *concentration* and *psychomotor* (MI = 74.756, standardized EPC = 0.201) were all iteratively flagged. The MI and EPC values did not merely exceed the cutoff values, but far surpassed them, showing the strength of these residual correlations. The strong pairwise relationships between related fatigue items (sleep problems and fatigue) and cognitive and functional impairment items (poor concentration and psychomotor symptoms) are in line with clinical theory in that the wording of the questions and the underlying concepts are similar. An association between feeling depressed and guilt, both affective symptoms of depression, also has a theoretical basis.

Importantly, including the three pairwise residual correlations (Figure 6.3b) in the one factor model leads to an improved model fit, relatively similar to the two factor model (Table 6.1) [16,17]. Equivalent multifactor models can still be derived for this one factor model with correlated residuals. However, this particular one factor solution using correlated residuals maintains the unidimensional interpretation of a single depression factor.

6.7 R^2

In traditional linear regression analysis, the R^2 value, the coefficient of determination, is interpreted as the amount of variation in the response that can be explained by the regressors in the model. R^2 and adjusted R^2 are used in traditional linear regression analysis as goodness of fit measures. These measures are also especially useful when comparing nested models, though in theory, apply to non-nested models as well. In the SEM setting, within a multi-equation model, each equation has a different R^2 or adjusted R^2. Therefore, examining R^2 for magnitude can be both context and equation specific, depending on the set of explanatory variables with respect to that outcome.[5] Thus, typically, other indices as described in Chapter 4 are preferred for use as more global measures of goodness of fit. In the context of model re-specification, a researcher can compare the R^2 values for a particular outcome across competing models and then evaluate for the model with the highest value.

R^2 can be extended for latent variable models with the interpretation of measuring the amount of variation accounted for in the endogenous constructs by the exogenous constructs. In a structural equation model with ordered-categorical variables and latent response variates, R^2 values are computed for the continuous latent variables underlying the ordered-categorical variables. These R^2 values represent the estimated proportion of the assumed continuous latent variables explained by the model [5].

---

[5] Defining R^2 in a non-recursive system is challenging since the residuals may be correlated with other predictors. One proposed solution is the reduced-form R^2 by Jöreskog (2000). Reference: Jöreskog, K.G., *Interpretation of R^2 revisited*. Retrieved from www.ssicentral.com/lisrel/techdocs/r2rev.pdf. 2000.

6.8 Akaike Information Criterion, Bayesian Information Criterion and Browne-Cudeck Criterion

Any test for model comparison in non-nested models is also applicable to nested models. However, the reverse is not true. For instance, without a nested structure, the chi-square tests of difference described above are not valid. Note that there are similar tests developed for model comparison in non-nested models, for example, Vuong [21] introduced a likelihood ratio test for non-nested models. Models under comparison can be nested or non-nested for both the *Bayesian information criterion (BIC)* and *Akaike information criterion (AIC)* [22,23]. Both BIC and AIC feature the model chi-square test statistic along with a penalty term.

AIC provides an asymptotically unbiased estimator of the expected *Kullback-Leibler divergence* between the generating (i.e. true) model and the fitted approximating model. The Kullback-Leibler divergence measures the discrepancy between two probability distributions [24]. More formally, it has an origin in *information theory* and is the expectation value of the logarithmic difference between the two probability distributions $p(x)$ and $q(x)$ for a random variable x where the expectation is taken with respect to $p(x)$. Martignon [25] defined information theory as "the mathematical treatment of the concepts, parameters and rules governing the transmission of messages through communication systems". See Kullback [24] for a thorough review of information theory and Kullback-Leibler divergence.

BIC can be derived from Bayesian theory. BIC provides a large-sample approximation of *Bayes factor*. Bayes factor is the Bayesian alternative to frequentist hypothesis testing; it is the ratio of the likelihood of two competing hypothesis (e.g. null hypothesis and alternative hypothesis). We give a brief overview of Bayesian SEM in Chapter 15.

As in Chapter 4, let χ^2_M be the chi-square test statistic for a substantive model of interest M. The BIC formula is

$$\text{BIC} = \chi^2_M + t \ln(N) \tag{6.5}$$

where t is the number of unknown parameters and N is the sample size. The model with the lower BIC value would be preferred. However, for small differences between two BIC values, since the model with more freely estimated parameters or a larger sample size will naturally have the larger value, model interpretation needs to be considered before deciding whether to exclude or include a regression path.

BIC values are dependent on sample size and model complexity. As a result, this can turn out to be a major limitation if we have too small of a sample, where BIC in formula (6.5) may automatically select the simplest model which may not be theoretically relevant.

AIC values do not depend on sample size in the penalty term. The AIC formula is

$$\text{AIC} = \chi^2_M + 2t \tag{6.6}$$

Similar to BIC, the model with the smallest AIC value is chosen, given a non-trivial difference. Relative correction for parsimony of the AIC still becomes smaller as the sample size increases [26]. The penalty term of BIC is more stringent than the penalty term of AIC (for $N \geq 8$, $t \ln(N)$ exceeds $2t$).

Neither BIC or AIC will identify if the model is a good fit. These criterion can be used to decide which is the "better" model given the observed data between a series of competing models.

The *Browne-Cudeck criterion (BCC)* [27] is a single sample *cross-validation* index which can be derived for each of the competing models under study. The BCC will give an indication of which models are stable under cross-validation. Cross-validation is a resampling procedure used to evaluate model performance. In cross-validation, data is split into training and test subsets. The average of model evaluation scores across the subsets is then used to summarize model performance. Cross-validation methods do not depend on parametric assumptions. There is a slight bias in cross-validation methods, in that the training sample is smaller than the actual data set. However, the effect of this bias will typically be conservative in that the estimated fit will be slightly biased in the direction suggesting a poorer fit [27]. See Hastie, Tibshirini and Friedman [28] for an overview of cross-validation techniques.

Similar to BIC and AIC, the lower the value of BCC, the better the fit. In general, BCC penalizes for model complexity (lack of parsimony) more than AIC or BIC.

In summary of using BIC, AIC and BCC for comparing between competing models:

- The lower the value of BIC, AIC and BCC, the better the fit.
- BCC penalizes for model complexity more than AIC and BIC.
- BIC penalizes for model complexity more than AIC.

One potential drawback of BIC, AIC and BCC is that all do penalize for model complexity. As a consequence, choosing a "best" model using these criteria may lead to results that are not in line with theoretical models that necessitate extraordinary complexity. These criteria should act more like guidelines, rather than strict codes dictating the "best" model.

Further, a researcher should understand the practical limits to measures, such as BIC, AIC and BCC, for model comparison in non-nested models. Recall, we stated in the introduction to this chapter we are considering competing models with the same set of variables. Now consider instead for the moment comparing a model with five variables to a non-nested model with 55 variables. BIC, AIC and BCC would likely be uninformative. That is, the introduction of additional variables that increase the complexity of models has a tendency to inflate these fit measures in an amount that is not necessarily evenly occurring with respect to the parsimony penalty.

Researchers may encounter formulas with different penalty terms for the BIC and AIC. For example, researchers could encounter versions of both formulas (6.5) and (6.6) replacing t with the model degrees of freedom. There are versions of these formulas with both t and the model degrees of freedom. In all the formulas for BIC and AIC, we are assessing the same relative change as a function of model complexity. Thus, different versions in these formulas when used for model comparison should not lead to meaningfully different conclusions. It is the difference in BIC and AIC between competing models that we evaluate, not the magnitude of a single BIC or AIC value.

There are also adjustments available to the penalty terms in BIC and AIC due to the noted limitations in these indices. For example, there is a *sample-size adjusted BIC (aBIC)* which replaces $\ln(N)$ in (6.5) with $\ln\left(\dfrac{N+2}{24}\right)$. That is,

$$\text{aBIC} = \chi^2_M + t\ln\left(\frac{N+2}{24}\right) \tag{6.7}$$

As a result, the sample-size adjusted BIC does not place as strict a penalty term for adding parameters based on sample size as the BIC [29]. There is also a *corrected AIC for small sample sizes (AICC)* that can be defined as

$$\text{AICC} = \text{AIC} + \frac{2t(t+1)}{N-t-1} \tag{6.8}$$

6.9 Residual Analysis

In the context of SEM, model residuals are useful for finding model misspecifications. Model residuals indicate overall model misspecifications [5]. MIs, as previously discussed, directly identify the troubling, restricted parameter [5]. Therefore, MIs are more useful for model modification. The *correlation residual* is the difference between the implied correlation and the observed correlation. *Fitted residuals* are the difference between the observed and implied covariances [11]. Fitted residuals can be standardized as a z-score by calculating the ratio of the fitted residual over its standard error [11]. Assuming asymptotic multivariate normality, standardized residuals can be tested under a null hypothesis that the population covariance residual is equal to zero [11]. Some rules of thumb are to flag absolute values of correlation residuals > 0.10 and standardized residual values > 2.0, indicating model misspecification [11].

Individual outliers and high leverage values can potentially lead to biased parameter estimates in SEM. However, individual case-level residuals are considerably more difficult to define due to the (1) presence of latent variables in the analysis and (2) multivariate nature of these models [30]. As a result, careful evaluation of case-level residuals in SEM through graphical displays and model diagnostics is still an area of research in development. There have been approaches proposed within SEM for evaluating case-level residuals such as Yuan and Hayashi [30,31].

6.10 Software-Based Specification Searches

Specification search procedures already built into software can prove to be very useful for researchers looking to cut labor time by running many model comparisons and tests at once. Specification searches are conducted with the intent to detect and correct specification errors between a proposed model and the unknown, true model characterizing the population and variables in a study [11]. Specification searches have been adapted by Marcoulides and Drezner based on genetic algorithms [32] and ant colony optimization [33] and in the TETRAD program [34].

An exploratory specification search is available in AMOS for choosing the "best" model among a series of competing models. The "best" model can be chosen on the basis of fit, parsimony and interpretability using the chi-square test statistic and significance level, chi-square test statistic minus the degrees of freedom, chi-square test statistic divided by the degrees of freedom, AIC, BIC and BCC [35]. We present an applied example corresponding to Figure 6.1 comparing metrics as provided by the AMOS 5.0 exploratory specification search.

The study consisted of 1,024 medical patients aged 45–64 recruited from two academic general internal medicine practices and two community health clinics in Chicago, IL, and Cleveland, OH. Twelve tests of physical performance across multiple domains (including balance, dexterity, upper and lower extremity strength, endurance and flexibility; cardiorespiratory endurance and measures of function, gait speed and climbing stairs) were administered and a global physical performance summary score was generated. Education was measured in years. In this analysis, we evaluated the model represented in Figure 6.1, depicting the possible relationships between education in years, neighborhood safety, social support, physical performance and self-reported physical functioning.

We specified education and neighborhood safety as exogenous variables with a non-casual association and direct causal effects on social support, physical performance and physical functioning. Social support is an endogenous mediator in the center of the model. All paths to and from social support were specified as "unknown" (dashed lines). The two primary outcomes (physical performance and self-reported physical functioning) were specified as having a "known" non-causal association.

In addition, neighborhood safety is specified as having direct causal effects on three indicators of the endogenous latent variable for self-report physical functioning. These dashed arrows signify the potential for a form of measurement bias (*differential item functioning*; Chapter 10) for the three items according to the level of neighborhood safety. However, within this model, these three paths are nonsensical and were deliberately included in the model to examine how the specification search would perform in investigating paths known by theory and prior evidence *not* to exist.

In the structural model in Figure 6.1 (not including factor indicators or model correlations), there are 11 regression paths; four of the paths are "known" while seven of the paths are "unknown." We define the unconstrained model (Model A) as the model for which all the "unknown" paths are specified as being present. Potentially $2^7 = 128$ models (or some subset of the 128 models) may now need to be evaluated for determining the single "best" model based on different potential combinations of these seven "unknown" paths. What a daunting computational task! These models include the unconstrained model, all models with six "unknown" path specified as being present, all models with five "unknown" paths specified as being present, …, fully constrained model.

In the specification search, AMOS fits every possible subset of the model both with and without each "unknown" path. Based on the fit function criteria, all or some may suggest the overall best-fitting model. Even if one or more statistical criterion suggests a better model than the initial model, ultimately the researcher is left to decide whether a model with improved fit advances prior theory and is consistent with prior evidence.

The unconstrained model (Model A) demonstrates relatively good overall model fit ($\chi^2_{(63)} = 476.33$; CFI = 0.95; TLI = 0.92; RMSEA = 0.07). We then performed the specification search and sorted all models by lowest to highest chi-square test statistic. Table 6.2 presents the description of the constraints used on the "unknown" paths for the seven models A through F, respectively, with the lowest chi-square test statistic. We also included the full constrained model (Model H) for comparison.

The results of the specification search for these eight models are presented in Table 6.3. We additionally report the R^2 values for each model with respect to the endogenous self-reported physical functioning latent variable.

The results in Table 6.3 give a mixed picture of how to specify the model. The least ambiguous finding across all of the fit indices is that the presence of the paths from neighborhood safety to PF1, PF2 and PF6 are not at all supported. Recall, these are the three paths known by theory and prior evidence *not* to exist. Results for the regression paths

TABLE 6.2

Description of the "Unknown" Paths Excluded (Constrained to Zero) in the Competing Models under Consideration after the Exploratory Specification Search in AMOS for Health Self-Ratings and Physical Performance Measures Example

Model	Constraints on "Unknown" Paths
A	Unconstrained
B	No path from neighborhood safety to PF1
C	No path from neighborhood safety to PF1 or PF2
D	No paths from neighborhood safety to PF1, PF2 or PF6
E	No paths from neighborhood safety to PF1, PF2 or PF6. No regression path from education to social support
F	No paths from neighborhood safety to PF1, PF2 or PF6. No regression paths from education to social support or from social support to physical performance index
G	No paths from neighborhood safety to PF1, PF2 or PF6. No regression paths from education to social support or from social support to physical performance index or from social support to self-reported physical functioning
H	Fully constrained

TABLE 6.3

Results in Models under Consideration after Exploratory Specification Search in AMOS for Health Self-ratings and Physical Performance Measures Example

Model	Params	χ^2	df	p	$\chi^2 - df$	AIC	BCC	BIC	χ^2/df	R^2
A	56	**476.336**	63	0	413.336	588.336	589.664	877.039	7.561	0.11
B	55	476.357	64	0	412.357	586.357	587.661	869.904	7.443	0.11
C	54	476.396	65	0	411.396	584.396	585.677	862.787	7.329	0.11
D	53	476.857	66	0	**410.857**	582.857	584.114	856.093	7.225	0.11
E	52	478.536	67	0	411.536	**582.536**	**583.769**	850.616	7.142	0.11
F	51	482.272	68	0	414.272	584.272	585.481	**847.197**	**7.092**	0.10
G	50	495.104	69	0	426.104	595.104	596.289	852.873	7.175	0.09
H	49	540.892	70	0	470.892	638.892	640.054	891.506	7.727	0.09

Bold values highlight the minimum value for the criterion in each column (where relevant) among the competing models under consideration in this table. Reported R^2 values are for the equation in each model with the endogenous self-reported physical functioning latent variable with the interpretation of total explained variance in self-reported physical functioning by the set of explanatory variables for self-reported physical functioning in the model. Params = the number of unknown parameters; χ^2 is the chi-square test statistic; df are the associated degrees of freedom and p is the associated model p-value; AIC = Akaike information criterion; BIC = Bayesian information criterion; BCC = Browne-Cudeck criterion.

were somewhat less clear. $\chi^2 - df$ criterion supports a model whereby social support mediates the effects of education and neighborhood safety on physical performance and physical functioning (Model D). AIC and BCC support the model (Model E) with an indirect effect of neighborhood safety on physical performance and physical functioning (no effect of education on social support). BIC and $\dfrac{\chi^2}{df}$ similarly support the model with an indirect effect of neighborhood safety on physical performance and physical functioning, but with the further subtraction of the direct path from social support to physical performance (Model F).

This applied example also provides an opportunity to examine how logic, theory and prior evidence can be used in a situation where empirical criteria provide conflicting evidence. As has been mentioned although Model A has the lowest overall chi-square test statistic, the paths from neighborhood safety to PF1, PF2 and PF3 were deliberately included, but should not be and have no basis in theory or logic. There remains conflicting evidence for models D, E and F, all of which suggest that models with the paths from neighborhood safety to PF1, PF2 and PF3 removed from the model have better fit, but differ with respect to the effect of education on social support and the effect of social support on physical performance.

A positive association between education and social support has been previously hypothesized. The reasoning here is that education increases social support by increasing the access that individuals have to forming supportive relationships across a wider variety of social networks [36]. This positive association has been found to exist in prior studies including the European Social Survey [37]; however, measurement of social support has focused on varied dimensions (e.g. instrumental vs. emotional) and some mixed results have been reported. In Model D, the estimate for the effect of education and social support is negative (in the opposite direction of prior work) and not statistically significant even in this relatively large sample. Thus, based on our consideration of logic, theory and the current and prior empirical evidence, we would likely decide to reject Model D in favor of Model E or Model F.

Conflicting evidence remains for the one parameter difference between Model E and Model F. Here, the path under consideration is the effect of social support on physical performance. The estimate here is positive (unstandardized = .25, standardized = .07) and of borderline significance ($p = .07$) in Model E thus further complicating the decision. AIC and BCC favor Model E, while BIC and $\frac{\chi^2}{df}$ favor Model F. R^2 is slightly higher for Model E. We have little to rely on from prior literature as we are aware of no other study that has measured social support and had subjects complete a full battery of physical performance tests. We do know that social support is associated with many other health outcomes and is generally protective; greater social support is associated with better health outcomes. The parameter estimate for the causal path between social support and physical performance in Model E is consistent with this prior work. Therefore, we would likely decide to reject Model F, which omits the path, in favor of Model E, which includes it.

Examination of the R^2 column showed little meaningful difference between the series of models we considered, with the "best" models explaining around 11% of the variation in physical functioning. Other criterion proved more useful in allowing us to decide between competing models in this study.

To demonstrate an alternative approach to the AMOS specification search procedure, MIs were estimated for the fully constrained model (Model H). We then revised the model by adding and freely estimating the "unknown" parameter with the highest MI, given the value was above five (regression path for social support to physical functioning; see Table 6.4). In this revised model we once again checked the MIs for the remaining "unknown" parameters and freed the parameter with the highest value above the cutoff of five (regression path for neighborhood safety to social support; see Table 6.4). Repeating this iterative procedure again we did not find any additional MIs above five. Thus, examination of the MIs suggested the addition of two regression paths to the fully constrained model: an effect from neighborhood safety to social support and an effect from social support to physical functioning; the identical model to Model F. Thus, in this example, there

TABLE 6.4

Modification Index Values above Five Iteratively Evaluated for Health
Self-ratings and Physical Performance Measures

Regression Path	MI	*p*
Social support → physical functioning	23.28	0.01
Neighborhood safety → social support	5.94	0.02

is agreement between information provided by an iterative procedure using MIs and the BIC value. However, as aforementioned, after careful consideration of additional empirical criterion and our theoretical and logical reasoning, we ended up choosing a slightly different model specification (Model E).

Conflicting model comparison results present a persistent challenge. Empirical criteria and codified rules of thumb alone can be particularly misleading if prior theories and sound logical arguments are not available to support model selection decisions. While further research on model specification decisions is warranted, how might researchers move forward with results such as those in our example? In our example, we used logic and prior evidence to reason our way past the conflicting evidence supporting Models D, E and F. If there is no prior evidence or logical argument to support the hypothesis of education influencing social support or of social support influencing physical task performance, we might be more inclined to accept Model F given all our empirical results. *Nevertheless, the authors of this textbook feel that perhaps the most important model specification guideline is to examine and report enough empirical criteria so as to allow other researchers to grasp the range of conflicting evidence.*

In our example, we were able to perform a reasonable specification search for the "best" model given seven "unknown" paths. However, a piecewise approach could be used for a model with a very large number of optional paths. The model could be broken down into smaller, more manageable pieces with fewer "unknown" paths. A specification search can be performed on one of these pieces first. The researcher can evaluate additional "unknown" paths in steps after previously optional paths have become designated as "known" paths to the model. The process is completed when a final model is identified after all optional paths have been tested by the researcher.

6.11 Conclusions

There are unique strengths and limitations to criteria and tests used for choosing a "best" model among competing models. No single measure should be rigidly employed for such a task. Researchers are advised to consider the results of several of the different measures discussed in this chapter that are appropriate for a particular study in order to make more sound decisions. Specification searches can be useful for making comparisons between models with several different constraints on "unknown" regression paths. As shown in our real-world data application to the health self-ratings and physical performance measures, empirical criteria used for model comparison can verify theory and steer a researcher away from illogical parameters, thus paving the way for rigorous hypothesis testing. However, similarly shown in the application is that regression paths that are not necessarily either supported or disproved by prior theory can lead to differing results among different empirical criteria.

This chapter is intended as an overview of model specification and re-specification. However, these procedures are consistently evolving with frequent additions in software packages so that specification becomes less labor intensive, with better rules governing how to choose between competing models. For example, in the field of Bayesian SEM methods (Chapter 15), the *deviance information criterion (DIC)* is used in addition to BIC [38].

MacCallum [1,2] has demonstrated the shortcomings of specification searches through simulation and real studies using goodness-of-fit indices and MIs. Unless sample size is sufficiently large, there can be difficulties in converging to a generalizable finding. The reliability of the measures as discussed in this chapter may be questioned with smaller sample sizes, as they may automatically favor the more parsimonious model. When results are data-driven, based at least in part from fitting the model to a particular sample, there is a non-trivial possibility that characteristics of the sample may influence the particular modifications that are performed. A conservative approach making few modifications with clear interpretability from an initial, theoretically derived model is certainly recommended [1,2].

Researchers employing SEM-based approaches often make assumptions about the cause and effect relationships between variables that cannot be tested and are based on theory and assumptions. Initial selection of causal directionality and which regression paths to include in a model for researchers must be in line with theory and prior evidence. When a number of models are plausible, empirical criteria can be used as scientific evidence for choosing one model over another. Results must be examined carefully and viewed in the context of theory, logic and prior evidence. This process can be seen as "abductive" rather than simply data-based or inductive [39]. In specifying models with seemingly infinite possible explanations for a particular social or biological process or set of observed relationships, we seek to "abduce" a single explanation (or small number of explanations) with the goal of eliminating many of the near-infinite possibilities and moving closer toward a true and clear solution.

References

1. MacCallum, R.C., M. Roznowski, and L.B. Necowitz, Model modifications in covariance structure analysis: The problem of capitalization on chance. *Psychological Bulletin*, 1992. **111**(3): p. 490.
2. McCallum, R., Specification searches in covariance structure modeling. *Psychological Bulletin*, 1986. **100**(1): pp. 107–120.
3. Kenny, D. Multiple latent variable models: Confirmatory factor analysis. 2016 [cited 2019 December 9]; Available from: http://davidakenny.net/cm/mfactor.htm.
4. Bentler, P.M. and A. Satorra, Testing model nesting and equivalence. *Psychological Methods*, 2010. **15**(2): pp. 111–123.
5. Muthén, L.K. and B.O. Muthén, *Mplus. The comprehensive modelling program for applied researchers: User's guide. Eighth edition*, 1998–2017, Los Angeles, CA: Muthén & Muthén.
6. Satorra, A. and P.M. Bentler, Corrections to test statistics and standard errors in covariance structure analysis, in Latent variables analysis: Applications for developmental research, A. von Eye and C.C. Clogg, Editors. 1994, Thousand Oaks, CA: Sage Publications, Inc., pp. 399–419.

7. Yuan, K.H. and P.M. Bentler, Three likelihood-based methods for mean and covariance structure analysis with nonnormal missing data. *Sociological Methodology*, 2000. **30**(1): pp. 165–200.

8. Satorra, A. and P.M. Bentler, A scaled difference chi-square test statistic for moment structure analysis. *Psychometrika*, 2001. **66**(4): pp. 507–514.

9. Satorra, A. and P.M. Bentler, Ensuring positiveness of the scaled difference chi-square test statistic. *Psychometrika*, 2010. **75**(2): pp. 243–248.

10. Joreskog, K. and D. Sorbom, *LISREL 8 user's reference guide*. 1996, Chicago, IL: Scientific Software.

11. Kline, R.B., Principles and practice of structural equation modeling, fourth edition. 2016, New York: Guilford Press.

12. Radloff, L.S., The CES-D scale: A self-report depression scale for research in the general population. *Applied Psychological Measurement*, 1977. **1**(3): pp. 385–401.

13. Saris, W.E., A. Satorra, and D. Sörbom, The detection and correction of specification errors in structural equation models. *Sociological Methodology*, 1987. **17**: pp. 105–129.

14. Brown, T.A., *Confirmatory factor analysis for applied research*. 2012, New York: Guilford Press.

15. Kroenke, K., R.L. Spitzer, and J.B. Williams, The Phq-9. *Journal of General Internal Medicine*, 2001. **16**(9): pp. 606–613.

16. Gunzler, D., et al., Disentangling multiple sclerosis & depression: An adjusted depression screening score for patient-centered care. *Journal of Behavioral Medicine*, 2015. **38**(2): pp. 237–250.

17. Gunzler, D.D. and N. Morris, A tutorial on structural equation modeling for analysis of overlapping symptoms in co-occurring conditions using MPlus. *Statistics in Medicine*, 2015. **34**(24): pp. 3246–3280.

18. Awang, Z., *A Handbook on SEM Overview of Structural Equation Modeling (SEM | Wan Mohamad Asyraf Wan Afthanorhan - Academia.edu*, 2012.

19. Brown, T.A., *Confirmatory factor analysis for applied research*. 2014, New York, NY: Guilford Publications.

20. Cohen, J., A power primer. *Psychological Bulletin*, 1992. **112**(1): p. 155.

21. Vuong, Q.H., Likelihood ratio tests for model selection and non-nested hypotheses. *Econometrica: Journal of the Econometric Society*, 1989. **57**(2): pp. 307–333.

22. Akaike, H., A new look at the statistical model identification. *IEEE Transactions on Automatic Control*, 1974. **19**(6): pp. 716–723.

23. Schwarz, G., Estimating the dimension of a model. *The Annals of Statistics*, 1978. **6**(2): pp. 461–464.

24. Kullback, S., *Information theory and statistics*. 1997, Mineola, NY: Dover Publications.

25. Smelser, N.J. and P.B. Baltes, *International encyclopedia of the social & behavioral sciences*. Vol. 11. 2001, Amsterdam: Elsevier.

26. Mulaik, S.A., *Linear causal modeling with structural equations*. 2009, Boca Raton, FL: CRC Press.

27. Browne, M.W. and R. Cudeck, Single sample cross-validation indices for covariance structures. *Multivariate Behavioral Research*, 1989. **24**(4): pp. 445–455.

28. Friedman, J., T. Hastie, and R. Tibshirani, *The elements of statistical learning*. Vol. 1. 2001, Berlin: Springer series in statistics Springer.

29. Kenny, D.A. Measuring model fit. November 24, 2015 July 18, 2018]; Available from: http://davidakenny.net/cm/fit.htm.

30. SAS Institute Inc., "The CALIS procedure." SAS/STAT® 13.1: User's Guide. 2013. Cary, NC: SAS Institute Inc.

31. Yuan, K.-H. and K. Hayashi, Fitting data to model: Structural equation modeling diagnosis using two scatter plots. *Psychological Methods*, 2010. **15**(4): p. 335.

32. Marcoulides, G.A. and Z. Drezner, Specification searches in structural equation modeling with a genetic algorithm, in *New Developments and Techniques in Structural Equation Modeling*, G.A. Marcoulides and R.E. Schumacker, Editors. 2001, New York: Psychology Press pp. 247–268.

33. Marcoulides, G.A. and Z. Drezner, Model specification searches using ant colony optimization algorithms. *Structural Equation Modeling*, 2003. **10**(1): pp. 154–164.

34. Scheines, R., Spirtes, P., TETRAD II: tools for causal modeling; user's manual and software. 1994, Hillsdale, NJ: Erlbaum.

35. Schumacker, R.E., Teacher's corner: Conducting specification searches with Amos. *Structural Equation Modeling*, 2006. **13**(1): pp. 118–129.

36. Ross, C.E. and M. Van Willigen, Education and the subjective quality of life. *Journal of Health and Social Behavior*, 1997. **38**(3): pp. 275–297.

37. Von dem Knesebeck, O. and S. Geyer, Emotional support, education and self-rated health in 22 European countries. *BMC Public Health*, 2007. **7**(1): p. 272.

38. Linde, A., DIC in variable selection. *Statistica Neerlandica*, 2005. **59**(1): pp. 45–56.

39. Peirce, C.S., Deduction, induction, and hypothesis. *Popular Science Monthly*, 1878. **13**(8): pp. 470–482.

7

Measurement Models for Patient-Reported Outcomes and Other Health-Related Outcomes

7.1 Introduction to Measurement Models for Patient-Reported Outcomes

Health and medical research and clinical practice frequently rely on self-report data or *patient-reported outcomes (PROs)*, where patients report on their own health and health-related outcomes. PROs have become integral to clinical trials and observational studies alike, and the National Institutes of Health (NIH) has invested heavily in developing reliable and valid PROs through the Patient-Reported Outcome Measurement Information System (PROMIS®) [1]. PROMIS® is a set of person-centered measures that evaluates and monitors physical, mental and social health in adults and children [1]. It was designed to be applicable to both the general population and individuals living with chronic conditions.

PROs can provide essential information from the patient's perspective for diagnoses, treatment and inferences about the effectiveness of treatments. However, PROs and other self-reported measures only indirectly measure outcomes. This is because the variables measured by the scales (e.g. depression or anxiety) are not directly observed by the researcher. With reflective constructs, which are the main constructs used in SEM and the focus of this chapter, the latent variable is responsible for and causes item responses (often symptoms). For example, feeling depressed may lead some individuals, unfortunately, to having thoughts about death. The more depressed an individual becomes, the greater the likelihood of thoughts about death. However, having thoughts about death does not generally precede and cause depression [2].

Often, the underlying phenomena can only be measured using subjective report and cannot be measured through direct observation. Because PROs only indirectly measure the latent variable of interest, they are imperfect measures. Thus, an individual's observed score will nearly always differ from their "true" score to some degree. This means that if a researcher examines the relationship between patients' observed reports on PROs and other variables, measurement error will attenuate the size of the true relationships [3]. Systematic measurement error especially (Chapter 10) leads to spurious findings in research or patient care.

SEM offers a method for understanding the relationship between patients' reports on their own health and one or more unobserved variables. It does this by explicitly formulating a measurement model as a part of the SEM equations. This model includes parameters for error so that one can more directly investigate the relationship between a latent variable and an outcome. Here, we use PROs as a framework for understanding the nomenclature, concepts and general procedures of measurement models, but it should be noted that one can fit a measurement model in any situation where one has multiple indicators that are conceptually caused by one or more latent variables (e.g. rater administered scales, multiple laboratory values). A model that only specifies a measurement model is a special case of SEM.

Before delving into measurement models in more detail, there is an important reason for a measurement model that warrants mentioning. Typically, PROs ask a set of questions about health outcomes. Throughout much of academic medicine's past, researchers and clinicians have "simply" aggregated responses to the questions into a composite descriptor of an individual's health (i.e. a score). A single summary score of responses often served as an estimate of the construct of interest. However, the possibility exists that, although a measure's developers intended a set of questions to measure a single construct, the questions actually measure more than one construct. Research based on a single score from these questions would lead to an inaccurate understanding of the relationship between the PRO and other variables. SEM allows one to explicitly test whether empirical data support a researcher's hypothesis about the specific way that a set of questions measures one or more latent variables.

In this chapter, we focus only on the measurement model within SEM and more concretely introduce it, especially as it relates to PROs. We detail the mathematical model for ordered-categorical variables, describe some reasons one needs to develop and test a measurement model using CFA, present some common and important hypothetical measurement models and introduce applications of the measurement model for health and medicine. In Appendix A, we present some discussion of treating ordered-categorical variables as continuous in a measurement model for analytical purposes, and in Appendix B, we introduce parceling.

In earlier chapters, we used the term latent variable to describe unobserved variables (or not directly observed phenomena). We note that throughout the literature different terminology is used synonymously such as latent trait, construct, factor, domain and dimension.

7.2 Measurement Model with Ordered-Categorical Items

Recall, that we have already represented the form of a measurement model in Chapter 3 for performing CFA for a vector of observed continuous items **y** in equation (3.1). Let us now consider a measurement model allowing for ordered-categorical items for performing CFA. We have previously discussed this latent variable model in Chapter 4 and now provide a formal description of this model.

Let y_{ij} equal the ith individual's score on the jth ordered-categorical item (question). Let the number of individuals equal N ($i = 1,2,\ldots,N$) and number of items equal p ($j = 1,2,\ldots,p$), and let the number of item responses range from 0 to s ($0,1,\ldots, s$). Consider all dichotomous items (i.e. responses no = 0 or yes = 1 on every item) as a special case.

The model assumes that a *latent response variate*, y_{ij}^*, determines responses. The variate corresponds to the idea that, although observed responses fall into discrete categories (e.g. no = 0/yes = 1), there is an underlying (latent) continuum "beneath" the possible responses. An *item threshold* value on the variate determines responses. An item threshold is the expected value of the construct (using a z-score) at which an individual endorses the next category. That is, if an individual's value on the latent response variate is less than the threshold, the individual won't endorse the item (i.e. will say "no"), but, if their value is greater than the threshold, they will endorse the item (i.e. will say "yes"). In total, the number of thresholds for each item is the number of categories minus one. For example, each PHQ-9 item consists of four categories (item responses 0,1,2,3) and has three thresholds; each dichotomous item has a single threshold.

Formally for the jth ordered-categorical item with item responses $0,1,\ldots, s$:

$$
\begin{aligned}
y_{ij} &= 0 \ \ \text{if } y_{ij}^* \leq \tau_{j,0} \\
y_{ij} &= 1 \ \ \text{if } \tau_{j,0} < y_{ij}^* \leq \tau_{j,1} \\
y_{ij} &= 2 \ \ \text{if } \tau_{j,1} < y_{ij}^* \leq \tau_{j,2} \\
&\ \vdots \\
y_{ij} &= s \ \ \text{if } \tau_{j,s-1} < y_{ij}^*
\end{aligned}
\tag{7.1}
$$

where $\tau_{j,0}, \tau_{j,1}, \tau_{j,2}, \ldots, \tau_{j,s-1}$ are the item threshold parameters. As noted earlier, one can use the thresholds to estimate the level of the construct at which individuals will likely endorse an item.

Let $\mathbf{y}_i$ be the vector of scores for the ith individual on all p ordered-categorical items. Now, suppose that some factor(s), η_i, causes item responses. Then, $\mathbf{y}_i^*$ the vector of latent response variates relates to the factor(s), assuming the familiar linear measurement structure, as follows [4]:

$$
\mathbf{y}_i^* = \mathbf{v}_y + \Lambda_y \eta_i + \varepsilon_i
\tag{7.2}
$$

$\mathbf{v}_y$ is a vector of the latent intercept parameters, Λ_y is a matrix of factor loadings, η_i is a vector of *factor scores* for the ith person and ε_i is a vector of the *unique factors* (error terms). *Factor scores* are individualized scores on the latent construct(s) and correspond to an individual's unknown "true" score on the construct. The loadings, like correlations, represent the degree to which an item relates to the factor(s). Higher factor loading values indicate a strong relation between the item and the latent variable. The loadings provide an indication of *reliability*. Reliability measures the overall consistency of a measure. In other words, reliability measures if a researcher repeated the study under the same conditions (i.e. study setting and context) would they obtain the same results. Greater reliability results when item responses relate strongly to the latent variable (i.e. large loadings). A commonly used rule of thumb is that factor loadings should have a standardized estimate >0.40 in absolute value to be considered as a substantial loading [5].

Intercept parameters give the expected value of the latent response variate when the value of the underlying factor(s) is zero. *Uniquenesses* (residual variances) include sources of variance not attributable to the factor(s). As a result, the uniquenesses also provide information about reliability. As a uniqueness value increases, the reliability of an item decreases [3,4].

A matrix worth noting in this context is ψ, the matrix of the factor variances and covariances. In a multidimensional model, Ψ includes the factor variances for each construct on the diagonal as well as the covariances between constructs in the off-diagonal. The matrix of the unique variances and covariances, Θ_ε, is typically assumed to be a diagonal matrix (i.e. error terms are not correlated). There are non-diagonal elements in this matrix if there are residual covariances in the measurement model.

Formally, the covariance matrix implied by the measurement model of the latent response variates $\mathbf{y}_i^*$ has the form

$$\Sigma^* = \Lambda_y \Psi \Lambda_y^T + \Theta_\varepsilon \tag{7.3}$$

where Σ^* is the population covariance matrix for this measurement model. In a unidimensional model, η_i is a scalar rather than a vector. And, similarly, there is only a single factor variance. One does not expect multiple factors in the unidimensional model.

The model in equation (7.2) is not identifiable without additional constraints. For example, it is necessary to fix the metric of the factor (Chapter 5). Unlike in CFA models with continuous items, it is also necessary to identify the uniquenesses [6].

In MPlus, when using robust WLS in the estimation procedure with latent response variates and ordered-categorical indicators, there are two different approaches to parameterization (i.e. setting the scale of the distribution of the latent response variates) to achieve identification. In the *delta parameterization*, which is the default parameterization, scale factors for the latent response variates are allowed to be parameters in the model, but residual variances are fixed. In the *theta parameterization*, residual variances are allowed to be parameters in the model, but scale factors are fixed. Mathematically, the *scale parameter* is the inverse of the standard deviation of the marginal distribution of the latent response variate for each indicator variable. The delta parameterization was found in the past to have computational advantages over the theta parameterization [7]. The theta parameterization allows one to estimate residual variances and some models cannot be run without it. The processing power of computers currently available makes the computational advantages of the delta parameterization moot.

Recall that in a unidimensional model one needs four indicators to identify the model sufficiently to evaluate fit. Statistically identifying multidimensional models with cross-loadings and/or correlated error terms can be complicated. Again we reference the classic SEM textbook by Bollen [4] for more detailed rules for determining identifiability of CFA models.

If the matrix of the factor variances and covariances Ψ is fixed to $\mathbf{I}$ (the identity matrix), assuming the factors are uncorrelated for identification in (7.3), then

$$\Sigma^* = \Lambda_y \Lambda_y^T + \Theta_\varepsilon \tag{7.4}$$

7.3 Internal Validity and Dimensionality

Proper interpretation of patient reported health outcomes depends on *valid* measurement. A scale or test is valid if it measures what it claims to measure. PROs frequently use sets of questions to measure one or more latent constructs. A single summary score of responses often serves as an estimate of each construct. This implicitly indicates that an investigator believes that the question set measures a single latent variable. The single latent variable also implicitly represents the intended dimension described collectively by the question set. For example, the investigator may believe that a question set describing symptoms of depression, affective, cognitive and somatic collectively measures depression. However, the possibility exists that, although a measure's developers intended a set of questions to measure a single construct, the questions measure more than one. Psychometricians call data measuring a single construct *unidimensional* and data measuring multiple constructs *multidimensional* [4,8]. If the questions measure multiple substantive constructs, one should not create a single score (or specify a single latent variable), as the single score would be an amalgamation of multiple constructs. Rather, one should create an individual score for each identified construct [8]. Thus, before specifying a single latent variable to be used in a model or generating summary scores based on a question set (or recommending that users create summary scores), investigators should first ask whether empirical data support the hypothesis that a question set is unidimensional [9,10].

In psychometrics, *internal validity* exists when responses to a set of questions measure a construct (or constructs) as expected. This differs from the more general concept of internal validity in research methods. In research methods, a study is internally valid when the research design rules out alternative explanations for a cause and effect relationship. Relatedly, in research methods, *external validity* relates to how generalizable the study findings are to a population beyond the study's sample.

With respect to a survey expected to measure a single, continuous construct (e.g. depressive symptomatology), internal validity would exist if the data support the expectation that the questions selected to measure the continuous construct do indeed measure a common continuous construct [8]. Too frequently, researchers have created measures and scores without empirically examining whether derived scores appear to measure the construct as intended [11]. Measurement model testing within SEM allows researchers to do this.

The measurement model uses equations to describe the relations among item responses (e.g. latent variable model described earlier). The equations' parameters provide empirical assessments of the questions' measurement properties. Model fit indices (Chapter 4) address the extent to which a hypothesized measurement structure is supported by the data. Fit indices allow one to make empirically based decisions about the validity of a hypothesized measurement structure (e.g. do ten items measure a single construct). One can review guidelines for evaluating acceptable to excellent fit in Chapter 4 on chi-square test statistic, CFI, TLI, RMSEA and SRMR. The parameters resulting from a good fitting model further allow one to make empirically based decisions about measurement quality. For example, if factor loadings from such a measurement model are substantial and consistent with a plausible interpretation of the factor structure, this provides considerable evidence that the items appear to measure the PRO reliably and validly. Later in this chapter, we will discuss different types of reliability and validity and how to formally assess the quality of a measurement model using multiple measures developed for this purpose.

If the model fit is unacceptable and the evidence fails to support unidimensionality, one may need to consider:

- multidimensional measurement models that specify multiple latent variables as an alternative
- allowing residual covariances among items (i.e. covariance between unique factors).

We discussed methods to evaluate residual covariances (i.e. using modification indices) in Chapter 6. Note that one can consider both of these approaches in tandem as they are not mutually exclusive.

7.4 Multidimensional Models

Multidimensional models allow for multiple factors. Typically, multidimensional models allow the factors to correlate. That is, the factors are not assumed to be independent constructs. In most research settings, including health and medicine, the assumption of correlated factors is more reasonable than independent (uncorrelated) factors. For example, we would not assume that the different dimensions of depression such as somatic and affective and cognitive would be independent.

7.4.1 Cross-Loadings

Single items can be allowed to load on multiple factors. Recall, this is termed cross-loading. A single cross-loading includes an additional item factor loading as a parameter, since the item loads onto two factors rather than one. However, cross-loadings can impede interpretation of what exactly an item measures (because it measures more than one variable) and cross-loadings can result in statistical identification challenges (see Bollen [4]). In scale construction having each item load onto only one construct translates readily to distinct dimensions (even if dimensions are correlated). It may be useful to omit or drop cross-loadings for the sake of simplicity. However, dropping a substantive cross-loading could also weaken analyses if including the cross-loading makes theoretical sense. In a reflective construct, the domains we infer from the scale are assumed to influence the indicators and not the other way around. Some of the item content may overlap in abstraction of these constructs. Thus it may be reasonable to specify an item loading onto multiple constructs in using all of the relevant information present at the indicator level to estimate the constructs [12].

7.4.2 Multidimensional Model Development

One can often specify a multidimensional model that fits the data well. There are several approaches to evaluating the structure of the data to determine such a multidimensional model. One approach would be to examine the modification indices that result from the unidimensional model. Iterative evaluation of the modification indices for residual correlations between modification indices for residual correlations between the error terms will reveal potential patterns indicative of factors. For example, let us assume we have specified a one factor model using 15 indicators $Y_i, i = 1, ..., 15$. If modification indices indicated that indicators Y_1, Y_2 and Y_6 all have correlated errors, and theoretically these indicators described a distinct dimension, then we could consider adding a factor on which Y_1, Y_2 and Y_6 load.

One could also conduct an EFA (Chapter 8) and develop a multidimensional model based on the EFA output. Whenever possible, one should use separate data (e.g. randomly splitting the data set in half or two different samples) for conducting EFA and CFA. This increases confidence in the model because replication helps rule out the possibility that the initial model reflects sample specific relationships.

Another model development strategy is examining item content and theory to develop a multidimensional model [13]. This approach relies on a research framework to identify factors. One can use the entire data set with this strategy and evaluate the validity of the model using model fit criteria.

In practice with real data, it can be challenging to assess the dimensionality of PROs, especially if they are not developed with a theoretical measurement model in mind. Some PROs fail strict tests of unidimensionality (e.g. less than acceptable fitting model with RMSEA and SRMR >0.10; CFI and TLI<0.90) but, simultaneously, identified multidimensionality may not be substantively meaningful [11,14–16]. For example, consider a measure of depression, generally considered a single (unidimensional) construct [17]. The measure may ask several questions specifically related to cognitive aspects of depression and several related to somatic aspects of depression. Each smaller set will include wording related to cognitive and somatic symptoms and this can lead to "smaller," specific factors. These item clusters may result in a model with several "smaller" factors. In a strict sense, the evidence supports multidimensionality. This would argue against a single score. However, responses to the questions may still measure a single depression construct (a *general factor*) and the item clusters may measure "specific," substantively unmeaningful factors. Essentially the scale does measure a single construct. The multidimensionality reflects "specific" factors (also labeled "grouping" and "nuisance" factors). These can occur because of shared item content and/or other methodological effects [13].

When specific factors occur in the presence of a single general factor and are uncorrelated with each other and the general factor, one can more validly create a single score from the entire item set [11,14–16]. This is because the data are sufficiently unidimensional [15,18,19]. Covariation in the items not explained by the unidimensional construct can be explained by the specific factors. From an interpretation (and scoring) perspective, when data fail unidimensionality tests the question becomes: does the scale "essentially" measure one construct (as well as one or more specific factors) or does it measure multiple meaningful constructs? If it sufficiently measures one construct, this provides evidence for the validity of a single factor or score. If it measures multiple meaningful constructs, one has evidence in favor of multiple scores rather than a single score.

In order to create valid scoring systems, one should always conduct empirical analyses to address whether a scale's measurement structure is consistent with a single construct, multiple constructs or single construct with specific factors. We describe four general types of measurement models (also described as factor models)

- pure unidimensional
- multidimensional
- *second order factor*
- *bifactor*

One can use SEM to examine the extent to which these models are more or less consistent with the data. Second order factor and bifactor models are both special types of multidimensional models. Unlike uni- and multidimensional models, second order factor models and bifactor models have been underutilized in health and medical research.

In Figure 7.1, we display a general example of each of the four models using items Y_1-Y_{10}. We label F as a unidimensional latent construct for the intended underlying trait measured by these ten items. However, multidimensional models consider that items Y_1-Y_3 can be grouped in the domain G_1, items Y_4-Y_6 can be grouped in the domain G_2 and items Y_7-Y_{10} can be grouped in the domain G_3. The three factor model allows the factors G_1, G_2 and G_3 to correlate with each other. The second order and bifactor models do not. In the second order model, G_1, G_2 and G_3 are conditionally independent of each other given F. In the bifactor

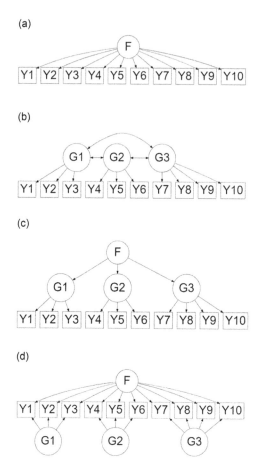

FIGURE 7.1
Four types of measurement models. (a) One factor model, (b) three factor model, (c) second order factor model and (d) bifactor model.

model, each observed item is an indicator of both F and one grouping factor, G_1, G_2 or G_3 and grouping factors are conditionally independent.

A bifactor model [20] is similar to a multidimensional model in that it specifies more than one factor. However, it differs from multidimensional models described so far because it specifies two types of factors: (1) a general factor, on which all of the items load, and (2) specific factors, on which only a smaller set of items load. Moreover, none of the specific factors are allowed to correlate with each other nor are they allowed to correlate with the general factor. This specification allows one to unambiguously interpret scores on the general factor because they are not uninfluenced by the specific factors. A bifactor model is shown in Figure 7.1d. In this figure, we consider a bifactor model with a single general factor. All items load on the general factor. And, each item loads on one of the specific factors (though not all items need to load on a specific factor in practice). Thus, when a bifactor model fits well, the item set's data structure is consistent with a single overarching construct and scores from the entire item set measure that construct. However, the overarching factor does not explain all of the covariance among the items. Specific factors help account for some of the covariance among the items. Sometimes these specific factors may result from a methods effect (e.g. common wording). Other times these specific factors may result from "sub-domains" and one *might* be able to create subscale scores on them. Though we do not go into detail here, Reise [21] and Rodriguez et al. [22] describe methods for evaluating the psychometric properties of the specific factors in bi-factor models.

A second order factor model [20] is also similar to a multidimensional model in that it specifies more than one factor. Yet, it differs from the multidimensional models described so far because, in second order models, the factors at one level are themselves caused by a "higher order" factor (or factors). In these models, a set of factors measure another, higher order factor (or factors). See Figure 7.1c for a visual depiction of the structure of a second order factor model with a single second order factor. In the figure, all of the items load on one of the first order factors. These first order factors then load onto the second order factor. The second order factor model does not allow any of the first order factors to correlate. This specification allows one to make the assumption that given the second order factor, the first order factors are independent of each other and one can unambiguously interpret scores on each first order factor given the level of the second order factor.

If one has fit a multidimensional model with good fit, one may be interested in whether covariance among the factors is accounted for by a higher order factor (in the same way one may be interested in whether the covariance among items can be accounted for by an underlying factor). One can compare the model fit (i.e. chi-square test statistic, CFI, TLI, RMSEA, SRMR) of a second order model to that of the multidimensional single order model.[1] One might conclude that the covariance among the first order factors is accounted for by a higher order if the second order model has a good model fit and is theoretically reasonable, the factors in the multidimensional single order model are highly correlated and if the second order model fits relatively well or better in comparison to the multidimensional model [23].

One should note that the initial choice to use a multidimensional (first order factor) model, second order factor model or bifactor model may be theoretical in nature. For example, if evaluating the factor structure of a set of items a unidimensional or multidimensional model (e.g. Figure 7.1a and b) is likely suitable. However, given attention to both a certain trait (e.g. depression, stress, happiness) and unique sub-dimensions, it may be more theoretically reasonable to evaluate a second order factor model or bifactor model. The initial choice between a second order factor model or bifactor model depends on the hypothesized relationship between two factor layers of interpretation and the observed indicators. However, the acceptance of the model will depend on empirical evidence for the model. We now move on to an example.

7.5 Dimensionality and Bifactor Model Example

Many examples of health and medical research use sum scores for scales and fail to address internal validity or use measurement models to investigate dimensionality generally, and the bifactor model specifically. This is unfortunate because (when appropriate) the bifactor model can resolve potentially thorny dimensionality issues [11,14–16,24] and subsequent difficulty regarding the interpretability of PROs and their relationship to other variables in a more complex structural equation model. Consider the following empirical example

---

[1] Note, however, that the higher order factor itself in our simplistic example in Figure 7.1c is just-identified with three first order factors (similar to a single factor model with only three indicators). Thus for the model represented in Figure 7.1c model fit is the same as the three factor model represented in Figure 7.1b.

that examines the internal validity of specifying a single "depression" factor from a set of items intended to measure depression in a large, nationally representative sample of the non-institutionalized US population. Generally, researchers analyzing these data consider depression a single construct [17]. However, as we have discussed, depression encompasses at least several specific areas of symptomatology (e.g. cognitive/affective aspect of depression and somatic aspects). As such, the data may not support a single summary depression score. The example uses data from the National Epidemiologic Survey on Alcohol and Related Conditions (NESARC) [25].

7.5.1 Methods

Participants: Participants (n = 11,678) were a subset of the 2001–2002 NESARC data designed and sponsored by the National Institute for Alcohol Abuse and Alcoholism. The original sample consisted of 43,093 individuals 18 years and older representing the non-institutionalized US adults. The complex, multistage design oversampled Black, Hispanics and adults aged 18–24. Sample weights adjust the data to make it representative [25]. This example analyses included all participants with complete data who reported on their depressive symptomatology in the past 12 months.

Measures: Depression is marked by a 2-week period that includes either (1) depressed mood most of the day, nearly every day or (2) markedly diminished interest or pleasure in daily activities. In addition, it includes at least three of the following nearly every day: (1) significant weight loss, or significant weight gain, or decrease in appetite, or increase in appetite; (2) insomnia or hypersomnia; (3) psychomotor agitation or retardation; (4) fatigue or loss of energy; (5) feelings of worthlessness or excessive or inappropriate guilt; (6) diminished ability to think or concentrate or indecisiveness; (7) recurrent thoughts of death, recurrent suicidal ideation without a specific plan or a suicide attempt or plan [17]. The NESARC's Alcohol Use Disorder and Associated Disabilities Interview Schedule-IV [26–33] uses 19 dichotomous items (0 = Yes, 1 = No) to operationalize these criteria. The analyses reported below used all items.

Analytical Approach: The analyses proceeded in steps. First, to test whether responses appeared to measure a single depression construct, we tested a unidimensional model's fit. Second, given the failure of the unidimensional model to fit well, we sought to develop a bifactor model (see Figure 7.2).

Analyses in this study considered a subset of the available model fit indices (RMSEA, CFI and TLI) to determine acceptable to excellent fit. We used Mplus (Version 6.1) [34], its theta parameterization and robust WLS estimator (WLSMV option) [35].

7.5.2 Results

Unidimensional Model: In this model, each item loaded on only a single factor. For statistical identification, the model had a factor mean of zero and factor variance of one. The model allowed no correlations among the error terms. This model did not fit well (RMSEA = 0.12; TLI = 0.64; CFI = 0.68) indicating that a single depression factor did not well account for the covariance among the item responses. Subsequently, analyses turned to developing and comparatively examining the fit of a bifactor model.

Bifactor Model: The current analyses took the approach of examining item content and theory to develop a multidimensional model. By definition to measure depression [17], one will require several questions to get at each of the specific content areas (e.g. restlessness, weight and appetite loss). Thus, the item content was a "good" place to start.

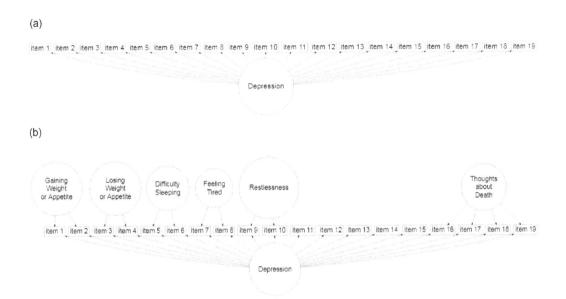

FIGURE 7.2
Models for *Depression* from the National Epidemiologic Survey on Alcohol and Related Conditions (NESARC) ($N = 11{,}678$). (a) One factor model and (b) bifactor model.

The 19 small rectangles represent observed responses to the items. In the unidimensional model, the presence of a single circle indicates that the responses measure one and only one factor. In the bifactor model, one circle as labeled represents a general depression factor. However, six circles as labeled represent specific factors that measure narrower facets of depression (e.g. questions asking about thoughts about death). In both models, the arrows from the circles to the rectangles indicate that the item responses measure the latent variables (for simplicity's sake and to minimize clutter, this figure does not include all of the measurement parameters e.g. uniquenesses, item thresholds).

Analyses estimated a bifactor model that included a general depression factor and that included six specific factors we identified after discussion with an expert panel in a team science strategy; one for gaining weight or appetite; one for losing weight or appetite; one for difficulty sleeping; one for feeling tired; one for restlessness; and one for thoughts about death. The thoughts about death specific factor included four items. The remainder included two items each (see Figure 7.2). Five of the items did not fit within any of these identified sub-dimensions and were not specified to load onto any of these specific factors. This model fit the data relatively well (RMSEA = 0.051; TLI = 0.94; CFI = 0.95).

7.5.3 Dimensionality Discussion

Confirmatory unidimensional and bifactor models addressed the internal validity of using a single factor to account for responses to the 19 depression questions on the NESARC. The results provide evidence that, despite some multidimensionality (as modeled by specific factors), responses to the questions do seem to measure a general depressive symptomatology construct. These results provide evidence that investigators can use responses to these questions to form a single depressive symptomatology construct and derive a single depression score from the item set.

Accordingly, researchers should empirically examine the apparent dimensionality of data resulting from scales. Despite the best efforts of experts, a set of survey questions may not measure a construct (or constructs) as expected [36]. Scoring systems following theoretical rather than empirical measurement structures (when they differ) may result in spurious and invalid conclusions. In these data, one can see that the initially hypothesized structure of a single domain did not appear to describe question responses well, suggesting users may not be able to validly create a single depression score. However, the bifactor findings indicated that, while responses to some of these questions seem to measure six specific factors each measuring relatively specific facets of depression, the evidence does support deriving a single depression score from item responses. Given the potential for real data to fail to correspond to theoretical expectations, investigators should always evaluate dimensionality in multi-item PROs under study.

The interpretability and validity of scores derived from measurement instruments depend upon whether the questions included in a composite score measure a single coherent construct. If developers or users of a scale intend to measure a single construct, but a priori theory and research and analytical results suggest a measurement structure more consistent with multiple substantive constructs and not a bifactor structure, one should not create a single summary score from the entire set of questions. This can lead to spurious results and invalid conclusions. Rather, one should create subscale scores for each of the constructs measured by the questions on the scale [4,14–16,20,24,36].

Before concluding this section, we note some limitations. First, one should not consider this brief treatment as a definitive step-by-step guide. For the interested reader, see Reise [21] and Rodriguez et al. [22] for details on how to more fully evaluate bifactor models. Rather, one should see this as an applied perspective on the importance of evaluating dimensionality and the use of bifactor model in that pursuit. Second, this chapter up to this point has focused on specifying a measurement model and using CFA, with an eye toward using the evidence to score a PRO. Although sum scores can provide construct estimates, other methods (e.g. item response theory or factor scores) generally provide more precise estimates. Finally, before making strong conclusions about a model's general acceptability, researchers should attempt to replicate findings in a separate sample.

7.6 Factor Scores

Factor scores can be of particular clinical interest, as they may represent meaningful measurements of patient characteristics on a construct of interest. For example, knowing that a patient has a high level of depression or has a low level of happiness (where *depression* and *happiness* are unidimensional constructs) might be clinically actionable. Since an individual's true level of a factor is an unobservable quantity, one needs an approach to predict an individual's level of a factor using the observed data and a model's parameters. These predictions are called *factor scores*.

A widely used approach to calculate factor scores is to apply Bayes' theorem to calculate the posterior distribution of the factor scores given the observed data (which incorporates the estimates of the model parameters). Then, one can predict factor scores by choosing the values which maximize the posterior distribution. An interested reader can refer to the technical appendices on the MPlus website (http://www.statmodel.com/techappen.shtml) for more details regarding this approach [37].

Factor scores can be output using this method through MPlus into another data file using a few lines of code in the SAVEDATA section. For example, saving factor scores into a csv file on the C drive called FScores can be performed using the following coding in Box 7.1 (when observed dependent variables are continuous):

BOX 7.1

```
SAVEDATA: FILE IS C:\FSscores.csv;
SAVE IS fscores;
```

Using this approach, the distribution of the factor scores will depend on the ability of the items to measure the full range of the factor, the items' measurement parameters, and the mean and variance specified in the model. It is worth noting that, as a result, even though the underlying factor may be normal, the distribution of factor scores may not be.

As noted earlier, multi-item PROs are commonly summarized in total scores. Research may have established guidelines for clinical interpretation. For example, the nine PHQ-9 items (Chapter 2, Figure 2.2) for an individual are typically summed into a total score within a 0–27 range [38,39]. A threshold of 10 has been used as a cutoff for screening positive for depression. Because factor scores are not on a total score metric, they are not directly interpretable in terms of the original scale (e.g. PHQ-9). One may want to transform a factor score to the metric of the original scale for a more interpretable score.

An approach has been adapted by two of the authors of this book (Gunzler and Perzynski) along with collaborators for transforming a factor score into a more meaningful scale with a large sample [5,40]. This method uses a probability integral transformation to retain the same empirical distribution of the original data. We describe this approach below (see Appendix C for code for the transformed _ scores function in R program).

To transform factor scores into original scale scores [5,40]:

1. Use a kernel density estimator to estimate the density of the scores for the original scale in the study sample.
2. Obtain the cumulative distribution function by numerical integration.
3. Numerically invert the cumulative distribution function for the original scale scores.
4. Repeat steps (1) and (2) for the factor scores.
5. Transform the factor scores of each individual into an original scale score by transforming the cumulative distribution function for the factor scores using the inverse of the cumulative distribution function for the original scale scores.

7.7 Types of Reliability and Validity of Measurement

We have described generally assessing reliability and internal validity of a measurement model using model fit criteria and factor loadings. Measures have been developed for evaluating particular types of reliability and validity when using CFA. We start with measures of reliability.

7.7.1 Reliability

An observed score is equal to the true score (i.e. as captured by the latent construct) plus measurement error according to classical test theory. Reliability is defined as the ratio of the true score variance to the observed score variance [41]. *Composite (or construct) reliability*, more specifically, is a measure of internal consistency in the observed indicators that load on a latent construct.

Cronbach's alpha (or *coefficient alpha*) is a routinely used measure of internal consistency in health and medicine that can be used to evaluate composite reliability of a measurement model [42]. The coefficient *omega* is another widely used measure of composite reliability. Cronbach's alpha is calculated using observed item covariances and depends on the assumption of *tau-equivalence*. With tau-equivalence, all unstandardized factors loadings are equal (i.e. each indicator contributes equally to the construct). Omega is calculated using factor loadings and variance and relaxes the assumption of equal factor loadings. Thus, omega, given the more practical assumptions for CFA, is widely considered to be a more useful measure in the context of assessing composite reliability of a measurement model.

Different versions of omega are available. One version uses the *congeneric measurement model*. A congeneric measurement model does not allow cross-loadings or correlated error terms [43,44]. The congeneric model does assume that, for a unidimensional construct, each individual item measures the same latent construct with possibly different scales, degrees of precision and amounts of error [45]. The congeneric model is the most commonly used measurement model and has desirable properties for ease of interpretability and analysis since each item loads onto only one factor.

A second version of omega allows for cross-loadings and correlated errors [46,47]. The two versions of omega discussed already both assume the model-implied covariance matrix perfectly explains the item relationships. A third version of omega, referred to as *hierarchical omega* (see McDonald [8]), is more conservative with continuous observed indicators in using the observed covariance in place of the model-implied covariance matrix.

Coefficient omegas can be calculated for ordered-categorical items (see Green and Yang [48]) by accounting for both item covariances and item thresholds. As a guideline, 0.70 has been used as an acceptable threshold for both alpha and omega coefficients, with higher values being more desirable. However, one should always evaluate a given threshold relative to how one intends to use the measure. For example, while a value of 0.70 may be acceptable for correlational-based research for coefficient alpha, this value is likely far too low when making clinical judgments at the individual level. Then, a value of 0.90 is preferable for coefficient alpha.

7.7.2 Validity

The term *factorial validity* has been used in particular to describe internal validity of a multi-item scale in its relationship with a factor (or factors) as determined by factor analysis. For factorial validity, the number of factors determined should reflect the intended number of dimensions of the scale, and the scale items should substantially load on the factors they were intended to load on. If the fit of the model is less than acceptable or the interpretation of the factor structure does not seem reasonable to the researcher, then the scale has poor factorial validity.

Average variance extracted (AVE) measures *convergent validity* in testing the degree to which a construct is well explained by its indicators. AVE is a measure of the amount of variance due to the construct itself in relation to the amount of variance due to measurement error. As a guideline, 0.50 is considered an acceptable threshold for AVE.

We have discussed discriminant validity, the degree to which measures of different constructs are unrelated in a multidimensional model, in Chapter 6. AVE can be used to assess discriminant validity in that the AVE of a factor should be higher than the highest squared correlation with any other factor. In Chapter 6, we discussed instead a rule that does not use AVE is that a high correlation between factors of $\rho \geq 0.85$ may imply poor discriminant validity [5,49]. Aforementioned, poor discriminant validity suggests that a more parsimonious factor solution is preferred [5,49]. A second order factor model or a bifactor model is also a useful alternative (since correlations between multiple factors are constrained to zero in specifying these models) to modeling the structure of a set of factors in a multidimensional model showing high correlation between factors.

Construct validity encompasses validity of measurement; it is the degree to which a construct measures the concept it was supposed to measure [49]. If one can demonstrate evidence for convergent and discriminant validity, as subcategories of construct validity, then one has demonstrated evidence for construct validity. Factorial validity is a type of construct validity as evaluated using factor analysis.

The *Multitrait-Multimethod Matrix (MTMM)* is an approach to assessing the construct validity. In MTMM, a set of traits (e.g. emotional, social and general intelligence) is measured by a set of methods (e.g. self, friend, parent and teacher ratings). The approach was originally developed by Campbell and Fiske [50]. The number of traits and methods can be equal or can vary from each other. However, each trait should be measured by each method. For strong convergent validity, correlation between measures of the same trait should be high. For strong discriminant, validity methods should adequately distinguish between different traits. See the textbook on CFA by Brown [49] for more details regarding MTMM.

7.7.3 An Illustrative Example Assessing Reliability and Validity of a Measurement Model

The National Health and Nutrition Examination Survey (NHANES) is a program of the National Center for Health Statistics that began in 1960. The objective of the NHANES is to assess the health and nutritional status of individuals in the United States. The NHANES is a cross-sectional collection of surveys and other health examination data for a nationally representative sample of the resident, civilian, non-institutionalized US population with approximately 5,000 individuals sampled each year [51,52]. We used data from 2015 to 2016 in our study for 5,134 individuals. The inclusion criteria for our study was having a recorded PHQ-9 total score and being 18 or older.

R program has a function `reliability` in the `lavaan` package to evaluate composite reliability (alpha and omega coefficients) and convergent validity (AVE) for different types of estimators (e.g. robust ML or robust WLS) and data (e.g. continuous or ordered-categorical). As of yet, MPlus does not have the availability of such a built-in function.

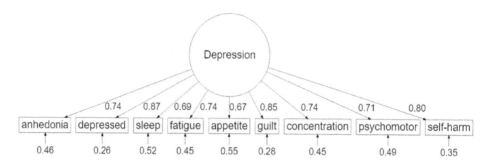

FIGURE 7.3

Measurement model of *Depression* using the PHQ-9 items and NHANES, 2015–2016 ($N = 5{,}134$).

Model fit: chi-square 583.77 (27) $p<0.001$, CFI = 0.976, TLI = 0.968, RMSEA (90% CI) = 0.063 (0.059, 0.068), SRMR = 0.045. CFA for this example was performed using lavaan package in R program. Figure includes the standardized factor loadings and the estimated residual variances (i.e. uniquenesses). We used a robust WLS estimator.

Therefore, we performed CFA in R program in the R Studio environment using the lavaan package for a unidimensional measurement model for the PHQ-9 using NHANES data (see Figure 7.3). The model describes the relationship between the nine PHQ-9 items and an underlying *depression* factor.

Due to a floor effect in the items of the PHQ-9 in this large, nationally representative, US sample and to account for the ordinal responses of the items included in the model we used a robust WLS estimator (similar to WLSMV option in Mplus). The one factor solution was a reasonably acceptable fit (see Figure 7.3). We note the RMSEA value was a little higher than acceptable levels. The standardized factor loadings ranged from 0.67 to 0.87, thus all well above criterion (i.e. >0.40) for a substantial loading. The estimated unexplained, residual variances (i.e. uniquenesses) ranged from 0.26 to 0.55. There is evidence for factorial validity given the reasonably acceptable fit, high standardized factor loading values and meaningful interpretability of the unidimensional construct.

Then, we used the reliability function to evaluate different types of reliability and validity, given corrections in the omega calculations for ordered-categorical items. In this example coefficient alpha = 0.920. The first and second versions of omega were the same = 0.849. The third version of omega, hierarchical omega = 0.858, calculated slightly higher composite reliability. Finally, the AVE = 0.577. Values of alpha and omega were high relative to the guidelines listed in this section, indicating good composite reliability and the AVE exceeded the threshold indicating acceptable convergent validity.

7.8 Formative Constructs

In the measurement models we have discussed thus far in this chapter, we have assumed each construct is *reflective*. In a reflective model, change on the items "reflects" change on the factor. As a result of this expectation, the indicators load onto the construct in reflective models. We have assumed the latent variable causes item responses. The hypothesized causal directionality of a reflective construct is a reasonable assumption for many traits in health and medicine. For example, an individual's *depression* levels cause the affective, somatic and cognitive symptoms that they report on in a measure of depression. However, for other phenomena, one may instead hypothesize that a construct is *formative* because it is the effect (not the cause) of the observed indicators. A formative construct can be viewed as composite variable that summarizes the common variation in a collection of indicators.

Cardiovascular risk or socioeconomic status can be hypothesized to be formative constructs. One may have a high cardiovascular risk due to the presence of a set of risk factors like high blood pressure, high total cholesterol and being a smoker. One does not develop high blood pressure, high total cholesterol and become a smoker because of one's internal cardiovascular risk levels. Rather, one has high cardiovascular risk because of the risk factors. Cardiovascular risk does not "cause" one to smoke. Rather, smoking increases cardiovascular risk. In this context, cardiovascular risk can be viewed as a composite index. It is a formative measure and should be modeled as such.

Formative constructs are often used in the context of prediction and explanation in relation to outcomes (either observed outcomes or reflective constructs). In current methodology in the SEM framework, a path from a formative construct to one or more observed and/or reflective constructs is one of the necessary constraints to make a formative model identifiable. Further identifiability constraints are also necessary. Some typical constraints are that one of the paths from an observed indicator (e.g. blood pressure) to the formative construct (e.g. cardiovascular risk) is constrained to one and the error term for the construct is constrained to zero. See the textbook on CFA by Brown [49] for more details regarding these constraints.

The error term in a formative construct is more accurately described as a disturbance term (part of the formative construct independent of the observed indicators) as opposed to measurement error. Thus, constraining it to zero would indicate that there is no part of the formative construct independent of the observed indicators (or it is defined precisely by the observed indicators).

In Figure 7.4, we identify the formative construct for metabolic risk (consisting of continuous indictors of five risk factors commonly used to define metabolic syndrome). We achieve this by constraining the disturbance term to zero and the indicator for waist circumference to one and regressing observed hemoglobin A1c and cardiovascular event outcomes on the formative construct. In the model, we hypothesize that metabolic risk has a direct effect on both observed indicators for hemoglobin A1c (higher levels above 6.5% serving as a proxy for type 2 diabetes) and time to first cardiovascular event (i.e. myocardial infarction, stroke or cardiovascular-related mortality). Also, there is an indirect path from metabolic risk to cardiovascular event via hemoglobin A1c.

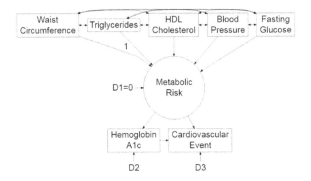

FIGURE 7.4
Model with a formative construct of *Metabolic Risk*.

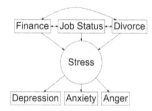

FIGURE 7.5
Mixed formative and reflective measurement model of *Stress*.

Metabolic risk is assumed to be composed of independent, albeit correlated risk factors in this example. However, these correlations among risk factors are not necessary for identification; indicators of a formative construct can be specified as uncorrelated with each other if it is theoretically plausible.

We typically evaluate the goodness of fit of a formative construct in influencing an outcome in SEMs using R-squared, which is reasonable given an aim of using the construct for prediction and explanation. This is similar to assessing a set of independent variables in traditional multiple linear regression. Model fit for a structural equation model with a formative construct on a global and incremental level can still be assessed using the typical criteria as discussed in Chapter 4 (e.g. chi-square test, RMSEA, CFI, TLI, SRMR).

Formative constructs can be used in complex models in health and medicine. For example, a systems-based model for evaluating risk factors for cardiovascular event outcomes with large observational data could include formative constructs for socioeconomic status and cardiovascular risk.

7.9 Mixed Formative and Reflective Constructs

In a reflective construct, *all* indicators are assumed to be caused by the latent trait. In a formative construct, *all* indicators are assumed to be the causes of the latent trait. A latent construct can also be a mixed formative and reflective construct. Level of stress (see Figure 7.5) may be assumed to be influenced by level of financial problems, loss of a job or divorce (i.e. formative indicators). Stress may also be an underlying trait that influences level of depression, anxiety and anger (i.e. reflective indicators). This type of mixed formative and reflective measurement model is structurally equivalent to a MIMIC model (i.e. reflective measurement model with covariates). We discuss MIMIC models in the context of measurement bias in Chapter 10.

7.10 Conclusions

In sum, health and medical researchers face a number of challenges with respect to measurement, particularly patient reported measurement. The illustrative examples in this chapter show the importance of examining dimensionality and establishing a valid measurement model. We used CFA for these purposes. Researchers should carefully consider the constructs they intend to measure. Do they expect responses to the questions to measure one or more constructs? Once one has identified a hypothetical measurement model, one should test the validity of the proposed measurement model. The results will either support the proposed measurement model, or they will prove useful in guiding the development of a modified, empirically based and theory-driven alternative measurement model.

Appendix

A. Notes on Treating Ordinal Variables as Continuous Variables in the Measurement Model

The guidelines for when it is tolerable to treat a set of ordered-categorical items each with four or more categories as approximating an interval scale are a source of debate, even among seasoned applied SEM researchers. Some researchers maintain that it is never truly acceptable and always a limitation of a study in which a researcher analyzed ordered-categorical data in this manner. Given modern technology and computational efficiency, there is little to be gained computationally from approximating an interval scale using ordered-categorical items.

Some other researchers contend that using continuous indicators provides flexibility and familiarity in the analyses and does preserve the ordering of the variable. These researchers might assert that given a large sample size and a reasonable distribution of the sample within different categories, approximating a continuous scale for estimation purposes may be reasonable [38,40,53–55]. Data analysis can be performed and interpreted in a manner readily understood by most researchers. For example, treating measures as continuous tends to simplify the interpretation of a model intercept and slope in linear regression models.

On the limitation side, this approach is approximating the relationship between categories in making the assumption that the distance is equal between each unit. This may be reasonable for certain ordered-categorical scales and less reasonable for other scales. For example, in a three category scale for income, if the categories are $0–$25K, $25–$50K and >$50K the distance is equal between the first two categories, but not in the third category. Ordered-categorical data showing a strong floor or ceiling effect (Chapter 4), respectively, decreases or inflates mean estimates and all such data decreases variance estimates; as a result, one should treat ordered-categorical data showing a strong floor or ceiling effect as ordered-categorical for estimation purposes.

We treated the PHQ-9 items within our MS-depression example as continuous for estimation purposes [38,40,53–55] (Chapter 4). The sample size was large ($N = 3,507$) and each item had four categories of an equal distance to each other. The individual items (with the exception of the item for self-harm) did not have high values in skewness and kurtosis and a robust ML estimator appeared to be a reasonable choice. We do note that some researchers may disagree with this approach and contend that these items should have been treated as ordered-categorical variables.

As a conservative approach, we examined the potential for bias based on variable distributions by re-running the analyses in Mplus in treating the PHQ-9 items as ordered-categorical variables. If there was discrepancy in the results, then we would have considered it appropriate to treat the items as ordered-categorical, given the nature of the items. However, all results were indeed verified in re-running analyses treating the items as ordered-categorical and using the WLSMV option.

B. Parceling Data

A researcher may wish to model one or more latent constructs but have a relatively high ratio of observed variables relative to sample size (e.g. 50 items and a sample size of 300). In such a case, *parceling* may be a useful technique. In parceling, a pre-modeling step, observed variables are combined and these combined variables are used as the indicators of the latent construct [56]. Parcels are created by calculating the sum or mean of a subset of items that are correlated and share similar content. One can then create several parcels (e.g. five) out of all the items (e.g. 50) for use in factor analysis. See Matsunaga [56] for a primer on parceling, including a discussion of the pros and cons of the technique.

C. The `tranformed_scores` Function in R Program to Calculate Transformed Scores Using a Probability Integral Transformation Approach

Input information for the function includes

- *PRO*: a vector of the total score for the original scale for each individual in the sample
- *F*: a vector of factor scores for each individual in the sample
- *a*: lower bound for the root finding function
- *b*: upper bound for the root finding function

Function then returns a vector of transformed scores in the original scale for each individual in the sample

Notes:

    a and *b* can be values chosen just outside of the range of PRO

    After running the `transformed_scores` function the user should:

1. truncate values out of range for the distribution of the original scale
2. round scores to the same type of number (e.g. integer) of the original scale

```
Packages to install:
library(cubature)
library(cmna)
transformed_scores <- function(PRO, F, a, b)
{
#get density of PRO
pdfPRO <- density(PRO)
# Interpolate the density of PRO
fPRO <- approxfun(pdfPRO$x, pdfPRO$y, yleft=0, yright=0)
# Get the cdf of PRO by numeric integration
cdfPRO <- function(x){
cubintegrate(fPRO, -Inf, x)$integral
}
# Use a root finding function to invert the cdf (e.g. bisection method)
invcdfPRO <- function(q){
bisection(function(x) {cdfPRO(x) - q}, a, b)
}
#get density of factor scores
```

```
pdfF <- density(F)
# Interpolate the density of factor scores
fF <- approxfun(pdfF$x, pdfF$y, yleft=0, yright=0)
# Get the cdf of factor scores by numeric integration
cdfF <- function(x){
cubintegrate(fF, -Inf, x)$integral
}
#perform probability integral transformation
transform=function(d) return(invcdfPRO(cdfF(d)))
tF = sapply(F, transform)
return(tF)
}
```

References

1. Cella, D., et al., The Patient-Reported Outcomes Measurement Information System (PROMIS) developed and tested its first wave of adult self-reported health outcome item banks: 2005–2008. *Journal of Clinical Epidemiology*, 2010. **63**(11): pp. 1179–1194.
2. Arsenault-Lapierre, G., C. Kim, and G. Turecki, Psychiatric diagnoses in 3275 suicides: A meta-analysis. *BMC Psychiatry*, 2004. **4**(1): p. 37.
3. Carle, A., Mitigating systematic measurement error in comparative effectiveness research in heterogeneous populations. *Medical Care*, 2010. **48**(6): p. S68.
4. Bollen, K., *Structural equations with latent variables*. 1989, New York: Wiley.
5. Gunzler, D.D. and N. Morris, A tutorial on structural equation modeling for analysis of overlapping symptoms in co-occurring conditions using MPlus. *Statistics in Medicine*, 2015. **34**(24): pp. 3246–3280.
6. Li, C.-H., *The performance of MLR, USLMV, and WLSMV estimation in structural regression models with ordinal variables*. 2014, East Lansing, MI: Michigan State University.
7. Muthén, B. and T. Asparouhov, Latent variable analysis with categorical outcomes: Multiple-group and growth modeling in Mplus. *Mplus Web Notes*, 2002. **4**(5): pp. 1–22.
8. McDonald, R.P., *Test theory: A unified treatment*. 1999, Mahwah, NJ: Erlbaum.
9. Reise, S., J. Morizot, and R. Hays, The role of the bifactor model in resolving dimensionality issues in health outcomes measures. *Quality of Life Research*, 2007. **16**: pp. 19–31.
10. Carle, A.C. and R. Weech-Maldonado, Validly interpreting patients' reports: Using bifactor and multidimensional models to determine whether surveys and scales measure one or more constructs. *Medical Care*, 2012. **50**: pp. S42–S48.
11. Carle, A.C., et al., Advancing PROMIS's methodology: Results of the Third Patient-Reported Outcomes Measurement Information System (PROMIS®) Psychometric Summit. *Expert Review of Pharmacoeconomics and Outcomes Research*, 2011. **11**(6): pp. 677–684.
12. Asparouhov, T., B. Muthén, and A.J. Morin, *Bayesian structural equation modeling with cross-loadings and residual covariances: Comments on Stromeyer et al.* 2015, Los Angeles, CA: Sage Publications.
13. Carle, A.C. and R. Weech-Maldonado, Validly interpreting patients' reports: Using bifactor and multidimensional models to determine whether surveys and scales measure one or more constructs. In Press.
14. Reise, S.P., et al., Bifactor and item response theory analyses of interviewer report scales of cognitive impairment in schizophrenia. *Psychological Assessment*, 2011. **23**(1): pp. 245–261.
15. Reise, S., T. Moore, and M. Haviland, Bifactor models and rotations: Exploring the extent to which multidimensional data yield univocal scale scores. *Journal of Personality Assessment*, 2010. **92**(6): pp. 544–559.

16. Reise, S.P., J. Morizot, and R.D. Hays, The role of the bifactor model in resolving dimensionality issues in health outcomes measures. *Quality of Life Research: An International Journal of Quality of Life Aspects of Treatment, Care and Rehabilitation*, 2007. **16** Suppl 1: pp. 19–31.
17. APA, *Diagnostic and statistical manual of mental disorders*, Fourth Edition. 1994, Washington, DC: American Psychiatric Association.
18. Lai, J.-S., P.K. Crane, and D. Cella, Factor analysis techniques for assessing sufficient unidimensionality of cancer related fatigue. *Quality of Life Research*, 2006. **15**(7): pp. 1179–1190.
19. Reeve, B.B., et al., Psychometric evaluation and calibration of health-related quality of life item banks: plans for the Patient-Reported Outcomes Measurement Information System (PROMIS). *Medical Care*, 2007. **45**(5 Suppl 1): pp. S22–S31.
20. Holzinger, K.J. and F. Swineford, The bi-factor method. *Psychometrika*, 1937. **2**(1): pp. 41–54.
21. Reise, S.P., The rediscovery of bifactor measurement models. *Multivariate Behavioral Research*, 2012. **47**(5): pp. 667–696.
22. Rodriguez, A., S.P. Reise, and M.G. Haviland, Evaluating bifactor models: Calculating and interpreting statistical indices. *Psychological Methods*, 2016. **21**(2): p. 137.
23. Byrne, B.M., Factor analytic models: Viewing the structure of an assessment instrument from three perspectives. *Journal of Personality Assessment*, 2005. **85**(1): pp. 17–32.
24. Reise, S., T. Moore, and A. Maydeu-Olivares, Target rotations and assessing the impact of model violations on the parameters of unidimensional item response theory models. *Educational and Psychological Measurement*, 2011. **71**(4): pp. 684–711.
25. Grant, B.F., et al., *Source and accuracy statement for wave 1 of the 2001–2002 national epidemiologic survey on alcohol and related conditions*. 2003, Bethesda MD: National Institute on Alcohol Abuse and Alcoholism.
26. Hasin, D. and A. Paykin, *Alcohol dependence and abuse diagnoses: Concurrent validity in a nationally representative sample*, Vol. 23. 1999, Alcoholism: Clinical and Experimental Research, pp. 144–150.
27. Grant, B.F., Convergent validity of DSM-III-R and DSM-IV alcohol dependence: Results from the national longitudinal alcohol epidemiologic survey. *Journal of Substance Abuse*, 1997. **9**: pp. 89–102.
28. Grant, B.F., Theoretical and observed subtypes of DSM-IV alcohol abuse and dependence in a general population sample. *Drug and Alcohol Dependence*, 2000. **60**(3): pp. 287–293.
29. Harford and B.O. Muthén, The dimensionality of alcohol abuse and dependence: A multivariate analysis of DSM-IV symptom items in the National Longitudinal Survey of Youth. *Journal Studies of Alcohol*, 2001. **62**: pp. 150–157.
30. Grant, B.F., et al., The Alcohol Use Disorder and Associated Disabilities Interview Schedule (AUDADIS): Reliability of alcohol and drug modules in a general population sample. *Drug and Alcohol Dependence*, 1995. **39**(1): pp. 37–44.
31. Hasin, D.S., B. Grant, and L. Cottler, Nosological comparisons of alcohol and drug diagnoses: A multisite, multi-instrument international study. *Drug and Alcohol Dependence*, 1997. **47**: pp. 217–226.
32. Grant, B.F., et al., The Alcohol Use Disorder and Associated Disabilities Interview Schedule-IV (AUDADIS-IV): Reliability of alcohol consumption, tobacco use, family history of depression and psychiatric diagnostic modules in a general population sample. *Drug and Alcohol Dependence*, 2003. **71**(1): pp. 7–16.
33. Grant, B.F., D.A. Dawson, and D.S. Hasin, *The Alcohol Use Disorder and Associated Disabilities Interview Schedule-DSM-IV Version (AUDADIS-IV)*. 2001, Bethesda, MD: National Institute of on Alcohol Abuse and Alcoholism.
34. Muthén, L.K. and B.O. Muthén, *Mplus: The comprehensive modeling program for applied researchers: User's guide. Eighth edition*, 1998–2017, Los Angeles, CA: Muthén & Muthén.
35. Little, R. and D.B. Rubin, *Statistical analysis with missing data*, Vol. 2. 2002, New York: John Wiley.
36. Carle, A.C., et al., Advanced psychometric methods for developing and evaluating cut-point-based indicators. *Child Indicators Research*, 2011. **4**: pp. 1–26.
37. Muthén, B.O., *Mplus technical appendices*. 2004, Los Angeles, CA: Muthén & Muthén.

38. Huang, F.Y., et al., Using the Patient Health Questionnaire-9 to measure depression among racially and ethnically diverse primary care patients. *Journal of General Internal Medicine*, 2006. **21**(6): pp. 547–552.

39. Kroenke, K., R.L. Spitzer, and J.B. Williams, The Phq-9. *Journal of General Internal Medicine*, 2001. **16**(9): pp. 606–613.

40. Gunzler, D., et al., Disentangling multiple sclerosis and depression: An adjusted depression screening score for patient-centered care. *Journal of Behavioral Medicine*, 2015. **38**(2): pp. 237–250.

41. Raykov, T. and G.A. Marcoulides, *Introduction to psychometric theory.* 2011, Abingdon: Routledge.

42. Cronbach, L.J., Coefficient alpha and the internal structure of tests. *Psychometrika*, 1951. **16**(3): pp. 297–334.

43. Bollen, K.A., Issues in the comparative measurement of political democracy. *American Sociological Review*, 1980. **45**: pp. 370–390.

44. Raykov, T., Estimation of congeneric scale reliability using covariance structure analysis with nonlinear constraints. *British Journal of Mathematical and Statistical Psychology*, 2001. **54**(2): pp. 315–323.

45. Raykov, T., Estimation of composite reliability for congeneric measures. *Applied Psychological Measurement*, 1997. **21**(2): pp. 173–184.

46. Bentler, P., A lower-bound method for the dimension-free measurement of internal consistency. *Social Science Research*, 1972. **1**(4): pp. 343–357.

47. Bentler, P.M., Alpha, dimension-free, and model-based internal consistency reliability. *Psychometrika*, 2009. **74**(1): p. 137.

48. Green, S.B. and Y. Yang, Reliability of summed item scores using structural equation modeling: An alternative to coefficient alpha. *Psychometrika*, 2009. **74**(1): pp. 155–167.

49. Brown, T.A., *Confirmatory factor analysis for applied research.* 2014, New York: Guilford Publications.

50. Campbell, D.T. and D.W. Fiske, Convergent and discriminant validation by the multitrait-multimethod matrix. *Psychological Bulletin*, 1959. **56**(2): p. 81.

51. Centers for Disease Control and Prevention (CDC) and National Center for Health Statistics (NCHS). National Health and Nutrition Examination Survey Questionnaire (or Examination Protocol, or Laboratory Protocol). 2006. http://www.cdc.gov/nchs/nhanes.htm.

52. Brody, D.J., L.A. Pratt, and J.P. Hughes, Prevalence of depression among adults aged 20 and over: United States, 2013–2016. *NCHS Data Brief*, 2018. **303**: pp. 1–8.

53. Johnson, D.R. and J.C. Creech, Ordinal measures in multiple indicator models: A simulation study of categorization error. *American Sociological Review*, 1983. **48**: pp. 398–407.

54. Zumbo, B.D. and D.W. Zimmerman, Is the selection of statistical methods governed by level of measurement? *Canadian Psychology/Psychologie Canadienne*, 1993. **34**(4): p. 390.

55. Hansson, M., et al., Comparison of two self-rating scales to detect depression: HADS and PHQ-9. *British Journal of General Practice*, 2009. **59**(566): pp. e283–e288.

56. Matsunaga, M., Item parceling in structural equation modeling: A primer. *Communication Methods and Measures*, 2008. **2**(4): pp. 260–293.

8

Exploratory Factor Analysis

8.1 Introduction to Exploratory Factor Analysis

Exploratory factor analysis (EFA) is typically used to explore whether one or more constructs account for the variance-covariance among a set of observed indicators. Objectives in performing EFA might be to:

- help an investigator determine the number of dimensions (i.e. latent factors or constructs) underlying a set of observed indicators
- describe the item content in a scale or other set of observed indicators under study by assigning meaning to latent constructs.

EFA output may provide initial evidence for that a scale measures a unidimensional construct and that a single score is valid. Alternatively, EFA output may indicate multidimensionality is more appropriate.

In the last chapter, we discussed measurement models and CFA. An important distinction between EFA and CFA is that when using EFA one does not specify the measurement model (i.e. relationships between the items and factors) prior to conducting exploratory data analysis. This is why it is described as exploratory rather than confirmatory. EFA freely allows for all possible cross-loadings of items. CFA is nearly always more restrictive with respect to cross-loadings in order to achieve an identifiable model.

In a typical application of EFA, one explores a series of models that differ only in the number of factors specified [1]. For example, one might start with an EFA model specifying one factor and move through models with an increasing number of factors until reaching a model with five factors. Typically, each item loads on each of the factors. Sometimes the factors are specified as correlated in an EFA and sometimes they are specified as independent. In this chapter, we discuss quantitative and subjective criteria one can use to help determine how many factors to retain for a given study.

8.2 Common Factor Model

The *common factor model* is the basic mathematical model used for both exploratory and confirmatory factor analysis. The form of the common factor model was given in Chapter 3 (equation 3.1 for either of the two equations, as an example for **y**) for continuous variables and Chapter 7 (Equation 7.2) for ordinal-categorical variables. In EFA, the only constraints specified in the model are those necessary for statistical identification. To this end, the mean and variance of each factor are typically set to zero and one respectively, and the matrix of unique variances and covariances is specified as diagonal. However, this is insufficient to statistically identify the model. Thus, additional constraints are needed, as we discuss in the next section.

8.3 Factor Rotation

To statistically identify the model in EFA, different *factor rotation* methods exist that impose restrictions on the factor model equations. These rotations aim to produce "interpretable" loadings, in addition to statistically identifying the model. Generally, solutions are considered more interpretable when any given item loads relatively strongly on only one factor and relatively weakly on the remaining factors. Rotations differ in whether the factors are allowed to correlate and they differ in terms of the criteria that are maximized or minimized. They are called rotations because, geometrically, a rotation is a change of the positioning of the axes of the geometric space spanned by the factors.

Consider *the varimax rotation*. This is an *orthogonal rotation* technique that specifies uncorrelated factors and rotates the axes in order to maximize the variance of the squared loadings on each factor, hence its name (maximum variance). In orthogonal rotations, the original factor space is rotated while independence (perpendicularity) is preserved. In many situations it may be more reasonable or theoretically justified to assume that the factors will be correlated and select a different rotation.

In an oblique rotation, the new axes in the rotated factor space are allowed to cross at an angle different than 90°, allowing an interrelationship between factors. *Geomin* is an example of an *oblique rotation* technique. With Geomin, the factors are assumed to be correlated with each other.

Commonly, when performing EFA with multiple-item PROs, one uses an oblique rotation technique under the assumption that factors are correlated. For example, one would not assume somatic, affective and cognitive dimensions of depression to be completely independent. These dimensions are associated with capturing domains of depression.

In Figure 8.1, we display a general example of an EFA model using an oblique rotation. The model retains two factors G_1 and G_2 that correlate with each other. All items Y_1-Y_6 in the EFA model freely cross-load onto both factors. The variances of the error terms e_1-e_6 are the uniquenesses.

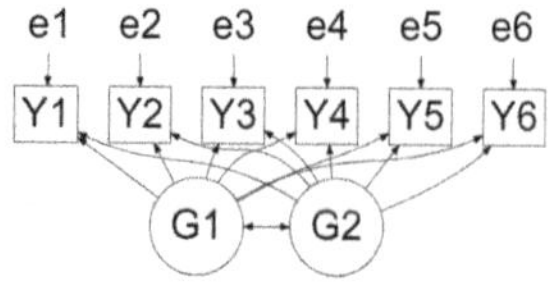

FIGURE 8.1
EFA model (oblique rotation).

8.4 When to Use EFA

EFA in itself can be classified as an alternative to an unsupervised learning technique, using machine learning language parlance. As the nomenclature "exploratory" suggests, EFA is performed under no hypotheses about the nature of the underlying factor structure of a set of indicators. One may be interested in applying EFA to a new scale. Recommended quantitative criteria in the literature, to be discussed later in this chapter, are used by researchers to determine the optimal number of factors for the observed data.

Typically, a researcher also incorporates subjective criteria when conducting EFA. That is, a researcher uses logic, theory and prior literature when evaluating EFA output to help determine plausible groupings of indicators and assign meaning to underlying dimensions. The subjective criteria act as a guide rather than a definitive road map. The researcher is typically uncertain, prior to conducting EFA, of how many factors to retain and which items load onto which factors.

If a researcher has a hypothesis about the number of underlying dimensions of a set of items *and* the factor structure then focus can be on evaluating measurement properties using CFA. CFA can also be conducted to compare a series of plausible measurement models with different, prespecified factor structures or to revise an initial model with a prespecified factor structure.

Exploratory structural equation modeling (ESEM) [2,3] provides a flexible framework to perform CFA, allowing for manipulation of constraints (or paths) among specific residual covariances, while also allowing for the cross-loading of all items across all factors as in EFA. ESEM includes techniques by which an EFA measurement model with rotations can be used in a structural equation model [2]. A researcher may employ ESEM, among many reasons, to avoid having restrictions on the cross-loadings or due to strong prior theory about the number of underlying dimensions, but not about which items load onto which factor. We briefly discuss and illustrate ESEM later in this chapter.

We summarize some recommendations in Box 8.1 of when to conduct EFA, CFA and ESEM given different levels of theory regarding the number of underlying dimensions of a set of indicators and the nature of the relationships between indicators and factors. The bullet points in Box 8.1 should be interpreted as general, flexible guidelines, rather than strict rules. In practice, background knowledge and theory regarding scale dimensionality and item content can be anywhere in the range of limited to extensive. The weight put on quantitative as compared to subjective criteria will also likely differ for each study.

BOX 8.1

- Conduct EFA to compare a series of plausible models each retaining a different number of factors, given none to weak prior theory regarding the number of factors to retain and factor structure

- Use ESEM if one has strong prior theory regarding the number of factors to retain, but none to weak prior theory regarding the factor structure

- Use CFA if one has strong prior theory regarding the factor structure (or several plausible possibilities to compare).

In this chapter, we will present an illustrative example using the PHQ-9 and NHANES survey data and conduct EFA. There was classical depression theory to consider regarding the factor structure of a two factor model for the PHQ-9 items. However, we were looking to evaluate the utility of solutions retaining more than two or even three factors, given there was theoretical reasoning and empirical advantages in considering such solutions. We used a contemporary research framework as a guide. We also subsequently conduct both CFA and ESEM analysis for this illustrative example.

8.5 Empirical Criteria for Exploratory Factor Analysis

8.5.1 Descriptive Analysis Prior to Conducting EFA

Assume a set of observed item responses to be used for EFA. As with all SEM techniques, one should begin by examining the data distribution and summary statistics for each of these items. For example, for continuous variables, statistics of interest include the mean, median, standard deviation, interquartile range, minimum, maximum, skewness and kurtosis. This preliminary step helps identify the range of variability of each item or indicator, checking for outliers, and missing data, to verify sample size and test normality of data. Frequency tables can be used to study categorical data.

One should also review the correlation matrix between items and evaluate for patterns of high correlation among the items prior to performing EFA. Correlations between items should not be so high, e.g. >0.80, indicative of multicollinearity. If a particular bivariate correlation between items is higher than such a threshold, a researcher should consider removing one of these items before performing EFA. Each item should provide some unique information in determining the underlying dimensions of a multi-item scale.

In studying the frequency table of the nine PHQ-9 items using NHANES, 2013–2014 ($N=5,397$), a floor effect was observed in most items. Thus, for conducting EFA for this sample, due to a floor effect and to account for the ordered-categorical responses of the items, we use a robust WLS estimator (WLSMV option) in Mplus.

Spearman correlation of the nine PHQ-9 items revealed item correlations ranging from 0.18 to 0.56 (see Table 8.1). No item correlations appeared to be so high (e.g. >0.80) as to be indicative of multicollinearity.

8.5.2 Determining the Number of Factors to Retain after Conducting EFA

Analyses of EFA output typically begin with examination of the *eigenvalues*. Eigenvalues are the variance accounted for by each underlying factor. The proportion of explained variance for each factor can be calculated as the corresponding eigenvalue for that factor divided by sum of all eigenvalues for all factors. The number of eigenvalues ≥1 represents unique factors according to Kaiser's rule [4].

A *scree plot* is a line graph that depicts the relationship between the eigenvalues on the vertical axis and number of factors on the horizontal axis. A scree plot has an elbow shape, with higher values on eigenvalues spread farther apart than lower values as one moves across the x-axis. The number of factors above the elbow indicates the optimal number of factors for the model.

TABLE 8.1

Spearman Correlation Matrix of the Nine PHQ-9 Items Using NHANES, 2013–2014 ($N = 5,397$)

	Anhedonia	Depressed	Sleep	Fatigue	Appetite	Guilt	Concentration	Psychomotor	Self-harm
Anhedonia	1.00	0.51	0.36	0.43	0.37	0.40	0.40	0.36	0.21
Depressed	0.51	1.00	0.36	0.42	0.39	0.56	0.42	0.38	0.32
Sleep	0.36	0.36	1.00	0.48	0.37	0.30	0.33	0.32	0.18
Fatigue	0.43	0.42	0.48	1.00	0.40	0.35	0.35	0.31	0.19
Appetite	0.37	0.39	0.37	0.40	1.00	0.35	0.34	0.31	0.19
Guilt	0.40	0.56	0.30	0.35	0.35	1.00	0.38	0.36	0.37
Concentration	0.40	0.42	0.33	0.35	0.34	0.38	1.00	0.43	0.24
Psychomotor	0.36	0.38	0.32	0.31	0.31	0.36	0.43	1.00	0.25
Self-harm	0.21	0.32	0.18	0.19	0.19	0.37	0.24	0.25	1.00

We performed EFA in MPlus on the NHANES 2013–2014 data for the PHQ-9 [5]. We used the geomin (oblique) rotation and, as previously mentioned, the WLSMV option in treating the items as ordered-categorical. In the output, only the first factor (eigenvalue=5.619) had an eigenvalue greater than one. Thus the proportion of variance explained by this factor is high at $\dfrac{5.619}{9} = 0.624$. The second factor had an eigenvalue of 0.762 and only explains $\dfrac{0.762}{9} = 0.085$ proportion of the variance. In the scree plot in Figure 8.2, only the first eigenvalue is above the elbow. Thus, the eigenvalue and scree plot analyses suggest a unidimensional depression factor.

There is sampling error involved in analyzing eigenvalues; sampling variability may produce eigenvalues greater than one even if all eigenvalues of the population correlation matrix are exactly one and no large components exist [6]. A simulation based analysis termed *parallel analysis*[1] can be performed to help account for this sampling error [6,7]. In parallel analysis, eigenvalues are computed from a random data set with the same numbers of indicators and observations as the original data set. This process is repeated to compute eigenvalues across a number of simulated random data sets and record the average eigenvalues. Since eigenvalues are relatively robust from data set to data set, the number

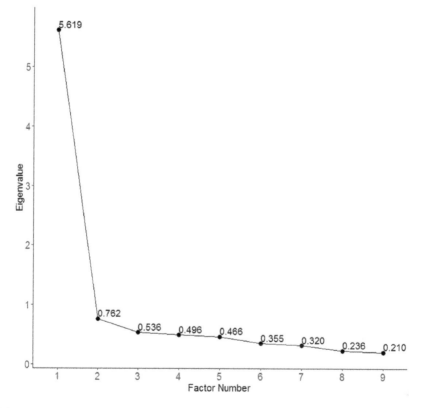

FIGURE 8.2
Scree plot for EFA of the nine PHQ-9 items ($N=5{,}397$).

---

[1] In MPlus, the PARALLEL = option can be added to the ANALYSIS section to perform parallel analysis. For example, specifying PARALLEL = 50 means simulating 50 random data sets for parallel analysis and recording the average eigenvalues over those 50 data sets.

of random data sets can be small (e.g. 50). When the average eigenvalues from the random data are smaller than the reported eigenvalues for the EFA, then the factors should be retained. When the eigenvalues from the random data are larger than the reported eigenvalues for the EFA, then the factors can be attributed to random noise. MPlus can provide parallel analysis for continuous data. MPlus does not provide parallel analysis for ordered-categorical data as of yet after exploration suggested poor performance with tetrachoric and polychoric correlations [8].

In addition to analyses involving eigenvalues, the number of factors can also be determined through examination of model fit indices (e.g. chi-square test statistic, CFI, TLI, RMSEA, SRMR). Increasing the number of factors improves model fit. One could evaluate for the number of factors necessary to reach criteria for an acceptable or excellent fitting model. One must keep in mind that an acceptable fitting model with a factor structure that has no substantial meaning is not an improvement over a model with less factors, but a meaningful factor structure. Also, a solution that reaches criteria for an acceptable fitting model may only minimally improve model fit compared to the model with one less factor; thus one wants to evaluate for nontrivial model fit improvement. For example, an improvement of CFI from 0.899 to 0.900 is interpreted as trivial; an improvement of CFI from 0.899 to 0.980 is viewed as non-trivial.

Mixed results according to the analyses of eigenvalues and model fit are common in health and medicine (as well as other fields). For example, if we considered eigenvalues (and a scree plot) and model fit criteria (see Table 8.2) equally in the NHANES data example with the PHQ-9, we can justify multiple solutions.

The one factor model was the preferred solution based on analyses of eigenvalues and the scree plot. Model fit, however, improves between one and two factors. The one factor solution is reasonably acceptable, with a slightly high RMSEA value (i.e. >0.05). We reach criteria for an acceptable to excellent fit for two factors. We further improve and reach criteria for an excellent fit for four factors. Model fit criteria in chi-square, RMSEA and SRMR still improve meaningfully from the three factor solution to four factor solution, making these differences empirically nontrivial. The chi-square test of difference indicates

TABLE 8.2

Model Fit Statistics and Indices from EFA for PHQ-9 for NHANES Survey Data, 2013–2014 ($N = 5,397$)

	Number of Factors				
	1	2	3	4	5
Chi-square	642.89 (27)	185.50 (19)	83.46 (12)	8.13 (6)	0.694 (1)
	$p<0.001$	$p<0.001$	$p<0.001$	$p=0.229$	$p=0.405$
Chi-square difference test[a]		381.43 (8)	96.55 (7)	70.66 (6)	7.40 (5)
		$p<0.001$	$p<0.001$	$p<0.001$	$p=0.192$
CFI	0.977	0.994	0.997	1.000	1.000
TLI	0.970	0.988	0.992	1.000	1.000
RMSEA (90% CI)	0.065	0.040	0.033	0.008	0.000
	(0.061, 0.069)	(0.035, 0.046)	(0.027, 0.040)	(0.000, 0.021)	(0.000, 0.034)
SRMR	0.053	0.029	0.021	0.007	0.002

We used the WLSMV option for this analyses.

[a] Chi-square difference test for the evaluating for a difference between the current solution with *k* factors and the previous solution with *k-1* factors. Adapted from Gunzler et al. Identify depressive phenotypes by applying RDoC domains to the PHQ-9. *Psychiatry Research*, 2020. **29**, p. 112872.

preference for the four factor solution: comparison of the three factor solution against four factor solution was significant ($p<0.001$) and four factor against five factor ($p=0.192$) was not significant.

8.6 How to Use Subjective Criteria to Help Determine the Optimal Number of Factors

Given the acceptable fit of the competing models in the previous section (i.e. one to four factor solutions), one may be left wondering how to select a model from among these four. Each solution can be interpreted. Subjective criteria in evaluating the different solutions (one solution may be more plausible than others) can help one make such a decision.

In interpreting a proposed rotation, each observed indicator should have a factor loading with a standardized estimate ≥ 0.40 on at least one factor for a substantial loading. This criteria for a factor loading (when squared) can be interpreted as $\geq 16\%$ of variance in that observed indicator is explained by the factor.

One can consider removing problematic indicators one at a time and re-run the EFA if this condition is not met for even the one factor model. Once again, however, we want to consider this criterion on the minimum value for a standardized factor loading as a guideline as opposed to a definitive threshold. Depending on theory and logic, one might still consider a loading <0.40. A multi-item scale or questionnaire may not be complete in content if one removes an item. Analytically, a consequence of having a lower value on a standardized factor loading is that a lower percent variance in that observed indicator is explained by the factor.

In Table 8.3, we display the output of EFA for the one to four factor models. We include in the table standardized factor loadings, estimated residual variances (uniquenesses) and factor correlations. Consider each of these four solutions.

8.6.1 One Factor Model

The one factor solution is straightforward to interpret as a unidimensional depression construct. The one factor model has a reasonably acceptable model fit. All factor loadings are high in magnitude and range from 0.70 to 0.86. Scree plot and eigenvalue examination also supported the one factor model. Many researchers, as a result, would favor this one factor solution. At the very least, we could now conclude based on these results that screening and monitoring for depression in the sample using a single depression score is likely useful in most circumstances.

8.6.2 Classical Depression Theory and the Two and Three Factor Models

The model fit criteria also reached an acceptable to excellent level at the two factor solution. The two factor solution has a basis in classical depression theory with affective and somatic (and cognitive) dimensions. According to this theory, we would describe PHQ-9 items for anhedonia, depressed mood, guilt and self-harm as affective symptoms and sleep, fatigue and appetite as somatic symptoms. Items for psychomotor and concentration are cognitive symptoms that could also be considered somatic symptoms. Classical depression theory suggests independence of affective and somatic dimensions, while the cognitive items might be included in either dimension [9,10].

TABLE 8.3

Exploratory Factor Analysis of the PHQ-9 Using NHANES, 2013–2014 (N=5,397)

PHQ-9 Item	One Factor		Uniqueness
	Depression		
Anhedonia	0.770*		0.408
Depressed	0.856*		0.266
Sleep	0.696*		0.516
Fatigue	0.757*		0.427
Appetite	0.706*		0.502
Guilt	0.825*		0.320
Concentration	0.761*		0.421
Psychomotor	0.762*		0.420
Self-harm	0.767*		0.412

PHQ-9 Item	Two Factor (Factor Correlation = 0.764)		Uniqueness
	Affective	Somatic (and Cognitive)	
Anhedonia	0.395*	0.426*	0.406
Depressed	0.764*	0.150*	0.219
Sleep	−0.122*	0.858*	0.409
Fatigue	0.017	0.789*	0.356
Appetite	0.187*	0.562*	0.488
Guilt	0.869*	0.006	0.236
Concentration	0.401*	0.410*	0.419
Psychomotor	0.362*	0.449*	0.418
Self-harm	0.873*	−0.070	0.327

PHQ-9 Items	Three Factor			Uniqueness
	Affective	Somatic	Cognitive	
Anhedonia	0.324*	0.401*	0.093	0.409
Depressed	0.772*	0.188*	−0.041	0.202
Sleep	−0.146*	0.857*	0.003	0.436
Fatigue	0.003	*1.087***	−0.301*	0.291
Appetite	0.130*	0.564*	0.047	0.492
Guilt	0.826*	0.010	0.047	0.241
Concentration	0.147	0.088	0.599*	0.362
Psychomotor	0.002	−0.009	0.855*	0.279
Self-harm	0.854*	−0.066	0.025	0.324

Factor Correlation Matrix			
	Affective	Somatic	Cognitive
Affective	1		
Somatic	0.786*	1	
Cognitive	0.788*	0.865*	1

TABLE 8.3 (*Continued*)

Exploratory Factor Analysis of the PHQ-9 Using NHANES, 2013–2014 (*N*=5,397)

| | Four Factor | | | | |
PHQ-9 Items	Negative Valence and Externalizing	Negative Valence and Internalizing	Arousal and Regulatory	Cognitive and Sensorimotor	Uniquenesses
Anhedonia	0.835*	0.011	0.021	0.084	0.159
Depressed	0.295*	0.643*	0.033	−0.010	0.221
Sleep	−0.064*	−0.055*	0.733*	0.154	0.406
Fatigue	0.087	0.073	0.757*	−0.062	0.318
Appetite	0.072	0.167*	0.425*	0.123	0.492
Guilt	0.050	0.856*	−0.017	0.023	0.200
Concentration	0.091	0.166	0.075	0.527*	0.378
Psychomotor	0.006	0.013	−0.005	0.858*	0.247
Self-harm	−0.107*	0.876*	0.014	0.032	0.287

| | Factor Correlation Matrix | | | |
	Negative Valence and Externalizing	Negative Valence and Internalizing	Arousal and Regulatory	Cognitive and Sensorimotor
Negative Valence and Externalizing	1			
Negative Valence and Internalizing	0.654*	1		
Arousal and Regulatory	0.702*	0.702*	1	
Cognitive and Sensorimotor	0.680*	0.754*	0.752*	1

* Statistically significant at the 5% level. We used the geomin (oblique) rotation in MPlus and WLSMV option.

The item loadings do not precisely lead to this interpretation of the dimensions in Table 8.3. Items for both concentration and anhedonia loaded onto both factors. EFA is used to *help* determine the factor structure. Therefore, we might use this information and specify a measurement model loading items for anhedonia, depressed mood, guilt and self-harm onto Affective and sleep, fatigue, appetite, concentration and psychomotor onto Somatic (and Cognitive). The loading of psychomotor on Affective was 0.36, which is relatively sizeable, if not quite substantial. Therefore, we could also likely use the EFA output in this example to interpret the dimensions as Cognitive/Affective and Somatic, with the cognitive items (concentration and psychomotor) loading onto Cognitive/Affective. A more classical understanding regarding depression theory could favor such a two factor model with some variation of Affective, Cognitive and Somatic (possibly with item cross-loading).

In the three factor model, we can generally interpret the factors as Affective, Somatic and Cognitive. One may note again that the item for anhedonia, using this interpretation, is out of place loading onto the Somatic factor instead of the Affective factor. In a successive measurement model, we would make this revision and specify the loading for the item for anhedonia on Affective instead of Somatic because the loading of anhedonia on Affective was 0.32.

There is a loading (italicized in Table 8.3) in the three factor model greater than one (standardized factor loading of 1.09). A standardized factor loading greater than one may be due to a negative residual variance. Negative residual variances are typically referred to as *Heywood cases*. A solution with a negative residual variance is inadmissible and could indicate an incorrectly specified model.[2] It is also possible there is little to no measurement error in the indicator because it is nearly perfectly correlated with the underlying factor. In that case, sampling variance might lead to a standardized factor loading estimate greater than one. This would result in a Heywood case but would not necessarily mean the model is misspecified.

A possible approach in lieu of this loading would be to use a different solution. In the example, we might only consider the one, two and four factor models. One could also remove the item with the loading greater than one and re-run EFA. In the example, considering the factor structure of the PHQ-9 without the item for fatigue seems theoretically unreasonable. Another possibility is just accepting that the factor loading is greater than one, which would indicate the item is strongly related to the factor as noted above. See Jöreskog [11] for a more in depth discussion of this topic regarding factor loadings greater than one. A negative residual variance can be constrained to zero (given it is close to zero) in CFA, which might then reduce the standardized factor loading less than one.

In the example with the NHANES data, however, the factor loading was greater than one *and* the corresponding residual variance for the item for fatigue was positive (0.29). Therefore, we would be more inclined to accept the solution if we determined it was the optimal model.

In the three factor model, using the oblique rotation, there was a high factor intercorrelation between Somatic and Cognitive ($\rho=0.87$). However, one should not over interpret this factor intercorrelation, since it was estimated under the arbitrary assumptions used to find meaning in the factor loadings in the oblique rotation. In confirmatory data analysis, discriminant validity is evaluated for a measurement model using CFA. However, one could still note that under this rotation and solution, these factors exhibit multicollinearity. Using subjective criteria and quantitative information, we could reduce the three factor model into a two factor measurement model. We move anhedonia to the first factor and then combine the second and third factors. This leads to the familiar variant of the two factor measurement model that includes Affective (items for anhedonia, depressed mood, guilt and self-harm) and Somatic (items for sleep, fatigue, appetite, psychomotor and concentration).

8.6.3 Research Domain Criteria and the Four Factor Model

We can use a contemporary research framework as a guide to help interpret the four factor model [5]. Research Domain Criteria (RDoC) uses knowledge about major systems of emotion, cognition, motivation and social behavior [12].

RDoC framework encourages research to be structured around six major domains. There is interaction and overlap among each domain. These domains include Negative Valence Systems, driving reactions to aversive stimuli; Positive Valence Systems, driving reactions to positive stimuli; Cognitive Systems, including various mental processes; Social Processes, responsible for interpersonal behavior and cognition; and Arousal and Regulatory Systems, involved in context-based and homeostatic regulation or neural systems [13]. Additionally, Sensorimotor Systems are responsible for the control and execution of motor behaviors, and their refinement during learning and development.

---

[2] There are other potential reasons for obtaining a negative residual variance, such as outliers in the data or the model is not identifiable.

In the four factor model, given four dimensions and expected overlap and interaction among domains, RDoC is a useful framework. Anhedonia substantively loads by itself onto a factor (Negative Valence and Externalizing). We use the descriptors "Externalizing" and "Internalizing" to help distinguish between two constructs that include Negative Valence Systems. Higher endorsement on anhedonia describes negative reactions to aversive stimuli and the externalizing of negative emotions. Externalizing behavior and symptoms are also evident in interpersonal situations. Thus Negative Valence and Externalizing describes items of the PHQ-9 that overlap among the RDoC domains of Negative Valence Systems and Social Processes.

Higher endorsement on depressed, guilt and self-harm items also describe negative reactions to aversive stimuli. These three items describe the relationship of the individual to their own emotional state, the internalizing of negative emotions.

Sleep, fatigue and appetite items describe somatic symptoms that are inherent in arousal and regulation. The factor is named accordingly Arousal and Regulatory Systems. Concentration and psychomotor items describe both mental process symptoms (Cognitive Systems) and motor behavior (Sensorimotor Systems). Thus, we name this factor Cognitive and Sensorimotor Systems using both domains.

We do note the loading of depressed mood on the first factor, Negative Valence and Externalizing, was 0.30, which again is relatively sizeable, if not quite substantial. Subjective reasoning suggests there is evidence that this item should cross-load onto the first factor. That is, item 1 for anhedonia and item 2 for depressed mood both should influence the same factor. These two items are used together in pre-screening for depression in clinical practice as the PHQ-2. Further, the item 2 for depressed mood, in addition to describing the internalizing of negative emotions, also describes the externalizing of negative emotion. The item in theory and interpretation loads onto both the first and second factor. We mentioned in Chapter 7 that dropping a substantive cross-loading could weaken an analyses if including the cross-loading makes theoretical sense.

8.6.4 Which Model Should We Choose?

If we were to determine the number of factors to retain based solely on the scree plot and eigenvalues, we would choose the one factor model. This model had a relatively acceptable model fit. Weighing the decision more on classical depression theory would lead us to choose a two factor model (e.g. Affective and Somatic), which had an acceptable to excellent model fit. The three factor model had some added complexities and did not offer meaningful advantages. Finally, if were to use the RDoC research framework as a guide, we would favor the four factor model, which had an excellent model fit [5].

8.6.5 Evaluating Factor Intercorrelations for Discriminant Validity

Now assume that we reviewed the EFA output and considered pertinent subjective criteria and decided upon a multifactor measurement model (e.g. four factor model). In specifying a CFA model, one must explicitly indicate the relationships between items and constructs. We used 2013–2014 NHANES survey data for EFA in the example. We have available the 2015–2016 NHANES survey data for CFA. We use these two cross-sectional samples under the assumption that sample characteristics are similar across the data sets.[3]

---

[3] While we do not go off topic into the details, this was verified through examination of descriptive statistics and the empirical cumulative distribution functions for the PHQ-9 data. See Gunzler, D., et al., Identify depressive phenotypes by applying RDoC domains to the PHQ-9. *Psychiatry Research*, 2020, **29**: p. 112872.

After performing CFA, the measurement model may need to be revised if the constructs have poor discriminant validity. For example, even an acceptable to excellent fitting two factor model may not be distinct from a unidimensional model if the factor intercorrelation is high (e.g. >0.85). These two factors could potentially be combined into a single factor.

One should keep in mind, however, that multiple factors, if they are different aspects of the same underlying phenomenon, would be expected to correlate in nature, possibly even to a very high degree. Further, we have mentioned other potential reasons for high factor intercorrelations, such as an unmodeled cross-loading. As a result, it is context dependent to determine the best course of action if one finds that factor intercorrelations are high in terms of leaving the model alone or revising the model.

An alternative possibility is to use either a second order or bifactor model. The *second order model* can be used to postulate both a single second order factor and multiple first order factors that are conditionally independent of each other. The *bifactor model* is different in the structure of the relationships between items and factors from the second order factor model (Chapter 7). The bifactor model can be used to postulate both a single general factor and multiple specific factors that are conditionally independent of each other. Both second order and bifactor models provide an approach to handle potential multicollinearity between factors, since lower level or specific factor intercorrelations are constrained to zero (given the second order or general factor).

The goal may be to evaluate underlying, but not necessarily independent, dimensions of a PRO. In addition, theory and evidence may indicate that two constructs are separate (e.g. depression and anxiety) yet correlate strongly. Studying such constructs, even if they correlate to a high degree, may enhance the understanding of the item content of the scale and/or increase external validity. However, this is achieved at the risk of reduced precision (reduced statistical power) due to multicollinearity. There is still an arbitrary cutoff for the intercorrelation between factors to which point researchers might cite poor discriminant validity is a possibility and that the multicollinearity is problematic (for example, the cutoff of 0.85).

8.6.6 Developing a Successive Measurement Model for the Four Factor Solution

We performed CFA in MPlus using a four factor model using the confirmatory sample, NHANES survey data, 2015–2016 (N=5,164).[4] Recall we conducted CFA for the one factor model for this sample in Chapter 7.

In Figure 8.3, we present the standardized factor loadings, factor intercorrelations and residual variances for the measurement model. We used the WLSMV option and the THETA parameterization to obtain estimates of the residual variances. In line with the EFA results, there was a low factor loading (standardized estimate=0.27) of the cross-loaded item 2 for depressed mood on the factor for Negative Valence and Externalizing. However, as noted previously, in consideration that this cross-loading is subjectively meaningful to the model, we would still maintain this cross-loading. All other factor loadings range between 0.69 and 0.95, showing substantial loading onto the factors.

The model fit reaches acceptable to excellent criterion and shows strong internal validity (see Figure 8.3). However, certain factor intercorrelations were high, potentially indicative of poor discriminant validity. The factor intercorrelation of 0.85 between Cognitive and Sensorimotor and Arousal and Regulatory may be especially high. The lowest

---

4 Note that with the lavaan package in R program (Chapter 7) the number of observations used was 5,134 but in Mplus the number of observations used was 5,164 for NHANES survey data, 2015-2016.

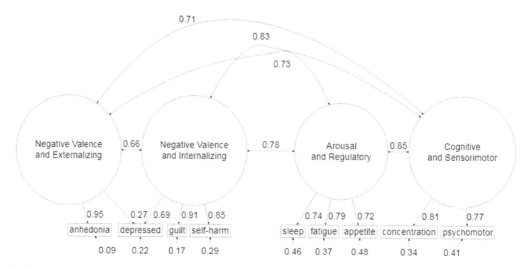

FIGURE 8.3
CFA model using NHANES survey data 2015-2016 ($N = 5,164$).

Model fit: chi-square 56.334 (20) $p < 0.001$, CFI = 0.998, TLI = 0.997, RMSEA (90% CI) = 0.019 (0.013, 0.025), SRMR = 0.011. We report on the figure standardized factor loadings, factor intercorrelations and residual variances.

factor intercorrelation for this model is between Negative Valence and Externalizing and Negative Valence and Internalizing, providing evidence that these dimensions each have unique aspects (with the modeled cross-loaded item).

In using this model specification, we would have to find it acceptable to have some naturally occurring multicollinearity between factors. In doing so we would be equally weighing subjective criteria in tandem with quantitative output.

8.6.7 Second Order Factor Model

Alternatively, we could consider the aforementioned second order factor or bifactor models. Both of these models would (1) utilize both the single factor and multifactor solutions in the form of a first order or general factor for depression and four second order or specific factors and (2) avoid potential multicollinearity between factors in the model specification.

We showcase the second order factor model in Figure 8.4.

In the second order factor model, the nine items load onto four first level factors and the four first level factors load onto a single depression second level factor. The correlation among the four first level factors is accounted for by the second level factor. In the model, Depression is hypothesized to predict Negative Valence and Externalizing, Negative Valence and Internalizing, Arousal and Regulatory and Cognitive and Sensorimotor but with some degree of error captured by the disturbance terms [14]. We provide the standardized solution for the second order factor model in Figure 8.3 using the WLSMV option and THETA parameterization in MPlus. All secondary factor loadings are high (ranging from 0.84 to 0.94) while first order factor loadings are all above 0.40 with the exception of the factor loading for the cross-loaded item depressed for Negative Valence and Externalizing.

The model fit is acceptable to excellent and only trivially worse than the first order factor model represented in Figure 8.3. Also, the fit of both of these models is improved

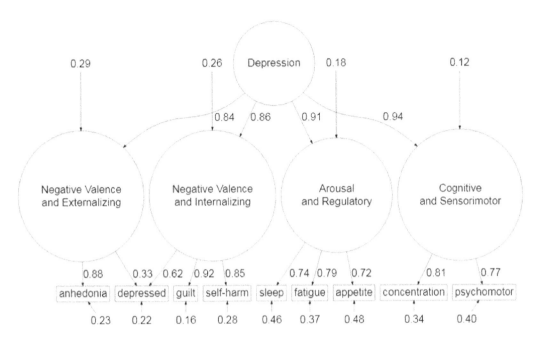

FIGURE 8.4
Second order factor model using NHANES, 2015-2016 ($N=5,164$).

R^2 for the first order factors given in parenthesis for Negative Valence and Externalizing (0.71), Negative Valence and Internalizing (0.74), Arousal and Regulatory (0.83) and Cognitive and Sensorimotor (0.88). Model fit: Chi-square=68.491 (22); $p<0.001$; CFI=0.998; TLI=0.997; RMSEA=0.020 (90% CI=0.015, 0.026); SRMR=0.012. We report on the figure standardized estimates of model parameters (factor loadings, factor correlations, residual variances).

compared to the unidimensional model (Chapter 7). Thus, there is strong evidence in favor of the application of this second order factor model if we deem it theoretically appropriate.

R^2 values can be calculated for a second order factor model to examine the explanatory value for second order factors on first order factors. In this example, given a single second order factor, R^2 values can be calculated as the square of the factor loadings for the first order factors. These R^2 values are high (see Figure 8.3) showing strong explanatory value for the second order factor on each of the first order factors.

8.7 Exploratory Structural Equation Modeling

A researcher can incorporate an EFA measurement model in a structural equation model (e.g. MIMIC model) when using ESEM, given the model is identifiable. In this section, we focus on the EFA measurement model using NHANES 2015–2016 to illustrate the technique. The interested reader can refer to Marsh et al. [3] for recommended ESEM applications and Asparouhov and Muthen [2] for some of the basic theory of ESEM.

Here we will assume there are four factors to retain, but we are uncertain of the factor structure and would like to model all cross-loadings. That is, for this section, suppose we have some theory about the dimensionality of the scale (given overlap and interaction

BOX 8.2

MODEL:
F1–F4 By PHQ9_Q1-PHQ9_Q9 (*1);

among domains of human functioning in depression screening we postulate four dimensions), but not precisely about how the items relate to the factors. We expect some cross-loading. Select model syntax in MPlus is in Box 8.1 in which four correlated factors are specified using an oblique rotation (F1–F4) using the nine PHQ-9 items (PHQ9_Q1-PHQ9_Q9). F1–F4 are one set of EFA factors with the label 1 (*1).

The four factors after ESEM analysis could be named similarly as before (Table 8.4). The model fit (Table 8.4) was almost trivially strong in allowing for all cross-loadings. The item for depressed mood had a loading ≥0.40 on both Negative Valence and Externalizing and Negative Valence and Internalizing using ESEM.

The factor intercorrelations are reported in Table 8.4. While the factor intercorrelations could still be considered relatively high, they were lower than in the four factor model via CFA as shown in Figure 8.3. Further, the highest factor intercorrelation in this model was 0.784, less than the 0.85 threshold that might be indicative of poor discriminant validity (see Table 8.4).

Note that there are alternative specifications using ESEM in which select items can only load onto select factors (e.g. PHQ_Q1, PHQ9_Q2, PHQ_Q6 and PHQ_Q9 can only load onto F1 and F2, while PHQ_Q3, PHQ9_Q4, PHQ_Q5, PHQ_Q7 and PHQ_Q8 can only load onto F3 and F4). Thus, one can specify some more constraints on the relationships between the items and the factors if theoretically justified.

TABLE 8.4

Factor Loadings from Exploratory SEM (ESEM) Using the Specification in Box 8.1 for a Four Factor Structure of Depression Using the PHQ-9 and the NHANES Survey Data 2015–2016 ($N=5{,}164$)

	1	2	3	4
Items	Negative Valence and Externalizing	Negative Valence and Internalizing	Arousal and Regulatory	Cognitive and Sensorimotor
Anhedonia	0.652	0.008	0.089	0.118
Depressed	0.448	0.578	−0.025	−0.019
Sleep	−0.026	0.000	0.622	0.171
Fatigue	0.051	0.001	0.826	−0.031
Appetite	0.028	0.106	0.404	0.216
Guilt	−0.003	0.861	0.064	0.014
Concentration	0.059	0.064	0.110	0.603
Psychomotor	0.004	−0.008	−0.020	0.827
Self-Harm	0.009	0.783	0.008	0.064

Model fit: Chi-square=6.621 (6) $p=0.357$; CFI 1.000; TLI=1.000; RMSEA=0.004 (90% CI=0.000, 0.019); SRMR=0.005.

Correlation between factors via ESEM: Negative Valence and Externalizing WITH Negative Valence and Internalizing (0.719), Arousal and Regulatory (0.685) and Cognitive and Sensorimotor (0.706); Negative Valence and Internalizing WITH Arousal and Regulatory (0.676) and Cognitive and Sensorimotor (0.733); Arousal and Regulatory (0.676) WITH Cognitive and Sensorimotor (0.784).

CFA is used far more often in health and medical research than ESEM. Understanding the factorial complexity of the items in a scale and evaluating the effect of all cross-loadings when using ESEM can be challenging [15]. Partial loadings invariance (Chapter 10) in multigroup analyses is currently not allowed with ESEM. This is because during the rotation a set of unequal parameters will result in a different set of unequal parameters [8].

8.8 Conclusions

EFA can help one determine the number of dimensions and factor structure of a group of items in a scale, questionnaire, test or other instrument under study. We have highlighted the usage of subjective criteria along with empirical criteria when conducting EFA. EFA is used in the context of exploratory data analysis given uncertainty about the number of factors to retain and the factor structure of a set of indicators. If a researcher has a priori theory regarding both the underlying dimensions and factor structure of a set of indicators, then there is little advantage to use EFA rather than CFA. The researcher can then examine the measurement properties, such as the internal validity, of the CFA model.

References

1. Preacher, K.J., et al., Choosing the optimal number of factors in exploratory factor analysis: A model selection perspective. *Multivariate Behavioral Research*, 2013. **48**(1): pp. 28–56.
2. Asparouhov, T. and B. Muthén, Exploratory structural equation modeling. *Structural Equation Modeling: A Multidisciplinary Journal*, 2009. **16**(3): pp. 397–438.
3. Marsh, H.W., et al., Exploratory structural equation modeling: An integration of the best features of exploratory and confirmatory factor analysis. *Annual Review of Clinical Psychology*, 2014. **10**: pp. 85–110.
4. Costello, A. and J. Osborne, Best practices in exploratory factor analysis: four recommendations for getting the most from your analysis. *Practical Assessment, Research and Evaluation*, 2005. **10**(7). http://pareonline. net/getvn. asp.
5. Gunzler, D., et al., Identify depressive phenotypes by applying RDoC domains to the PHQ-9. *Psychiatry Research*, 2020. **29**: p. 112872.
6. Franklin, S.B., et al., Parallel analysis: A method for determining significant principal components. *Journal of Vegetation Science*, 1995. **6**(1): pp. 99–106.
7. Horn, J.L., A rationale and test for the number of factors in factor analysis. *Psychometrika*, 1965. **30**(2): pp. 179–185.
8. Muthén, L.K. and B.O. Muthén, *Mplus: The comprehensive modeling program for applied researchers: User's guide. Eighth edition*, 1998–2017, Los Angeles, CA: Muthén & Muthén.
9. Cheng, H.-T., M.-C. Ho, and K.-Y. Hung, Affective and cognitive rather than somatic symptoms of depression predict 3-year mortality in patients on chronic hemodialysis. *Scientific Reports*, 2018. **8**(1): pp. 5868–5868.
10. Patel, J.S., et al., Measurement invariance of the patient health questionnaire-9 (PHQ-9) depression screener in U.S. adults across sex, race/ethnicity, and education level: NHANES 2005–2016. *Depression and Anxiety*, 2019. **36**(9): pp. 813-823.
11. Jöreskog, K.G., *How large can a standardized coefficient be.doc (statmodel.com)*. 1999.

12. Insel, T., et al., Research domain criteria (RDoC): Toward a new classification framework for research on mental disorders. *American Psychiatric Association*, 2010. **167**: p. 7.

13. Carcone, D. and A.C. Ruocco, Six years of research on the national institute of mental health's Research Domain Criteria (RDoC) initiative: A systematic review. *Frontiers in Cellular Neuroscience*, 2017. **11**: p. 46.

14. Byrne, B.M., Factor analytic models: Viewing the structure of an assessment instrument from three perspectives. *Journal of Personality Assessment*, 2005. **85**(1): pp. 17–32.

15. Elsworth, G.R., S. Nolte, and R.H. Osborne, Factor structure and measurement invariance of the Health Education Impact Questionnaire: Does the subjectivity of the response perspective threaten the contextual validity of inferences? *SAGE Open Medicine*, 2015. **3**: p. 2050312115585041.

9

Mediation and Moderation

9.1 Introduction to Structural Models for Health and Medical Studies

The structural model in the SEM framework can be used to model real-world, complex relationships in health and medicine. For example, in Figure 9.1, we depict the hypothesized relationships between multiple sclerosis (MS) characteristics, functional impairment and depression and fatigue in persons living with MS (see Figure 9.1).[1] The corresponding systems-based model was developed by MS specialists using logic, theory and information from prior studies [1–4].[2]

In the example, we are interested in addressing *if and how* MS characteristics influence depression and fatigue. We hypothesize that a progressive (compared to a relapsing) MS type and a longer time since MS symptom onset leads to higher levels of functional impairment (hand function and mobility impairment) which lead to higher levels of depressive symptoms and fatigue. In general, evaluating potential mechanisms of change between an independent variable and an outcome is the focus of many studies in health and medicine.

Mediation analysis is an approach for testing a hypothesis of mediation. Recall that a mediator is an intermediate variable that helps explain how or why an independent variable influences an outcome [5–8]. Both logical and temporal causal assumptions are utilized in mediation studies. An independent variable is hypothesized to precede and influence a mediator which is hypothesized to precede and influence an outcome. A complex model with hypothesized mediation relationships such as in Figure 9.1 includes many model parameters. Large sample sizes are necessary for any study analyzing similarly complex models.

Baron and Kenny [8] distinguished mediation from moderation, in which a third variable affects the strength or direction of the relationship between an explanatory variable and a response variable. For example, older persons may be hypothesized to respond differently than younger persons to a particular intervention for lowering blood pressure. In this case, age is a moderator. Moderation analysis helps generalize results by testing if relationships hold for different groups in the study population. Mediation and moderation can be implemented together. In a mediation model, different levels of the moderator can influence the pathways between an independent variable and an outcome.

---

[1] In this first figure for this chapter, we distinguish a scale that captures symptoms of fatigue as MS-related from other scales that may also capture fatigue in the context of depressive symptoms. When we mention fatigue throughout the rest of this chapter, we are referring to MS-related fatigue unless denoted otherwise.

[2] Cognitive impairment is a third component of the multiple sclerosis functional composite (see Reference: Rudick, R.A., et al., Assessing disability progression with the multiple sclerosis functional composite. *Multiple Sclerosis Journal*, 2009. **15**(8): pp. 984-997.) along with hand function and mobility impairment. However, for illustration purposes and given the measurement properties of the scales in our available data, we focused on hand and mobility impairment only in assessing functional impairment in this chapter.

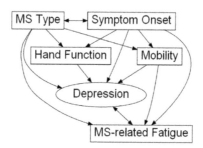

FIGURE 9.1
Multiple mediator multiple outcome Multiple Sclerosis (MS)-depression and fatigue model.

Time since symptom onset and MS type (relapsing or progressive) describe individual-specific disease characteristics for persons living with MS. Hand function (upper extremity) and mobility (lower extremity) impairment describe functional impairment. Depression is a latent variable with effect indicators (not shown) of
symptoms of depression. MS-related fatigue is a measure of fatigue as a symptom of MS. While left out of the
model, a correlation between hand function and mobility might be theoretically reasonable and could potentially be added at the discretion of a research team.

We provide a list of some of the major advantages and limitations of using a SEM approach
to test for mediation and moderation effects in health and medical research studies.

ADVANTAGES

- Allows for the inclusion of latent variables as independent variables,
  moderators, mediators or outcomes.
- Can assess mediation and moderation using a multi-equation model in a
  single analysis.
- Allows one to evaluate multiple independent variables, moderators, media-
  tors or outcomes in a single analysis.
- Techniques are available to handle missing data under various assumptions.
- Provides model fit information about consistency of the model to the data.
- Nomenclature gives a rich language to express hypothesized causal relation-
  ships in mediation and moderation.

LIMITATIONS

- Causal assumptions are strong assumptions and must be grounded in theory
  and prior evidence.
- Typically requires a very large sample size; estimates of mediation and
  moderation effects may be inaccurate in low powered samples.
- Potential for model misspecification and unmeasured confounding.
- Conceptual model of interest may be non-identifiable.
- There may be plausible alternative models that are equivalent.

9.2 An Introduction to Mediation Analysis

Let us begin our formal discussion of mediation analysis with a simplified example. We first discuss a regression of a continuous outcome on an independent variable. This regression does not yet involve a mediator. We hypothesize that a progressive (compared to relapsing) MS type leads to a higher level of fatigue (Figure 9.2).

The structural equation corresponding to Figure 9.2 that regresses the outcome on the independent variable is as follows:

$$Y = i + cX + D \tag{9.1}$$

Here, Y (*Fatigue*) is the outcome and X (*MS Type*) is the independent variable, i is the intercept, c is the parameter for relating X to Y and D is the error term. In solving this equation, we could determine *if* MS type influences fatigue, but we could not determine *how (or via what mechanism)* MS type influences fatigue.

Figure 9.3 is an extension of Figure 9.2 after accounting for a continuous mediator. In Figure 9.3, we additionally hypothesize that a progressive (compared to relapsing) MS type leads to increased hand function impairment which leads to a higher level of fatigue. This hypothesis supposes the mechanism of change, hand function impairment, in which MS type influences the level of fatigue.

The corresponding model for this figure formalizes this mediation process with two structural equations:

$$Y = i_y + c'X + bZ + D_y,$$
$$Z = i_z + aX + D_z \tag{9.2}$$

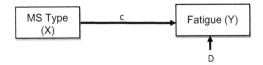

FIGURE 9.2
Regression of Y on X for MS-fatigue example.

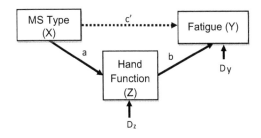

FIGURE 9.3
Mediation process for MS-fatigue example.

Z (*Hand Function*) is the mediator, i_y and i_z are intercepts, c' is the parameter relating X to Y controlling for the mediator Z, b is the parameter relating Z to Y controlling for X and a is the parameter relating X to Z and D_y and D_z are error terms.

Equations in (9.1) and (9.2) may be generalized to incorporate additional independent variables, nonlinearities and interaction terms [9]. Further, additional equations can be used to incorporate multiple mediators and outcomes. We describe some of these extensions from the basic representation later in the chapter.

In the case of a latent variable outcome and/or mediator in the structural equations above a further identifying constraint is necessary, such as the respective model intercept is constrained to zero. A typical assumption and identifying constraint is no residual correlation of the error terms D_y and D_x. Under this assumption, the error terms are assumed to be independent of each other and both continuous with zero mean and positive variance.

Recall in Chapter 2 we provided an introduction of the direct effect (DE), indirect (also termed mediation or mediated) effect (IE) and total effect (TE) (see Table 9.1).

The definitions in Table 9.1 can be linked to the path diagrams in Figures 9.2 and 9.3 and equations (9.1) and (9.2). Corresponding to the path diagram in Figure 9.3 and equation (9.2):

$$DE = c'$$

$$IE = ab \qquad\qquad (9.3)$$

$$TE = c' + ab$$

In equation (9.3) the indirect effect can be conceptualized through the product of a and b from the path diagram in Figure 9.3 and the equation in (9.2), termed the *product of coefficients method*. Alternatively, in the *difference in coefficients method*, one estimates the mediation effect based on the difference between $c - c'$ from the path diagrams in Figures 9.2 and 9.3 and equations (9.1) and (9.2). The difference in coefficients is the difference between the unadjusted effect of the independent variable on the outcome and the effect of the independent variable on the outcome controlling for the mediator. The product of coefficients and difference in coefficients formulas should be approximately equal with continuous data under similar assumptions.

The point estimate of the mediated effect can be corrected when a and b are correlated. If r is the correlation between a and b, then the indirect effect can be calculated as

$$IE = ab + rSE_a SE_b \qquad\qquad (9.4)$$

SE_a and SE_b are the standard errors of a and b, respectively. In mediation models with a latent variable or variables, the covariance between a and b is nonzero [10]. However, this correlation is expected to be small in most cases [10].

TABLE 9.1

Basic Definitions of Direct, Indirect and Total Effects

Direct effect (DE): is the pathway from the independent variable to the outcome while controlling for the mediator.
Indirect effect (IE): is the pathway from the independent variable to the outcome through the mediator.
Total effect (TE): is the sum of the direct and indirect effects and consists of all paths from the independent variable to the outcome.

We used observational data on 3,507 persons with MS to estimate the effects (a, b, c and c') in equations (9.2) and (9.3) for the MS-fatigue example[3] using the ML option[4] in MPlus (Box 9.1). A physical performance test (operationalized as an observed variable measured as time to complete the test), the 9-hole peg test, was used for hand function impairment. The Fatigue domain of the Performance Scales© [11] was used for MS-related fatigue.

BOX 9.1

REGRESSION OF *FATIGUE* ON *MS TYPE*

$$\text{Fatigue} = 2.046 + 0.402 \text{ MS Type}$$

$$(0.027)\,(0.063)$$

MEDIATION EQUATIONS

$$\text{Fatigue} = 1.468 + 1.482 \text{ Hand Function} + 0.226 \text{ MS Type,}$$

$$(0.137)\,(0.355) \qquad\qquad (0.079)$$

$$\text{Hand Function} = 0.390 + 0.119 \text{ MS Type}$$

$$(0.004)\ \ (0.015)$$

PRODUCT OF COEFFICIENTS

$$DE = c' = 0.226$$

$$IE = ab = 0.119 \times 1.482 = 0.176$$

$$TE = c' + ab = 0.226 + 0.176 = 0.402$$

DIFFERENCE IN COEFFICIENTS

$$DE = c' = 0.226$$

$$IE = c - c' = 0.402 - 0.226 = 0.176$$

$$TE = c = 0.402$$

Note for Box 9.1: These example results utilize unstandardized coefficients. Health and medical researchers generally examine both standardized *and* unstandardized coefficients when available. In many studies, standardized estimates are often reported and relied on for more straightforward interpretation.

---

[3] The 9-hole peg test used for hand function was scaled by 60 in changing the units to number of pegs placed per minute.

[4] MPlus calculates and tests the significance of the IE, DE and TE with the MODEL INDIRECT statement and IND option after the MODEL statement.

We report the bias-corrected (BC) bootstrap standard errors using 10,000 bootstrap replications under each path estimate in parenthesis. The positive direction of our regression path estimates for a and b are in line with our hypothesis that progressive MS leads to increased hand function impairment which leads to higher levels of MS-related fatigue. We obtain the same results for the product of coefficients and difference of coefficients methods for calculating the indirect effect in Box 9.1.

MS type is entered as a dummy variable with values of 0 for relapsing and 1 for progressive in MPlus. We do use FIML (Chapter 4) and include the mean and variance of MS type in the model to use all available cases. There was a large amount of missing data in this illustrative analysis for hand function impairment (<3% on *Fatigue* and *MS Type*, 40% on *Hand Function*).

9.2.1 Percent Mediated

Percent mediated explains how much of the effect of the independent variable on the outcome is due to the indirect effect. This can be calculated using either the product of coefficients or difference in coefficients method (see Box 9.2). In the example, using either approach, 43.8% of the total effect of MS type on fatigue was mediated by hand function impairment. Note that researchers will sometimes report *proportion mediated* (calculated as percent mediated divided by 100) instead of percent mediated, which merely converts the unit of measurement.

Percent mediated does not have much meaning if the total effect is small in magnitude (i.e. not substantively meaningful or statistically significant). We will soon discuss approaches for evaluating direct, indirect and total effects for statistical significance. Percent mediated also does not have much meaning with *inconsistent mediation*. In inconsistent mediation the indirect effect and the direct effect have opposite signs, reducing the size of the total effect as a sum total and inflating the percent mediated.

BOX 9.2

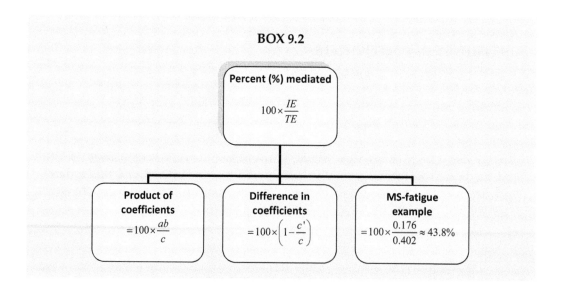

Percent (%) mediated

$$100 \times \frac{IE}{TE}$$

Product of coefficients	Difference in coefficients	MS-fatigue example
$=100 \times \dfrac{ab}{c}$	$=100 \times \left(1 - \dfrac{c'}{c}\right)$	$=100 \times \dfrac{0.176}{0.402} \approx 43.8\%$

9.2.2 Hypothesis Testing for Mediation

The null hypothesis in a mediation analysis is that the effect of the independent variable on the outcome is not broken (i.e. not mediated) by a change in the mediator. The alternative hypothesis is that the effect of the independent variable on the outcome is mediated. In a *full mediation* process, the effect of the independent variable on the outcome is 100% mediated by the mediator. That is, in the presence of the mediator, the pathway connecting the independent variable to the outcome is completely broken so that the independent variable has no direct effect on the outcome. In most applications, *partial mediation* is more common, in which case the mediator only mediates part of the effect of the independent variable on the outcome. That is, the independent variable has some residual direct effect on the outcome even after the mediator is introduced into the model. In partial mediation, this residual direct effect should be reduced in absolute value from the direct effect of the independent variable on the outcome before controlling for the mediator.

We drew a dashed line in our path diagram for the direct casual pathway c' in Figure 7.3 since one is evaluating if this pathway is broken by the mediator (and thus in the case of full mediation should be equal to zero). This dashed line is an optional feature in a path diagram for mediation analysis for clarity. In accordance with the simultaneous nature of the causal chain between the variables in a mediation process, testing for mediation in the SEM framework can be performed in a single analysis.

An interesting application of mediation in health and medicine is to evaluate the utility of a potential biomarker [12,13]. If a potential biomarker is a full mediator, in theory, it becomes a useful surrogate for measuring the effect of an intervention (or other independent variable of interest) on a health outcome. Several potential biomarkers can be simultaneously evaluated for partial mediation in a multiple mediator model. In general, if a potential biomarker is a partial mediator, then the indirect effect involving that measure should explain a sufficiently large proportion of the total effect between an intervention and a health outcome.

In applications of mediation analysis for discovery of a new biomarker, it is difficult to verify that a measure is truly a biomarker. For example, poor quality data or a model that is misspecified (e.g. omitted confounding variables, variables on inappropriate scales or lack of relevant interaction terms) may lead one to draw false conclusions about a biomarker that does not generalize to other settings.

9.3 Classic Approaches for Performing Mediation Analysis

In this section, we very briefly discuss some classic approaches used to conduct mediation analysis. We provide some explanations of why these approaches have generally gone out of favor. Baron and Kenny [8] in the most widely cited article for mediation methods recommended formal testing of a mediation hypothesis in four steps using a series of traditional regression models.

The Baron and Kenny approach includes testing for full mediation using the series of regression equations in (9.1) and (9.2) [14][5]:

1. X is significantly related to Y before accounting for the mediator Z.
2. X is significantly related to Z.
3. Z is significantly related to Y.
4. X is no longer significantly related to Y after accounting for the mediator Z.

For partial mediation, the first three steps should be met but not the fourth, and the estimate of the absolute value of the residual direct effect c' in step 4 should be reduced from the absolute value of the estimate of c in step 1.

Some researchers continue to this day to use the Baron and Kenny approach. The method has been shown as problematic since the required steps may lead to missing or falsely supporting mediation [15,16]. The steps may be too restrictive for evaluating mediation [16]. The interested reader should refer to the paper by Zhao et al. [16] for "a nontechnical summary of the flaws in Baron and Kenny logic".

Currently, many researchers follow the recommendation that having a significant indirect effect is enough to suggest mediation [16]. Under this guideline, a significant total effect is not necessary for mediation to occur [17–24]. Further, while one of the path estimates a or b for the indirect effect may not be significant, the indirect effect can still be significant. Simulations have also shown that the Baron and Kenny test has low power for detecting full mediation compared to a test of mediation based on the indirect effect [10].

In the next section in this chapter, we will discuss computer-intensive approaches for testing for mediation based on the indirect effect. First, we discuss some classic approaches for testing for mediation based on the indirect effect and why we generally do not recommend these approaches.

The Sobel test [25,26] is performed by comparing a test statistic calculated by dividing the indirect effect by its standard error to the normal distribution to determine its significance. Sobel calculated the standard error of the indirect effect using the product of coefficients method based on first derivatives using the delta method [10,25,26]. The delta method typically uses a first order Taylor approximation to expand a function of a random variable about its mean and then estimate the variance. An approximate 95% confidence interval can also be calculated for the indirect effect.

There are many variations of the Sobel method within the mediation literature, usually with negligible effects on test outcomes [17]. For example, a slight variation of the standard error formula has been derived based on the first- and second-order derivatives and exact variance under independence of a and b [8,27,28]. There are further variations of this formula taking into account the covariance between a and b [28]. Alternatively, a standard error and subsequent test or confidence interval could be calculated based on the difference in coefficients method.

The Sobel test and related variations assume a normal distribution for both the indirect effect and its standard error. In most health and medical research studies, the distribution of these statistics will rarely (if ever) meet this assumption. A false presumption of a symmetric distribution of the mediated effect leads to a conservative test that has low power [29].

---

[5] The four steps can be stated as (1) the total effect c is statistically significant; (2) the path estimate for a is statistically significant; (3) the path estimate for b is statistically significant; (4) c' is not statistically significant.

9.4 Computer-Intensive Approaches for Performing Mediation Analysis

A popular approach to assessing mediation in health and medicine is to use bootstrap methods to construct confidence intervals for the indirect effect [17]. Bootstrap methods are more robust and less conservative compared to the delta method. We described bootstrapping in the context of SEM in Chapter 4.

We now demonstrate how to use the percentile bootstrap approach to perform mediation analysis for the MS-fatigue example. First, we resample with replacement the original data set 10,000 times. An ML estimator is used to estimate model parameters a, b and c' in the mediation model for each bootstrapped sample (see Figure 9.4).

Then we calculate the indirect effect as the product of coefficients for each of these bootstrapped samples, corresponding to $IE_1^*, IE_2^*, \ldots, IE_{10,000}^*$ in Figure 9.4. We use the percentile method (Chapter 4) for constructing a 95% confidence interval around the average of these 10,000 indirect effects. That is, out of the 10,000 estimates of the indirect effect we find the 2.5th percentile estimate and the 97.5th percentile estimate, which leaves 95% of the estimates in the middle. As previously noted in Chapter 4, this confidence interval can be asymmetrical. It is based on an empirical estimation of the sampling distribution of the indirect effect, rather than on an assumption that the sampling distribution is normal [17].

In the example, the 95% bootstrap confidence interval around the indirect effect does not contain zero and is tight around the indirect effect (see Table 9.2). Likewise, 95% bootstrap confidence intervals around the direct effect and total effect do not contain zero and are reasonably tight around these effects. We can conclude partial mediation since both the indirect and direct effect bootstrapped confidence intervals do not contain zero.

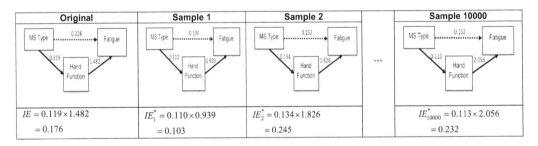

FIGURE 9.4
Bootstrap indirect effects for MS-fatigue example.

IE is the estimate of the indirect effect from the original sample. $IE_1^*, IE_2^*, \ldots, IE_{10,000}^*$ are the estimates of the indirect effects for each of the 10,000 bootstrapped samples.

TABLE 9.2

95% Bootstrap Confidence Intervals (Lower and Upper Limits) for the Direct, Indirect and Total Effects for the MS-Fatigue Example

Effect	Estimate	Percentile Bootstrap		Bias-Corrected Bootstrap	
		Lower	Upper	Lower	Upper
Direct	0.226	0.063	0.369	0.077	0.386
Indirect	0.176	0.103	0.277	0.095	0.266
Total	0.402	0.278	0.531	0.277	0.530

We further corrected for bias in the distribution of the bootstrap estimates and used the BC bootstrap (Chapter 4) in conducting mediation analysis for the MS-fatigue example. The confidence intervals for the indirect effect and direct effect are shifted, but about the same width as the confidence interval using the percentile method (see Table 9.2). The confidence interval for the total effect is relatively similar. Both bootstrap approaches, percentile and bias-corrected, lead to a similar conclusion of partial mediation.

Another computer-intensive approach, the *Monte Carlo approach* has been shown to perform reasonably well when compared to bootstrapping [30,31]. The Monte Carlo method has been recommended as a good alternative when the bootstrap is not readily available [30]. For example, in multilevel SEM, as of yet, there is no readily available bootstrap in most SEM software [30].

MONTE CARLO APPROACH FOR ASSESSING MEDIATION [30–33]

1. Assume normality for the estimates a and b in the regression equations in (9.2).

2. Define the sampling distribution for $a^* \sim N\left(a, \text{SE}_a^2\right)$ and $b^* \sim N\left(b, \text{SE}_b^2\right)$ where $N\left(\mu, \sigma^2\right)$ is the normal distribution with mean μ and variance σ^2.

3. Sampling distribution of the indirect effect a^*b^* is formed by repeatedly generating a^* and b^* (e.g. 10,000,000 times) from the random normal distributions defined above and computing their product.

4. Use the percentile method for confidence interval construction about the sample indirect effect.

Large sample assumptions (i.e. normality) are invoked for the distribution of a^* and b^*, but no assumptions are made about the distribution of a^*b^*. The joint sampling distribution for a^* and b^* can also include an off-diagonal non-zero covariance term if a and b are correlated.

Again, consider the MS-fatigue example. We describe the sampling distribution of the indirect effect a^*b^* using the Monte Carlo method from $a^* \sim N\left(a = 0.119, \text{SE}_a^2 = 0.015^2\right)$ and $b^* \sim N\left(b = 1.482, \text{SE}_b^2 = 0.355^2\right)$. We generate a^* and b^* 10,000,000 times. We obtain a slightly more conservative 95% confidence interval around the indirect effect using the Monte Carlo method $(0.088, 0.277)$[6] as compared to the bootstrap results in Table 9.2 for this example.

In general, we recommend researchers testing mediation to use a sufficiently large sample, and to use a bootstrap method, with the Monte Carlo approach as a viable alternative. Neither of these approaches makes assumptions about the distribution of the indirect effect.

One should keep in mind that despite our general recommendations, the field is still undergoing development. For example, a study by Fritz [34] found that for sample sizes

[6] Generated with R code using a similar function as Selig, J.P. and K.J. Preacher, Monte Carlo method for assessing mediation: An interactive tool for creating confidence intervals for indirect effects [Computer software], 2008. Available from: http://quantpsy.org/.

<2,500, the percentile bootstrap and numerical integration tests[7] have more accurate Type I error rates compared with the BC and accelerated BC bootstrap tests. Gunzler et al. [35] found that ML approaches may produce biased estimates of parameters and standard errors when parametric assumptions are violated in studies of longitudinal mediation using SEM with missing data under the MAR assumption.

9.4.1 Mediation Analysis with a Small Sample Size

Previously mentioned in Chapter 4, bootstrap approaches may still be unreliable on smaller samples and work best on at least a moderately large sample size [17]. However, there is as of yet no widespread agreement on the best approach for performing mediation analysis with a small sample size. Thus, many researchers continue to use bootstrapping techniques with smaller sample sizes [17,32]. Bayesian approaches to SEM or partial least squares-based SEM (PLS-SEM) [36] are also used with smaller sample sizes. See Chapter 15 for a brief overview of these methods. We note that researchers should be cautious about interpreting results of any analysis with a small sample size. Low statistical power and other concerns about possible selection bias may lead to inaccurate results, such as reduced chance of detecting a true indirect effect.

9.5 Mediation Analysis with a Systems-Based Model

Researchers in health and medicine have the exciting opportunity to use SEM for addressing research hypotheses with systems-based models and large observational data sets. The relationships among concepts in a particular system often depend on the direct and indirect pathways among latent and observed variables. Mediation analysis can be used to address hypotheses of interest in such models.

The path diagram in Figure 9.1 corresponds to a systems-based model of the pathways between MS characteristics and depression and fatigue. This model consists of two independent variables, two mediators and two outcomes, one of which is a latent variable. While factoring in other model relationships, including the correlation between the two outcomes, we are interested in assessing mediation between each independent variable and each outcome. For example, we would like to understand potential mechanisms of change between time since *symptom onset* and *depression*.

Figure 9.1 is an example in which multiple mediators operate simultaneously (or in parallel). These mediators are not causally related to each other. They are also specified as uncorrelated with each other.

Without loss of generality, let us consider a single independent variable X, two mediators (Z_1 and Z_2) and a single outcome Y. The path diagram in Figure 9.5a represents a simpler model based on the mediating relationships described above for Figure 9.1; two mediators occur simultaneously and are uncorrelated with each other.

---

[7] The numerical integration test was employed in PRODCLIN (see Reference: MacKinnon, D.P., M.S. Fritz, J. Williams, and C.M. Lockwood, Distribution of the product confidence limits for the indirect effect: Program PRODCLIN. *Behavior Research Methods*, 2007. **39**(3): pp. 384389.), a program available in Fortran, SAS, SPSS, and R formats, that can be used to construct asymmetric confidence limits while still using the distribution of the product approach.

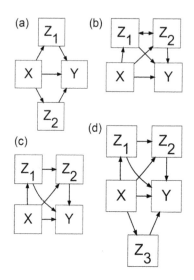

FIGURE 9.5
Multiple mediator models. (a) Uncorrelated mediators Z_1 and Z_2 occur simultaneously, (b) correlated mediators Z_1 and Z_2 occur simultaneously, (c) Z_1 influences Z_2, and (d) Z_3 occurs parallel to the sequence in which Z_1 influences Z_2.

There are other possible specifications of a multiple mediator model. For example, multiple mediators can have relationships with each other. The two mediators Z_1 and Z_2 can operate at the same stage, but be correlated with each other as in Figure 9.5b. The two mediators can also be linked sequentially (e.g. $Z_1 \rightarrow Z_2$) as in Figure 9.5c. In this example, the indirect effect of an independent variable X on a dependent variable Y operates through the chain of mediator variables Z_1 and Z_2. In Figure 9.5d, with an additional mediator Z_3, we represent a model with both simultaneous and sequential mediators. One can revise and extend these models represented in Figure 9.5 and create complex systems-based models with both simultaneous and sequential mediators and multiple independent variables and outcomes. Importantly, the specification for a multiple mediator model should be in line with theory, logic and prior evidence.

9.5.1 Specific Indirect Effects and Total Indirect Effects

One can evaluate both *specific indirect effects (SIEs)* and the *total indirect effect* (TIE) for the model represented in Figure 9.1. A SIE is the indirect effect for a particular mediator, controlling for the other mediators. The TIE is the summation of the SIEs (see Appendix). Depending on the application, one may only be interested in one or more SIE and/or the TIE.

In the application corresponding to Figure 9.1, we are interested in evaluating all the indirect pathways between each independent variable (*MS type* and *symptom onset*) and outcome (*depression* and *fatigue*). We are interested in assessing, separately, the SIEs of hand function and mobility impairment, to evaluate the individual contribution of each mediator. We are also interested in the TIE of functional impairment (*hand function* and *mobility impairment*) as a potential mechanism of change.

The reader should realize that it is possible for there to be significant mediation, but the TIE equals zero or near zero. For example, one can think of the special case with two mediators with two SIEs equal in effect size, but opposite in sign [29].

9.5.2 Testing Mediation Effects with the Multiple Mediator Multiple Outcome MS-Depression and Fatigue Model

Another physical performance test measuring mobility impairment (operationalized as an observed variable) in the data was the timed 25-foot walk. Depression was a latent variable with effect indicators of the nine items of the PHQ-9. We also used measures for fatigue, hand function impairment, MS type and time since symptom onset as previously described in this chapter in this data set.

In the structural model, we controlled for racial group (Caucasian or other), sex (male or female) and age in each regression equation. We used the ML estimator and the BC boot-strap with 10,000 replications in MPlus. Means, variances and covariances of the five exogenous variables (MS type, symptom onset, sex, race and age) were entered in the model to include all cases in the FIML procedure.

We reported standardized estimates to help evaluate the magnitude of the SIEs and TIEs given the vastly different scales for the measures under study. We determined that an effect should have at least a small effect size to signify some degree of clinical relevance. We denoted 0.10 as a small effect size. Thus, in order to report an effect size for some degree of clinical relevance, we would look to observe a standardized SIE (as the product of two pathways) of at least $0.10^2 = 0.01$ and a TIE of at least 0.02 (as the sum of two SIEs, while keeping in mind the contribution of each SIE).

The model did not show a good model fit according to the fit statistics and indices (see Table 9.3). The reader can review Chapter 4 for rule of thumb guidelines for the select measures reported in Table 9.3. Notably, RMSEA value was high (i.e. >0.08), and the CFI and TLI values were both low (i.e. <0.90). Therefore, a researcher should

- consider these results as exploratory
- modify the model and identify an alternative, better-fitting model before considering any findings as valid

Review Chapter 6 for recommended approaches to perform model modification using empirical criterion in conjunction with clinical theory.

The correlation between the two model outcomes *depression* and *fatigue* was moderately high (standardized estimate = 0.695). In Table 9.3 we present the statistically significant effects of interest.

The TIE for functional impairment (*hand function* and *mobility*) was statistically significant between each independent variable (*MS type, symptom onset*) and each outcome (*depression, fatigue*). The standardized TIE ranges from 0.024 to 0.046 (see Table 9.3). Thus, we can interpret this range as from small to slightly greater than small effect size [37]. In analyzing SIEs, *hand function* partially mediated the effects of both *MS type* and *symptom onset* on both *depression* and *fatigue*. *Mobility* was a partial mediator between *symptom onset* and *fatigue*, but the standardized SIE in this case was very small (0.008) and thus likely not

TABLE 9.3

Assessing Direct, Indirect and Total Effects for the Multiple Mediator Multiple Outcome MS-Depression and Fatigue Model

Pathway	Estimate	Lower	Upper
Symptom Onset → Depression			
Direct effect	−0.048	−0.092	−0.001
Total indirect effect	0.024	0.012	0.041
Specific Indirect Effect Via			
Hand function	0.020	0.010	0.035
MS Type → Depression			
Total effect	0.073	0.033	0.111
Total indirect effect	0.042	0.016	0.071
Specific Indirect Effect Via			
Hand function	0.036	0.014	0.062
Symptom Onset → Fatigue			
Total indirect effect	0.027	0.016	0.043
Specific Indirect Effects Via			
Hand function	0.020	0.010	0.033
Mobility	0.008	0.002	0.015
MS Type → Fatigue			
Total effect	0.079	0.043	0.114
Total indirect effect	0.046	0.022	0.072
Specific Indirect Effects Via			
Hand function	0.035	0.015	0.059

$\chi^2(92) = 2670.187$, $p \leq 0.001$; RMSEA (90% Confidence Interval) = 0.089 (0.086, 0.092); CFI = 0.862; TLI = 0.811; SRMR = 0.048. In the table, we reported only the 95% bias-corrected bootstrap confidence intervals (lower and upper limits) that do not contain zero. We used the ML option in MPlus. We used the STDYX option to report the standardized estimates involving the continuous independent variable Symptom Onset and the STDY option to report the standardized estimates involving the binary independent variable MS Type.

clinically relevant. In general, clinicians might consider high levels of functional impairment, with specific attention to hand function impairment, when tailoring care in patients with high levels of depressive symptoms or fatigue [31].

9.6 Noncontinuous Outcomes and Mediators

The formulas for assessing the total effect, indirect effect and direct effect defined above in this chapter apply for continuous mediators and outcomes. These definitions do not necessarily hold for non-continuous mediators and/or outcomes. For example, using logistic regression for a binary outcome or mediator, the product of coefficients methods and the difference of coefficients method are no longer equivalent. Since the residual variance is fixed in both logistic and probit regression, the scaling of the coefficients will also vary given binary mediators and/or outcomes. In the case of dichotomous mediators and/or outcomes, Mackinnon and Dwyer [27] recommended standardizing coefficients since coefficients become comparable under standardization. Then, using these standardized coefficients, the product of coefficients method and the difference of coefficients methods should lead to similar estimates of the indirect effect.

9.7 Causal Mediation Analysis

In addition to linear modeling assumptions, the classic paradigm for conducting mediation analysis in a treatment study assumes no treatment-mediator interaction. Many of the recent methodological advances in mediation have been developed using the causal inference framework for performing mediation analysis with nonlinearities and/or a treatment-mediator interaction.

Causal mediation analysis is the term for mediation analysis using causal inference methods. Typically, effects are defined for causal mediation analysis using the counterfactual framework and potential outcomes [38–44]. To very briefly explain counterfactuals, without loss of generality, consider a treatment-control study. One is assigned to only the treatment or control. As a result, the outcome is observed for each individual based on the level of assignment, either treatment or control. The counterfactual outcome for each individual is the outcome we cannot observe, based on the level not assigned. The interested reader can refer to the textbook by Morgan and Winship [45] for an introduction to counterfactuals and causal inference.

In causal mediation analysis, researchers can define mediation effects in a way that is not tied to a specific statistical model and identify them under certain assumptions of no unmeasured confounding [38–44]. In latent variable software programs such as MPlus, one can additionally include latent independent, mediator and outcome variables as continuous variables in a model used for causal mediation analysis [46].

In Table 9.4, we present some basic definitions for causal mediation analysis. In much of the literature, the independent variable (e.g. treatment variable) is referred to as the "exposure." The term "exposure" in epidemiology can be broadly applied to any factor that may be associated with an outcome of interest [47]. The binary exposure variable (X) used as the independent variable in Table 9.4 is a dummy variable for the intervention ($X = 1$) or control ($X = 0$). M is the mediator and Y is the outcome.

The reader should note that throughout the causal mediation analysis literature, as a growing field, there are many variations in the general nomenclature listed in Table 9.4.

9.7.1 No Unmeasured Confounding Assumptions for Causal Mediation

The *no unmeasured confounding* assumptions for identifying causally defined effects for mediation are strong. These assumptions include (1) no unmeasured exposure-outcome confounding, (2) no mediator-outcome confounding, (3) no exposure-mediator confounding and (4) no mediator-outcome confounder affected by exposure. Under assumptions (1)

TABLE 9.4

Definitions of Some Causally-Defined Effects for Causal Mediation Analysis

Controlled Direct Effect (CDE): Expected change in the outcome as the level of exposure changes from control to intervention when the mediator is set to a fixed level *m*.

Natural Direct Effect (NDE): Expected change in the outcome as the level of exposure changes from control to intervention when the mediator is set to a fixed level as it would have obtained under the control.

Natural Indirect Effect (NIE): Expected change in the outcome when the level of exposure is set to intervention and the mediator changes to the level it would have obtained under the intervention.

Total Effect (TE): is the expected change in the outcome as the exposure changes from control to intervention. Formally,

$$CDE = E[Y(1,m) - Y(0,m)]$$

$$NDE = E[Y(1,M(0)) - Y(0,M(0)]$$

$$NIE = E[Y(1,M(1)) - Y(1,M(0)]$$

$$TE = NDE + NIE = E[Y(1) - Y(0)]$$

(9.5)

For the outcome *Y*, the first index is 1 if *X* is the intervention and 0 if *X* is the control. The second index for the NDE and NIE is the value that the mediator obtains under the specified value of *X*. In the CDE, the mediator is set to a fixed level *m*. The TE can be calculated as the sum of the NDE and NIE.

and (2), the CDE is identified from the data [41,46]. Under all four assumptions, the NDE and NIE are identified from the data [41,46]. Even if a treatment is perfectly randomized, this still would not guarantee the assumption of no mediator-outcome confounding. In the typical experimental study, as mentioned in Chapter 1, one does not randomize based on levels of the mediator [41,46]. Under these strong assumptions it is then possible to well define causal mediation effects.

Sensitivity analyses have been developed to examine the robustness of the results under various scenarios of unmeasured confounding [44,46]. The interested reader should refer to Imai et al. [44] and Muthén and Asparouhov [46] for more discussion about sensitivity analyses in causal mediation analysis.

The CDE could be of interest in evaluating policy interventions (assessing pathways not through the mediator) [39,40,46]. The NDE and NIE, on the other hand, will be of greater interest in assessing mediation and for effect decomposition [46]. In defining causally defined effects in Table 9.4, for simplicity, we used a binary exposure variable as the independent variable. These definitions can be extended for a continuous independent variable [48]. In causal mediation analysis with linear models (and no exposure-mediator interaction term) as in equations (9.1) and (9.2), standard definitions hold as CDE = NDE = *c'* (independent of level *m*) and NIE = *ab*.

9.7.2 Exposure-Mediator Interaction

If the estimate of the direct effect varies across different levels of the mediator, then the exposure and mediator might interact in explaining the outcome [49,50]. Not modeling such an interaction that should be in the model compromises the examination of the indirect effect, potentially leading to incorrect causal conclusions [51].

Conceptually, however, there may not be a strong justification to include the exposure-mediator interaction term in many models in health and medicine. As a parallel, Muthén and Asparouhov [46] mention that in their experience the exposure-mediator interaction

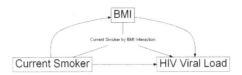

FIGURE 9.6
Smoking-HIV viral load mediation model for people living with HIV.

Model includes an exposure-mediator (i.e. current smoker by BMI) interaction term. We controlled for age in each of the structural equations in the model. BMI = body mass index.

effect is not often found in behavioral science applications [46]. Nevertheless, if this interaction is present then estimates of direct and indirect effects will be inaccurate if formulas are not adjusted for the presence of this interaction term [52].

9.7.3 Binary Outcome, Continuous Mediator Smoking-HIV Viral Load Example

Obesity has been linked with numerous deleterious health outcomes, including hypertension, diabetes, heart disease, myocardial infarction and stroke [53,54]. Cigarette smoking is associated with many of the same health risks as obesity, in addition to lung cancer.

Some past studies [55,56] have found possessing a heavier than normal BMI is associated with improved immunological health in HIV positive subjects. Cigarette smoking has been found to be associated with lower viral suppression rates (higher viral load) in HIV positive subjects [57]. Cigarette smoking has also been associated with lower BMI, due to appetite suppression among other factors, in HIV positive subjects [56].

In a study sample of 1,315 people living with HIV, we were interested in testing if being a current smoker (yes or no) leads to a lower BMI which in turn leads to lower viral suppression rates (see Figure 9.6). This data set consisted of complete cases extracted from an electronic health records data base (2012–2018) at a public health care system located in Cleveland, OH. The variable used for HIV viral load was binary of either detected ($\geq$200 copies/mL) or not detected (<200 copies/mL). In a person living with HIV, a not detected viral load means there is less HIV in one's body even though the virus is still present. We modeled the probability of a not detected HIV viral load. In each of the structural equations in the model, we controlled for age. We also included the interaction term between current smoker and BMI (exposure-mediator interaction term) for illustration purposes. Therefore, the two structural equations in the model included: (1) regression of HIV viral load on current smoker, BMI, age and the interaction of current smoker by BMI and (2) regression of BMI on current smoker and age.

A probit regression approach was used to estimate model parameters in MPlus. We used an ML estimator and the BC bootstrap with 10,000 replications.[8] The interaction of current smoker and BMI in explaining the outcome had a confidence interval that contained zero with an estimate = 0.022 (95% BC bootstrap confidence interval [CI] = −0.002, 0.047). The regression path estimate from current smoker to BMI had a confidence interval that did not contain zero with an estimate = −1.726 (95% BC bootstrap CI = −2.374, −1.016).

---

[8] MPlus can automatically calculate and test the significance of causally defined effects (for a single mediator and a single outcome) based on counterfactuals with the MODEL INDIRECT statement starting from Version 7.2. The IND option can be used when there is no moderation. The MOD option is used to specify these causally defined effects when there is moderation. The MOD option is necessary when one specifies an exposure-mediator interaction term.

The regression path estimate from BMI to HIV viral load had a confidence interval that did contain zero with an estimate = 0.009 (95% BC bootstrap CI = −0.007, 0.024).

Some selected MPlus output for this causal mediation analysis is in Box 9.3. We used the variable names *HIVVL* for HIV viral load and *SMK* for current smoker. The definitions for `Tot natural IE` (total natural indirect effect) and `Pure natural DE` (pure natural direct effect) correspond to our definitions of the NIE and NDE, respectively.

Box 9.3 includes the NIE, NDE and total effect point estimates and 95% BC bootstrap confidence intervals (lower and upper limits) for this analysis. The confidence interval for the NIE does not contain zero. This indicates a significant drop in the probability of a lower HIV viral load due to the indirect effect of being a current smoker. The confidence interval for the total effect also does not contain zero. However, the confidence interval does contain zero for the NDE. Odds ratio estimates are also provided in Box 9.3. For example, the odds ratio for the NIE is estimated as 0.903 and the confidence interval (0.825, 0.961) does not contain one.

In summary of these results, the total effect is significant, NDE is not significant and NIE is significant. We would have violated a condition for even partial mediation via the Baron and Kenny approach since the regression path estimate from BMI to HIV viral load is not statistically significant (i.e. Z is not significantly related to Y). Under a less restrictive approach, we would conclude that mediation is present since the NIE was statistically significant via the bootstrap method [16]. The regression path estimate from current smoker to BMI is negative, indicating that being a current smoker leads to a lower BMI. The NIE is negative. Thus, we can infer from these results that the indirect effect of being a current smoker leads a significant drop in the probability of a not detected HIV viral load.

This analysis was presented for illustration purposes, but for application we would have omitted the current smoker-BMI interaction term from our model. This could be argued in two ways:

- omitting the interaction term from the initial model based on theory
- testing the interaction term and then removing it since it was not statistically significant.

BOX 9.3

CONFIDENCE INTERVALS OF TOTAL, INDIRECT, AND DIRECT EFFECTS BASED ON COUNTERFACTUALS (CAUSALLY-DEFINED EFFECTS)

```
      Lower 2.5% Estimate Upper 2.5%
Effects from SMK to HIVVL

  Tot natural IE -0.020  -0.009  -0.004
  Pure natural DE -0.053  -0.020   0.008
  Total effect  -0.062  -0.029  -0.003

Odds ratios for binary Y

  Tot natural IE  0.825   0.903   0.961
  Pure natural DE 0.622   0.824   1.101
  Total effect  0.565   0.744   0.979
```

The latter case would suppose that we theorized that the interaction term should be included in the initial model and omitted it since it was not statistically significant. We did re-run the analysis with no interaction term and our findings were similar. However, the authors of this book might lean toward the first argument of omission from the initial model. We do not find a current smoker-BMI interactive term theoretically warranted in addition to the influence of current smoker on BMI.

9.8 Moderation Analysis

The risk of cardiovascular disease may be higher in people living with HIV compared to the general population [58]. Hypertension is a well-known traditional risk factor for cardiovascular disease [59]. We hypothesized that within our sample of people living with HIV, having a not detected (vs. detected) HIV viral load decreases the level of systolic blood pressure (SBP).

Chronological aging is also a traditional risk factor for both hypertension and cardiovascular disease [60]. However, there is also a precedent for a beneficial, modifying effect of older age for disease control. For example, adults with type 2 diabetes (DM2) of an older age may have better disease control compared to their younger counterparts [61–64]. This finding was not attributed to accumulated wisdom or due to shorter disease duration [61–64]. Some possible explanations are that certain subgroups of older aged individuals (1) have genetic and environmental factors that have allowed them to thrive over time despite having a serious physical condition or (2) experience a milder, later onset version of the physical condition. Another explanation could be that persons with poorer control are less likely to be present at older ages because their poor health status caused them to die earlier and not be present in the data.

In this example, we simply tested if age changes the strength of the relationship between HIV viral load and SBP. We hypothesized while older age increases SBP the interactive effect (moderation effect) of older age and a not detected viral load leads to a lower SBP.

An example of a path diagram with this hypothesized moderator for age is shown in Figure 9.7.

We used the same study sample as the smoking-HIV viral load example in the previous section for this analysis. The SBP variable contained additional missing values; thus here, N=1,267 after using listwise deletion. The corresponding fitted regression equation for Figure 9.7 using the ML estimator in MPlus included an interaction term between the moderator and independent variable:

$$SBP = 128.351 - 2.027 \text{ HIV Viral Load} + 0.236 \text{ Age} - 0.112 \text{ HIV Viral Load} \times \text{Age} \tag{9.6}$$

$$(0.827) \quad (0.987) \qquad\qquad (0.057) \quad (0.074)$$

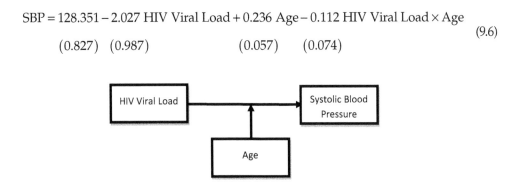

FIGURE 9.7
Relationship between HIV viral load and systolic blood pressure, moderated by age.

We reported the BC bootstrap standard errors using 10,000 bootstrap replications under each path estimate in parenthesis in equation (9.6).

We centered the continuous variable for age. The variable *age* in equation (9.6) is the variable for centered age. In centering age, we subtracted each subject's age by the mean age for the sample (Age = 41.651, SD = 12.588). As a result, the variable for centered age across the sample had a mean close to zero.

The centering of age was done for a more meaningful interpretation of the model intercept when including an interaction term in the model. The intercept in (9.6) can be interpreted as the predicted SBP for a subject of an average age in this sample with a detected HIV viral load. Only continuous independent variables should be centered for interpretation of the model intercept; it is not necessary to center categorical predictors or the dependent variable for this purpose. For simplicity, we do not control for any additional covariates in this illustrative example.

In Figure 9.8, we illustrate the moderation effect of HIV viral load on SBP. In the sample, we defined low centered age as −13 (one standard deviation below the mean), medium centered age as 0 (mean centered age) and high centered age as 13 (one standard deviation above the mean). This then roughly equated to low age = 29, medium age = 42 and high age = 55 within the study population. We classified each individual in the dataset into one of three age groups according to centered age: less than or equal to -13 (N=263), -13<centered age<13 (N=808), or greater than or equal to 13 (N=196). Then, we calculated the mean SBP in each age group at each level of viral load (detected, not detected). The figure shows that, on average, older subjects with a not detected viral load have a lower blood pressure than individuals with a detected viral load. The slope in the plot appears to decrease with a sharper decline for high age than for medium age or low age. The 95% confidence bands overlap in this figure for high and medium age.

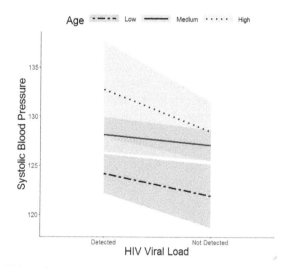

FIGURE 9.8

Plot of systolic blood pressure against HIV viral load by levels of age (*N* = 1,315).

In this figure, we define low age as −13 (one standard deviation below the mean), medium age as 0 (mean centered age) and high age as 13 (one standard deviation above the mean). This then roughly equated to low age = 29, medium age = 42 and high age = 55 within our sample.

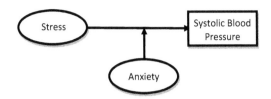

FIGURE 9.9
Relationship between *stress* and systolic blood pressure, moderated by *anxiety*.

In the regression analysis performed for this example, the 95% BC bootstrap confidence interval did contain zero for the interaction term (−0.258, 0.036) but not for the main terms for HIV viral load (−3.938, −0.100) and age (0.125, 0.349). In summary, we found that a lower HIV viral load and older age lead to a significant increase in SBP, but no overall moderation of the effect of HIV viral load by age on SBP. However, both the plot in Figure 9.8 and the model point estimate in (9.6) still indicate that high age as compared to other age groups may have some beneficial effect in lowering SBP for individuals with a not detected viral load.

Interaction terms in SEM can involve latent variables [65]. For example, we hypothesize that the level of *anxiety* moderates the relationship between *stress* and *SBP* (Figure 9.9). *Anxiety* and *stress* are latent variables, while *SBP* is an observed variable. The *latent moderated structural equations method* is one that is built into MPlus software for handling interaction terms between latent variables [65,66].[9]

9.9 Mediation Process Accounting for Moderation

A mediation process can account for moderation. For example, we present such a model in Figure 9.10a. In the model, we hypothesize an indirect relationship between socioeconomic position (SEP) and SBP through number of comorbidities [58].

In Figure 9.10a, we hypothesize that lower SEP leads to a higher number of comorbidities which leads to higher SBP. We also hypothesize lower SEP leads to a lower SBP. In Figure 9.10a, we account for the moderator age in this mediation process. In Figure 9.10a, age is hypothesized as a moderator of every relationship in the mediation process. We have a theoretical underpinning that higher SEP and younger age has a beneficial effect, leading to a lower number of comorbidities and lower SBP. Further, we hypothesize in Figure 9.10a that a lower number of comorbidities and younger age also lead to lower SBP.

In practice, one should hypothesize moderation for the regression paths in which it is theoretically warranted, which may be a subset of all paths. In Figure 9.10b, we omit hypothesized moderation of the mediator-outcome path. We may not have substantial theory to hypothesize an age by number of comorbidities interactive effect on SBP after accounting for other model relationships in Figure 9.10b. That is, we may hypothesize that having a higher number of comorbidities leads to higher SBP comparably across all age groups.

---

[9] XWITH is used to specify an interaction term between latent variables. For example, within the MODEL statement for performing analysis for the model corresponding to Figure 9.9, we could use a line of code to define an interaction term (which we will call sXa) between *stress* and *anxiety*: sXa | stress XWITH anxiety;

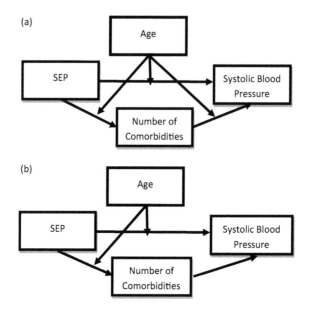

FIGURE 9.10
Mediation models accounting for moderation. (a) All paths moderated by age and (b) no moderation by age for the path between number of comorbidities and systolic blood pressure.

The moderator can be a variable outside of the mediation process, such as age in Figure 9.10. The moderator can also be a variable that is already part of the mediation process. In the section on causal mediation analysis, we discussed an interaction term between the exposure and mediator under the hypothesis that the strength of the relationship between the exposure and the outcome would vary by the level of the mediator.

9.9.1 Mediated Moderation and Moderated Mediation

In *mediated moderation,* the effect of the moderator is mediated. Mediated moderation involves an overall moderation of the exposure effect on the outcome [67]. The moderation of the exposure effect should be reduced in absolute value after accounting for the mediator (or equal to zero in the case of "full" mediated moderation) [67]. Consider the SEP-SBP example in both Figure 9.10a and b. For mediated moderation, initially, the interactive effect of SEP by age on SBP should be significant and substantively meaningful before accounting for the mediator number of comorbidities (i.e. overall moderation by age of the effect of SEP on SBP). Then, after accounting for the mediator in an appropriate model (e.g. model corresponding to Figure 9.10b), the interactive effect of SEP by age on SBP should be reduced in absolute value for mediated moderation.

In *moderated mediation,* the effect of the mediator is moderated. In moderated mediation, there is no overall moderation of the exposure effect on the outcome [67]. The prototype of moderated mediation is that the indirect effect of the exposure on the outcome still depends on the level of the moderator [67]. That is, the moderation of the exposure effect should be significant and substantively meaningful after accounting for the mediator. In the SEP-SBP example for moderated mediation, initially, the interactive effect of SEP by age on SBP is *not* significant and substantively meaningful before accounting for the mediator number of comorbidities (i.e. *no* overall moderation by age of the effect of SEP on SBP). However, for moderated mediation, the indirect effect of SEP on SBP through the mediator number of comorbidities depends on the level of age after accounting for the mediator, using the appropriate model (e.g. model corresponding to Figure 9.10b). The interested reader should refer to Muller et al. [67] for an introduction to mediated moderation and moderated mediation.

In a mediation model accounting for moderation, the indirect, direct and total effects are defined conditional on the level of the moderator. For example, age as a moderator could be categorized into low, medium and high age or, given a very large sample, as deciles of age. Then, one could explicitly calculate the conditional indirect, direct and total effect at each chosen level of the moderator. When the moderator is at level zero (e.g. centered variable Age = 0), given linear mediation and moderation, then the standard definitions for mediation analysis from (9.3) hold for the IE, DE and TE.

Stride has provided a helpful resource, a web page with links to Mplus code (http://offbeat. group.shef.ac.uk/FIO/mplusmedmod.htm), for testing different configurations of models for mediation, moderation and mediation accounting for moderation [68]. The web page includes derivations of the formulas for the indirect, direct and total effects in different configurations of models. Additionally, moderation analysis for a mediation process using causally defined effects can be performed using MPlus Version 7.2 and above[10] [66].

9.10 Moderation Analysis Using Multigroup Modeling

Multiple group (MG; also termed *multigroup*) models are stratified models. For example, MG models across sex would include Model MEN using data from men in a sample and Model FEMALE using data for females in a sample. One can use a multigroup framework for making group comparisons as appropriate for most of the models discussed in this book. In Chapter 10, we will discuss multigroup comparisons of a measurement model in the context of measurement equivalence and extensions to a structural model. Here we focus on multigroup path analysis.

Consider the MG approach to test for equality across groups of a structural model with only observed variables. In terms of notation, one either subscripts or superscripts regression parameters to allow for group differences. For example, for multigroup analysis to be conducted using continuous observed variables for h groups we can extend equation 3.4 in Chapter 3 and use the equations:

$$\mathbf{y}^{(g)} = \boldsymbol{\alpha}_y^{(g)} + \mathbf{B}^{(g)}\mathbf{y}^{(g)} + \boldsymbol{\Gamma}^{(g)}\mathbf{x}^{(g)} + \boldsymbol{\zeta}^{(g)} \tag{9.7}$$

where $g = 1, ..., h$.

Multigroup modeling can be used to perform moderator analysis with a categorical moderator such as sex or race/ethnicity. A sufficiently large sample size is necessary within each group of a strata variable used for multigroup modeling. As a result, typically researchers use only a handful of categories (e.g. dichotomous split) for a grouping variable. This makes a variable such as sex with male and female strata very practical for multigroup modeling. Under these sample size considerations, categorizing variables such as area deprivation index, number of comorbidities or age for multigroup analyses can

---

[10] See the addendum for MPlus Version 7.2 in the user's guide available at www.statmodel.com for code for using the MOD option in the MODEL INDIRECT statement for testing different configurations of models for a mediation process accounting for moderation [65].

be done. However, alternatively, given that these variables are continuous (or consist of many ordered categories), one could treat them as continuous moderators and study each moderator effect as an interaction. Note that one can also study the effect of a categorical moderator as an interaction and does not necessitate multigroup analysis.

Consider the simple regression of SBP on BMI (Figure 9.11). To evaluate for a moderation effect by sex, one could compare two nested multigroup models. In model M1, the regression slopes across the MALE model (γ_{MALE}) and FEMALE model (γ_{FEMALE}) are freely estimated. In model M2, these regression slopes are constrained to be equal ($\gamma_{MALE} = \gamma_{FEMALE}$) across the MALE model and FEMALE model. One can then test for equality across groups by using chi-square difference testing to test for differences between models M2 and M1.

We again used the study sample of people living with HIV to conduct multigroup path analysis for the model represented in Figure 9.11. We hypothesize that a higher BMI leads to increased levels of SBP and that the strength of this relationship may be differ by sex. After listwise deletion, the sample for this illustrative example consisted of 287 males and 984 females. We used the MLR option in MPlus to conduct this stratified analysis.

Model M1 is the saturated model with no informative fit measures. Model M2 had a Satorra-Bentler scaled chi-square statistic = 3.59 ($p = 0.058$; MLR correction factor = 0.984). Therefore, conducting the Satorra-Bentler scaled chi-square test for model M2 is equivalent to conducting the Satorra-Bentler scaled difference test in comparing model M2 to the saturated model. We can conclude that constraining the slope to be equal across groups does not lead to a worse fit (since $p > 0.05$) and there is equality in the slope across males and females (i.e. no significant moderation effect by sex). Also, we find that using model

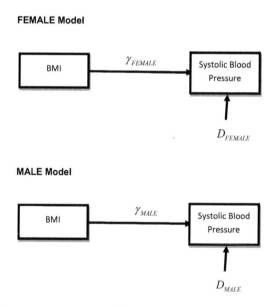

FIGURE 9.11
Relationship between body mass index and systolic blood pressure, moderated by sex. (a) FEMALE model and (b) MALE model.

Here γ_{FEMALE} is the slope for relating body mass index (BMI) to systolic blood pressure, D_{FEMALE} is the error term for the FEMALE model, γ_{MALE} is the slope for relating body mass index to systolic blood pressure and D_{MALE} is the error term for the MALE model. The MALE and FEMALE models also include intercepts (not shown).

M2 a one unit increase in the BMI leads to an increase in SBP ($\hat{\gamma}_{\text{MALE}} = \hat{\gamma}_{\text{FEMALE}} = 0.896$, S.E. $= 0.078$, $p < 0.001$).

The simple moderation model from this example can be extended in many flexible ways. For example, one could conduct mediation analysis accounting for moderation for a categorical moderator using the multigroup framework. A less restricted model can be specified in which one freely estimates parameters (given identification constraints) across groups. Then, a more restricted model constrains the indirect effect to be equal across groups. If the fit is worse (via chi-square difference testing or other multigroup model fit comparison standards) under the more restricted model, this would indicate group differences on the indirect pathway.

9.11 Conclusions

In this chapter, we discussed approaches for testing mediation and moderation in a structural model. A structural model can be specified for a specific research study and evaluated to address scientific goals. For example, these goals might include understanding mechanisms of change (mediators) in intervention research or research involving disease pathways and progression. The structural model is also commonly used to evaluate variables (moderators) that change the strength of an effect for more generalizable results.

Complex systems-based models in health and medicine may include latent variables and multiple independent variables, moderators, mediators and/or outcomes. These models can be used to test research hypotheses of interest of mediation and/or moderation with large observational data sets using approaches and extensions of approaches discussed in this chapter.

We did not discuss mediation analysis for longitudinal data in this chapter. We discuss this topic in Chapter 13 after introducing longitudinal models.

Appendix

Consider a model with a single independent variable and a single outcome and J mediators operating jointly at the same stage and uncorrelated with each other. One can calculate the total indirect effect (TIE) for this model as the summation of the J specific indirect effects:

$$\text{TIE} = \sum_{j=1}^{J} a_j b_j \qquad (9.8)$$

Thus, the total effect (TE) from an independent variable to an outcome in this model:

$$\text{TE} = c' + \sum_{j=1}^{J} a_j b_j \qquad (9.9)$$

For more on the classic theory for decomposition of direct, indirect and total effects see Alwin and Hauser [69].

References

1. Beal, C.C., A.K. Stuifbergen, and A. Brown, Depression in multiple sclerosis: A longitudinal analysis. *Archives of Psychiatric Nursing*, 2007. **21**(4): pp. 181–191.
2. Brown, R., et al., Longitudinal assessment of anxiety, depression, and fatigue in people with multiple sclerosis. *Psychology and Psychotherapy: Theory, Research and Practice*, 2009. **82**(1): pp. 41–56.
3. Krupp, L.B., *Fatigue in multiple sclerosis: A guide to diagnosis and management*. 2004, New York: Demos Medical Publishing.
4. Gunzler, D., et al., Disentangling multiple sclerosis and depression: An adjusted depression screening score for patient-centered care. *Journal of Behavioral Medicine*, 2015. **38**(2): pp. 237–250.
5. Kline, R.B., *Principles and practice of structural equation modeling, fourth edition*. 2016, New York: Guilford Press.
6. Bollen, K., *Structural equations with latent variables*. 1989, New York, NY: Wiley.
7. Gunzler, D., et al., Introduction to mediation analysis with structural equation modeling. *Shanghai Archives of Psychiatry*, 2013. **25**(6): pp. 390–394.
8. Baron, R.M. and D.A. Kenny, The moderator–mediator variable distinction in social psychological research: Conceptual, strategic, and statistical considerations. *Journal of Personality and Social Psychology*, 1986. **51**(6): p. 1173.
9. MacKinnon, D.P., A.J. Fairchild, and M.S. Fritz, Mediation analysis. *Annual Review of Psychology*, 2007. **58**: pp. 593–614.
10. MacKinnon, D., *Introduction to statistical mediation analysis*. 2012, Abingdon: Routledge.
11. Schwartz, C.E., T. Vollmer, and H. Lee, Reliability and validity of two self-report measures of impairment and disability for MS. North American Research Consortium on multiple sclerosis outcomes study group. *Neurology*, 1999. **52**(1): pp. 63–70.
12. Wu, X., et al., Potential mediating biomarkers underlying the association of body mass index or waist circumference with blood pressure: Results from three population-based studies. *Scientific Reports*, 2017. **7**(1): p. 5364.
13. Chaparro, M.P., et al., Neighborhood deprivation and biomarkers of health in Britain: The mediating role of the physical environment. *BMC Public Health*, 2018. **18**(1): p. 801.
14. Little, T.D., Card, N.A., Bovaird, J.A., Preacher, K.J., Crandall, C.S., et al., Structural equation modeling of mediation and moderation with contextual factors, in *Modeling contextual effects in longitudinal studies*, T.D. Little J.A. Bovaird, and N.A. Card, Editors. 2012, Abingdon, Mahwah, NJ: Lawrence Erlbaum Associates Publishers. pp. 207–230.
15. Krause, M.R., et al., Testing mediation in nursing research: Beyond Baron and Kenny. *Nursing Research*, 2010. **59**(4): pp. 288–294.
16. Zhao, X., J.G. Lynch Jr, and Q. Chen, Reconsidering Baron and Kenny: Myths and truths about mediation analysis. *Journal of Consumer Research*, 2010. **37**(2): pp. 197–206.
17. Preacher, K.J. and A.F. Hayes, Asymptotic and resampling strategies for assessing and comparing indirect effects in multiple mediator models. *Behavior Research Methods*, 2008. **40**(3): pp. 879–891.
18. Collins, L.M., J.J. Graham, and B.P. Flaherty, An alternative framework for defining mediation. *Multivariate Behavioral Research*, 1998. **33**(2): pp. 295–312.
19. Judd, C.M. and D.A. Kenny, Process analysis: Estimating mediation in treatment evaluations. *Evaluation Review*, 1981. **5**(5): pp. 602–619.
20. Kenny, D., D. Kashy, and N. Bolger, Data analysis in social psychology, in *The handbook of social psychology*, D. Gilbert, S. Fiske, and G. Lindzey, Editors, Vol. 1. 1998, Boston, MA: McGraw-Hill, pp. 233–265.
21. MacKinnon, D.P., Analysis of mediating variables in prevention and intervention research. *NIDA Research Monograph*, 1994. **139**: pp. 127–127.
22. Rose, J.S., et al., Contrasts in multiple mediator models, in *Multivariate applications in substance use research*, J.S. Rose, L. Chassin, C. Presson, and S J. Sherman, Editors. 2000, New York: Psychology Press. pp. 155–174.

23. MacKinnon, D.P., J.L. Krull, and C.M. Lockwood, Equivalence of the mediation, confounding and suppression effect. *Prevention Science*, 2000. **1**(4): pp. 173–181.
24. Shrout, P.E. and N. Bolger, Mediation in experimental and nonexperimental studies: new procedures and recommendations. *Psychological Methods*, 2002. **7**(4): p. 422.
25. Sobel, M.E., Asymptotic confidence intervals for indirect effects in structural equation models. *Sociological Methodology*, 1982. **13**: pp. 290–312.
26. Sobel, M.E., Some new results on indirect effects and their standard errors in covariance structure models. *Sociological Methodology*, 1986. **16**: pp. 159–186.
27. MacKinnon, D.P. and J.H. Dwyer, Estimating mediated effects in prevention studies. *Evaluation Review*, 1993. **17**(2): pp. 144–158.
28. Valente, M.J., et al., A note on testing mediated effects in structural equation models: Reconciling past and current research on the performance of the test of joint significance. *Educational and Psychological Measurement*, 2016. **76**(6): pp. 889–911.
29. Kenny, D.A. *Mediation*. 2018 [cited 2018 August 23]; Available from: http://davidakenny.net/cm/mediate.htm.
30. Preacher, K.J. and J.P. Selig, Advantages of Monte Carlo confidence intervals for indirect effects. *Communication Methods and Measures*, 2012. **6**(2): pp. 77–98.
31. Gunzler, D., Morris, N, Perznski A, Miller D, Lewis S, Bermel RA, Mediation analysis of co-occurring conditions for complex longitudinal clinical data. *SM Journal of Biometrics and Biostatistics* 2017. **1**(1): p. 1004.
32. MacKinnon, D.P., C.M. Lockwood, and J. Williams, Confidence limits for the indirect effect: Distribution of the product and resampling methods. *Multivariate Behavioral Research*, 2004. **39**(1): pp. 99–128.
33. MacKinnon, D.P., *Introduction to statistical mediation analysis*. 2008, Abingdon: Routledge.
34. Fritz, M.S., A.B. Taylor, and D.P. MacKinnon, Explanation of two anomalous results in statistical mediation analysis. *Multivariate Behavioral Research*, 2012. **47**(1): pp. 61–87.
35. Gunzler, D., et al., A class of distribution-free models for longitudinal mediation analysis. *Psychometrika*, 2014. **79**(4): pp. 543–568.
36. Hair, J.F., C. Ringle, and M. Sarstedt, PLS-SEM: Indeed a silver bullet. *Journal of Marketing Theory and Practice*, 2011. **19**: pp. 139–151.
37. Cohen, J., A power primer. *Psychological Bulletin*, 1992. **112**(1): p. 155.
38. Loeys, T., et al., Flexible mediation analysis in the presence of nonlinear relations: Beyond the mediation formula. *Multivariate Behavioral Research*, 2013. **48**(6): pp. 871–894.
39. Robins, J.M., *Semantics of causal DAG models and the identification of direct and indirect effects*. 2003, New York: Oxford University Press, pp. 70–81.
40. Pearl, J. Direct and indirect effects. Proceedings of the Seventeenth Conference on Uncertainty in Artificial Intelligence, Seattle, WA, 2001. Morgan Kaufmann Publishers Inc.
41. Valeri, L. and T.J. VanderWeele, Mediation analysis allowing for exposure–mediator interactions and causal interpretation: Theoretical assumptions and implementation with SAS and SPSS macros. *Psychological Methods*, 2013. **18**(2): p. 137.
42. Muthén, B., Applications of causally defined direct and indirect effects in mediation analysis using SEM in Mplus. Manuscript submitted for publication, 2011. https://www.statmodel.com/download/causalmediation.pdf
43. Pearl, J., Causal inference in statistics: An overview. *Statistics Surveys*, 2009. **3**: pp. 96–146.
44. Imai, K., L. Keele, and D. Tingley, A general approach to causal mediation analysis. *Psychological Methods*, 2010. **15**(4): p. 309.
45. Morgan, S.L. and C. Winship, Counterfactuals and causal inference: Methods and principles for social research, 2nd Edition. 2014, Cambridge: Cambridge University Press.
46. Muthén, B. and T. Asparouhov, Causal effects in mediation modeling: An introduction with applications to latent variables. *Structural Equation Modeling: A Multidisciplinary Journal*, 2015. **22**(1): pp. 12–23.
47. Velentgas, P., et al., *Developing a protocol for observational comparative effectiveness research: a user's guide*. 2013, Washington, DC: Government Printing Office.

48. Wang, W. and B. Zhang, Assessing natural direct and indirect effects for a continuous exposure and a dichotomous outcome. *Journal of Statistical Theory and Practice*, 2016. **10**(3): pp. 574–587.

49. VanderWeele, T., *Explanation in causal inference: Methods for mediation and interaction*. 2015: Oxford: Oxford University Press.

50. Liu, S.-H., et al., Implementation and reporting of causal mediation analysis in 2015: A systematic review in epidemiological studies. *BMC Research Notes*, 2016. **9**: p. 354.

51. Fairchild, A.J. and H.L. McDaniel, Best (but oft-forgotten) practices: Mediation analysis. *The American Journal of Clinical Nutrition*, 2017. **105**(6): pp. 1259–1271.

52. VanderWeele, T.J. and S. Vansteelandt, Conceptual issues concerning mediation, interventions and composition. *Statistics and Its Interface*, 2009. **2**(4): pp. 457–468.

53. Artham, S.M., et al., Obesity and hypertension, heart failure, and coronary heart disease-risk factor, paradox, and recommendations for weight loss. *The Ochsner Journal*, 2009. **9**(3): pp. 124–132.

54. Lavie, C.J., et al., Obesity and cardiovascular diseases: Implications regarding fitness, fatness, and severity in the obesity paradox. *Journal of the American College of Cardiology*, 2014. **63**(14): pp. 1345–1354.

55. Blashill, A.J., et al., Body mass index, immune status and virological control in HIV-infected men who have sex with men. *Journal of the International Association of Providers of AIDS Care*, 2013. **12**(5): pp. 319–324.

56. Obry-Roguet, V., et al., Risk factors associated with overweight and obesity in HIV-infected people: Aging, behavioral factors but not cART in a cross-sectional study. *Medicine*, 2018. **97**(23): p. e10956.

57. Pollack, T.M., et al., Cigarette smoking is associated with high HIV viral load among adults presenting for antiretroviral therapy in Vietnam. *PLoS One*, 2017. **12**(3): p. e0173534.

58. Okello, S., et al., Association between HIV and blood pressure in adults and role of body weight as a mediator: Cross-sectional study in Uganda. *The Journal of Clinical Hypertension*, 2017. **19**(11): pp. 1181–1191.

59. Rapsomaniki, E., et al., Blood pressure and incidence of twelve cardiovascular diseases: Lifetime risks, healthy life-years lost, and age-specific associations in 1· 25 million people. *The Lancet*, 2014. **383**(9932): pp. 1899–1911.

60. Dhingra, R. and R.S. Vasan, Age as a risk factor. *The Medical Clinics of North America*, 2012. **96**(1): pp. 87–91.

61. Partnership, B.H., Better Health Partnership's 18th Annual Report. 2017.

62. Cebul, R.D., et al., Electronic health records and quality of diabetes care. *New England Journal of Medicine*, 2011. **365**(9): pp. 825–833.

63. Sajatovic, M., et al., A preliminary analysis of individuals with serious mental illness and comorbid diabetes. *Archives of Psychiatric Nursing*, 2016. **30**(2): pp. 226–229.

64. Sajatovic, M., et al., Clinical characteristics of individuals with serious mental illness and type 2 diabetes. *Psychiatric Services*, 2015, **66**(2): pp. 197–199.

65. Maslowsky, J., J. Jager, and D. Hemken, Estimating and interpreting latent variable interactions: A tutorial for applying the latent moderated structural equations method. *International Journal of Behavioral Development*, 2015. **39**(1): pp. 87–96.

66. Muthén, L.K. and B.O. Muthén, *Mplus: The comprehensive modelling program for applied researchers: User's guide*. Eighth edition, 1998–2017, Los Angeles, CA: Muthén & Muthén.

67. Muller, D., C.M. Judd, and V.Y. Yzerbyt, When moderation is mediated and mediation is moderated. *Journal of Personality and Social Psychology*, 2005. **89**(6): p. 852.

68. Stride, C., et al., Mplus code for mediation, moderation and moderated mediation models, 2016, pp. 1–80.

69. Alwin, D.F. and R.M. Hauser, The decomposition of effects in path analysis. *American Sociological Review*, 1975. **40**: pp. 37–47.

10

Measurement Bias, Multiple Indicator Multiple Cause Modeling and Multiple Group Modeling

10.1 Introduction to Measurement Bias

The possibility exists that individuals respond to questions on surveys, questionnaires, scales and tests about themselves differently depending on their backgrounds (e.g. sociodemographic characteristics). Consider a multi-question (or item) self-reported health scale such as a patient-reported outcome (PRO). Typically, the answers to individual questions help describe symptoms; collectively, the answers to the questions help describe a person's health status. This scale should have equivalent psychometric properties across various subpopulations (e.g. men and women). Otherwise, symptoms and dimensions measured by this scale may have different meanings across groups.

For example, two people with equivalent alcohol dependence behavior levels may respond to questions about their alcohol use differently due to divergent beliefs about discussing their alcohol use. One may feel free to discuss their behavior, while the other is more reserved regarding their behavior. Thus, despite equivalent alcohol use, the two individuals would appear dissimilar based on their responses to these questions. As a result, efforts to understand individuals' health based solely on their responses to questions about their health would include systematic flaws.

A form of systematic measurement error often labeled *measurement bias* or *differential item functioning (DIF)* occurs when multiple persons with an identical underlying level on the outcome nevertheless respond to the individual questions asking about their health differently due to their different backgrounds.

Dissimilar socialization may result in men and women tending to interpret the same question differently. Socioeconomic status (SES) can be another contextual factor in which different levels of resources and prestige can lead to a different viewpoint on how to fill out a question. As a result, observed differences across groups of individuals (e.g. men and women, SES groups) may reflect measurement bias rather than true differences.

In much of health and medical research, this problem has not been adequately acknowledged and methods have not been adopted to evaluate and mitigate it. This leaves unclear whether the differences in health outcomes across subpopulations reflect true differences or systematic measurement error. Bias can obscure differences, decrease reliability and validity, and render group comparisons impossible [1,2]. The diagram in Figure 10.1 depicts the negative impact of measurement bias in evaluating health across White, Black and Hispanic race groups.

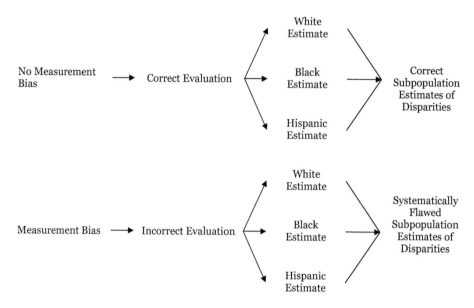

FIGURE 10.1
An example of measurement bias' influence on health measurement across race groups.

In this chapter, we will introduce a variety of methods to examine and account for measurement bias.

SEM offers a powerful set of tools that can tackle the challenges identified above and investigate the cross-group psychometric properties of PROs. Specifically, models and testing procedures can be used to investigate *measurement invariance* (or *measurement equivalence*). Within SEM, measurement invariance is also referred to as *factorial invariance* [3]. Measurement invariance refers to the statistical property that a scale has the same measurement properties across groups of interest or across time periods.

Without establishing equivalent measurement, researchers in the field of health and medicine cannot:

1. Draw strong conclusions about disparate outcomes between groups
2. Support evidence-based practice and policy
3. Address health disparities.

In this chapter, we will discuss *multiple group (MG)* and *multiple cause multiple indicator (MIMIC)* models and extensions which can all be used to evaluate measurement equivalence. MIMIC models are measurement models with covariates, or CFA with covariates, and can be used to evaluate DIF. The observed covariates explain the latent construct in the MIMIC model.

Aforementioned in Chapter 9, MG (also termed *multigroup*) models are stratified models. In the SEM framework, multigroup models allow for in depth analyses of differences between groups depending on where in the model the differences occur (e.g. differences in the item thresholds, factor loadings, residual variances) as we will describe later in this chapter.

We will also discuss applications of MIMIC and multigroup models in health and medicine, such as the hybrid *MG-MIMIC* models. MG-MIMIC models are MIMIC models within a multigroup framework.

SEM methods allow one to test for the presence of measurement bias by evaluating differences in relationships among latent and observed variables across levels of sources of potential measurement bias. This chapter addresses measurement bias and discusses how MIMIC, multigroup and MG-MIMIC models can be used to provide important insight into this issue.

10.2 Multiple Indicator Multiple Cause Models

MIMIC models expand the measurement model to include observed background covariate(s). These covariate(s) can directly influence the latent variable's measurement and the latent variable itself. One can use MIMIC analysis to assess if the mean of the latent variable is different at different levels of each covariate by evaluating the magnitude of relationship between the covariate(s) and latent variable.

A significant relationship between the covariate(s) and latent variable indicates the factor means are different at different levels of the covariate(s). Adding in DIF paths (direct relationships between the covariates and item indicators assumed to be affected by the latent variable) can then allow one to additionally assess if particular item responses are different at different levels of a covariate(s). We have crafted this discussion thus far around a single latent variable to introduce basic concepts. However, MIMIC models can be expanded to include several latent variables.

We use the notation from the measurement model for ordered-categorical items with underlying latent response variates in Chapter 7. A second structural equation allows the covariate to directly influence the measurement of the latent variable in the MIMIC model:

$$\mathbf{y}_i^* = \mathbf{v}_y + \mathbf{\Lambda}_y \mathbf{\eta}_i + \mathbf{\varepsilon}_i,$$
$$\mathbf{\eta}_i = \mathbf{\alpha}_\eta + \mathbf{B}\mathbf{\eta}_i + \mathbf{\Gamma}\mathbf{x}_i + \mathbf{\zeta}_i \tag{10.1}$$

As before in the structural model (Chapter 3), $\mathbf{\alpha}_\eta$ describes the latent variables' mean values, $\mathbf{\zeta}_i$ indicates residuals and $\mathbf{\Gamma}$ captures the influence of the covariates on the latent variable(s).

It is a straightforward exercise to express the general form of a MIMIC model for continuous items instead of ordered-categorical items as a special case of LISREL using similar notation from Chapter 3 (with no individual-level subscripts):

$$\mathbf{y} = \mathbf{v}_y + \mathbf{\Lambda}_y \mathbf{\eta} + \mathbf{\varepsilon}$$
$$\mathbf{\eta} = \mathbf{\alpha}_\eta + \mathbf{B}\mathbf{\eta} + \mathbf{\Gamma}\mathbf{x} + \mathbf{\zeta} \tag{10.2}$$

An extension of the measurement model allows covariates to directly influence the measurement of the latent variable (i.e. explicit modeling of DIF paths). For example, the measurement model in a MIMIC model for ordered-categorical items with underlying latent response variates can be written in the form:

$$\mathbf{y}_i^* = \mathbf{v}_y + \mathbf{\Lambda}_y \mathbf{\eta}_i + \mathbf{\Gamma}_y \mathbf{x}_i + \mathbf{\varepsilon}_i \tag{10.3}$$

In the more conventional applications of a MIMIC model, in the structural model, the covariates influence the latent variables, but latent variables do not influence each other:

$$\eta_i = \alpha_\eta + \Gamma x_i + \zeta_i \tag{10.4}$$

That is, if there are multiple latent variables in a MIMIC model, they may be correlated with each other (e.g. as the underlying dimensions of a multiple-item scale), but are not hypothesized to be causally related.

A limitation to using the MIMIC model as discussed thus far is that it tests for *uniform DIF* but not *non-uniform DIF* [7]. Uniform DIF is constant across a construct. Non-uniform DIF varies across the construct by levels of different groups. For example, age-based DIF may vary across a health construct for men and women. This limitation can be addressed through the MG-MIMIC model discussed later in this chapter. Different moderated models can also be used to investigate non-uniform DIF within the MIMIC framework (see for example Woods and Grimm [4] and Montoya and Jeon [5]).

10.2.1 Illustrative Example of MIMIC Analysis

In Figure 10.2, two observed continuous covariates (age, number of comorbidities) are shown that influence depression in an example of a MIMIC model. We hypothesize the factor mean for depression is different according to the level of age and medical comorbidities.

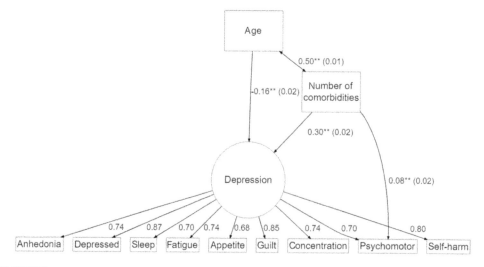

FIGURE 10.2
MIMIC model example for factor mean differences in *Depression* using NHANES, 2015–2016 ($N = 5,735$).

**$p < 0.001$. Model fit: chi-square = 619.131 (42), $p < 0.001$; RMSEA (90% CI) = 0.049 (0.046, 0.052); CFI = 0.977; TLI = 0.970; SRMR = 0.034. We used the WLSMV option and the DELTA parameterization in MPlus to perform these analyses. Standardized estimates (STDYX option) are reported on the figure. In the structural model, we also include estimates of the standard errors in parenthesis. Note that 571 cases were missing on all observed indicators except for age and number of comorbidities and thus included in this model in the procedure for handling missing data for the WLSMV option given covariates (Chapter 4). This explains the discrepancy between this sample size used for this analyses and previous analyses using MPlus for the measurement model for the PHQ-9 items with NHANES, 2015–2016 with no covariates ($N = 5,164$). Finally, we note that is a simplified example and figure to illustrate MIMIC model analysis. Not all paths and constraints are shown (e.g. residual variance constraints under DELTA parameterization) and additional paths of interest could be added at the discretion of a researcher.

Also, an increased number of comorbidities is hypothesized to lead to an increased level of psychomotor symptoms of depression. Thus, we hypothesize measurement bias in the PHQ-9 in this study population. Individuals with an identical underlying level of depression may have differences in the level of the item for psychomotor symptoms according to the level of the number of comorbidities. We note this is a simplified example to illustrate MIMIC model analysis and that the number of comorbidities can be hypothesized to have an effect on additional items (e.g. anhedonia, sleep, fatigue, appetite and concentration).

We performed this analyses using the WLSMV option and the DELTA parameterization in MPlus with the NHANES survey data 2015–2016 ($N = 5{,}735$). The DELTA parameterization was used so we could estimate the correlation between age and number of comorbidities in the model. Model fit was acceptable to excellent (see Figure 10.2).

We found a moderate effect of number of comorbidities on depression (standardized estimate = 0.30, SE = 0.02, $p < 0.001$). An increased number of comorbidities leads to a higher factor mean for depression. We found a small effect of age on depression (standardized estimate = −0.16, SE = 0.02, $p < 0.001$). Being older leads to a lower factor mean for depression. The number of comorbidities and age were largely associated (standardized estimate = 0.50, SE = 0.01, $p < 0.001$), as, on average, being older is correlated with increased number of comorbidities. Further, we found only a small DIF effect (standardized estimate = 0.08, SE = 0.02, $p < 0.001$). On average, having an increased number of comorbidities leads to an increased level of psychomotor symptoms, although this DIF effect is potentially not clinically meaningful due to the small size.

10.2.2 Item Response Theory

A traditional latent variable method with roots in test theory is *item response theory* (IRT). IRT is a theory of testing based on modeling the relationship between individuals' performances on a test item and the test takers' levels of performance on an overall measure of the ability that item was designed to measure. IRT models are also commonly referred to as *latent trait models*.

Traditionally IRT models were restricted to unidimensional structures; multidimensional IRT has been developed for a multifactor instrument [6]. Some popular one-parameter and two-parameter IRT models are also available in latent variable software such as Mplus [7]. This is because these IRT models are formally equivalent to CFA models for ordered-categorical data (given constraints). DIF detection in examining the validity of a test or questionnaire across subgroups (e.g. men and women) using IRT can be done within the MIMIC model framework [8]. The interested reader can see Nguyen et al. [9] for an introduction to IRT for PROs.

10.3 Multigroup Modeling

We have outlined how the MIMIC model can be used to make group comparisons in the factor means and item responses. MIMIC, however, assumes factor loadings are the same across groups. Multigroup modeling is another approach for investigating measurement invariance. Multigroup modeling allows for a researcher to evaluate many types of equivalence in measurement across groups (e.g. invariance of item thresholds, factor loadings, residual variances/covariances, factor means and factor covariances).

Now, consider the multiple group approach to investigating measurement bias. In terms of notation, one either subscripts or superscripts (depending on one's preference) the measurement parameters in a measurement model to allow for group differences. For example, for multigroup CFA to be conducted with ordinal categorical indicators and latent response variates for h groups, we can use the equation:

$$\mathbf{y}_i^{*(g)} = \mathbf{v}_y^{(g)} + \Lambda_y^{(g)'}\eta_i^{(g)} + \varepsilon_i^{(g)} \tag{10.5}$$

where $g = 1,...,h$.

One constrains some or most of the measurement parameters to equality across groups (given the model is identifiable) and tests the constrained model's fit compared to a less constrained model. If fit statistics and indices indicate the constraints' acceptability, measurement equivalence exists. If not, bias presents. Once one has developed a revised model, adjusting for group differences, one can use model-based estimates to compare the health of various groups. This analyses then accounts for the systematic measurement error that bias introduces. We soon provide details of how to conduct measurement invariance testing.

10.3.1 Measurement Invariance

Traditionally, measurement invariance has been evaluated using the multigroup CFA framework with a series of nested models. Each model increases the equality constraints. Measurement invariance studies for continuous models most often begin by testing for *configural invariance*. Configural invariance is a test of invariance across the configural model when performing separate analyses for each group. The configural model is specified with the same model across groups, but free estimation of parameters within each group (given some identifying constraints). *Weak or metric invariance* examines the equivalence of factor loadings across groups. *Strong or scalar invariance* examines the equality of intercepts across groups. *Strict invariance* examines the equivalence of residual variances. For an example of conducting measurement invariance testing (i.e. configural, weak, strong and strict) using the SF-36 health-related quality of life measure using multigroup CFA, see Sudano et al. [10].

An acceptable fit, according to the previously mentioned guidelines (Chapter 4) for chi-square test statistic, CFI, TLI, RMSEA and SRMR, for a configural model supports configural invariance [11–13]. If configural invariance is not established then one must either modify the model (sometimes by reducing the number of indicators) or assume that the construct in general is non-invariant and discontinue further invariance testing [13]. If configural invariance is established, then one can proceed in further measurement invariance testing for weak invariance. This procedure then continues for testing for strong invariance and strict invariance.

The models used for configural, weak, strong and strict invariance are all nested, and each model is more restricted (more constraints) compared to the previous model. For each subsequent model, if the model fit is significantly worse, then invariance under those restrictions is not established. If the model fit is relatively the same or better, then invariance is established.

The chi-square test of difference between each model and the previous model within this sequence can be used to test for invariance. For example, a non-significant chi-square test of difference between the model with constrained factor loadings and the configural model would support weak invariance. That is, the model fit is not significantly different when constraining factor loadings to be equal across the groups since the factor loadings do not vary across groups.

Some work has suggested that one can use the change in CFI between nested models of ≤ 0.010 [14]. Comparison of RMSEA values and 90% confidence intervals between nested models can be used as criterion; if the values fall within one another's 90% confidence intervals then invariance is established [15,16].

If invariance is not established, one can modify the model and specify *partial invariance*. In *partial invariance* testing, some but not all of the parameters are constrained to equality across groups in the testing of measurement equivalence [11]. Constrained parameters can be freed up with the highest modification index one at a time until criteria for invariance is reached. Thus, specific non-invariant parameters (e.g. factor loadings or intercepts) across groups can be identified as a source of measurement bias. The revised model should then be used before specifying any further constraints.

For example, suppose one fails to establish weak invariance. After freeing two factor loadings across groups, criteria for invariance are reached. The revised model includes the same restrictions as the model used for weak invariance testing, except these two factor loadings are freely estimated across groups. Intercepts are then constrained to be equal across groups using this revised model in order to test for strong invariance. This type of procedure for using revised models for further invariance will be shown in the illustrative example of MG-MIMIC modeling later in this chapter.

While similar invariance testing can be done with ordinal data, this language above was developed for continuous data. Models for ordinal data include item thresholds and thus while the levels of invariance can be described similarly as before, thresholds are the focus of scalar invariance tests instead of intercepts [17]. The chi-square difference test may also be the most useful test for evaluating invariance when using a robust WLS estimator [18]. See Bowen and Masa [17] for an overview of invariance testing with ordinal data.

10.3.2 Structural, Dimensional and Longitudinal Invariance

In a multidimensional model, one can also test for *structural invariance*. Structural invariance is equivalence across groups in the factor means, variances and/or covariances (given multiple factors with a nonzero correlation).

Structural invariance testing consists of additional nested models (beginning with the model that established strict invariance) under restrictions of equality between groups of the factor variances, covariances and means, respectively. Non-invariance of the structural parameters does not indicate a problem with the scale being studied [19]. Instead, it indicates heterogeneity among the comparison groups and is generally expected [19]. Measurement and structural invariance testing for second order factor / bifactor models includes sequentially testing for invariance of parameters related to both second order / general and first order / specific factors [20].

Dimensional invariance is equivalence across groups in the number of latent constructs and item-factor structure. EFA can be used to help test for dimensional invariance.

Invariance testing can be conducted to examine for measurement and structural equivalence over time (referred to as *longitudinal invariance*). See Widaman et al. [3] for an overview of factorial invariance within longitudinal SEMs.

10.3.3 Some Practical Considerations about the Steps for Testing for Measurement Invariance

We have been methodical in listing steps for testing for measurement invariance. We hope to continue to make clear throughout this textbook that SEM analyses in practice in health and medicine will often stray from such hard guidelines and methodical rules of thumb.

The multigroup model may be specified to be different across groups. For example, there may be residual correlations in one group model but not in the other group model. Establishing all types of invariance may not be of interest for a particular study. A researcher may decide to test for equivalence of the factor loadings only, given consideration that of theoretical interest is to determine specifically if a construct has the same meaning to individuals across groups.

Some constraints may be specified from the outset. For example, one might assume equivalence between groups in the item thresholds and factor loadings for particular indicators based on logic and theory.

10.4 MG-MIMIC Analyses

The MG-MIMIC approach simultaneously controls for differences in responses due to some variables (e.g. education and income) and allows an investigation of bias across another (e.g. race and ethnicity) [21,22]. MG-MIMIC models extend the MIMIC and multigroup models by specifying sets of structural equations for the measurement model incorporating background variables as covariates within each group [21–24]. Here we can express the mathematical model for the MG-MIMIC using ordinal categorical indicators with latent response variates as:

$$\mathbf{y}_i^{*(g)} = \mathbf{v}_y^{(g)} + \Lambda_y^{(g)}\eta_i^{(g)} + \varepsilon_i^{(g)},$$

$$\eta_i^{(g)} = \alpha_\eta^{(g)} + \mathbf{B}^{(g)}\eta_i^{(g)} + \Gamma^{(g)}\mathbf{x}_i^{(g)} + \zeta_i^{(g)}$$

(10.6)

The example below, again using data from the NESARC [25], describes a MG-MIMIC analysis. It shows how measurement bias as a function of income, educational attainment and minority status may lead to erroneous conclusions about alcohol dependence. It also shows how model-based estimates by accounting for measurement bias within the MG-MIMIC framework can mitigate this error [22].

10.4.1 Methods

10.4.1.1 Participants

Participants (16,109 non-Hispanic White (hereafter White), 4,072 non-Hispanic Black/African-Americans (hereafter Black) and 4,819 Hispanic) were a subset of the 2001–2002 NESARC data. These analyses included White, Black and Hispanic participants with complete data who reported on their alcohol consumption in the past 12 months.

10.4.2 Measures

Alcohol Dependence. Alcohol dependence is a maladaptive alcohol use pattern that leads to significant impairment or distress. It demonstrates at least three of seven criteria identified by the DSM-IV [26]. The NESARC's Alcohol Use Disorder and Associated Disabilities Interview Schedule-IV, [27–34] uses 27 dichotomous items (0 = Yes, 1 = No) to operationalize these criteria. These analyses used all 27 items.

Ethnicity. Five options coded race. A single item allowed Hispanic self-identification. Individuals were considered White if they identified as White and non-Hispanic, Black/African-American if they identified as Black/African-American and non-Hispanic, and anyone who self-identified as Hispanic was considered Hispanic.

Income. Participants reported their total past 12 months' personal and family incomes. From this, the NESARC estimated household income (hereafter income). Aforementioned in Chapter 9, as in regression [35] and analysis with an interaction term such as a moderator, centering a variable (i.e. subtracting the mean from all scores), can increase the interpretability of coefficients. By centering income, one can interpret bias attributable to this variable in terms of differences relative to those at average income level. Thus, the analyses used centered income.

Educational Attainment. The analyses used centered years of education.

10.4.3 Analytical Approach

The analyses examined measurement invariance for the MG-MIMIC model with binary indicators for alcohol dependence (see references by Millsap and Yun-Tien [36] Carle [22] and Woods [37].) This procedure involved using model fit criteria to establish an initial good fitting model across race groups and then chi-square difference testing to establish invariance given increasingly more restricted models. Constraints that led to significantly decreased fit identified bias. Subsequent models freed these constraints to develop a partial invariance model. All analyses used Mplus, its THETA parameterization and WLSMV option.[1] An overview of the models and summary of the results is provided in Table 10.1.

10.4.4 Results

10.4.4.1 Evaluating Internal Validity

Analyses first examined whether the question set measured a single construct across groups within the MG-MIMIC framework. This provided a test of whether data reflected the theoretical assumption that responses measured alcohol dependence only and whether alcohol dependence appears to be a single construct [30,38]. Thus, analyses tested a single factor alcohol dependence model (Model 1) across Whites, Blacks and Hispanics. Model 1 allowed income and educational attainment each to have direct effects on each of the items (within statistical identification limits) and allowed income and educational attainment

---

[1] Complex sampling design and weights were incorporated in Mplus for this example. See for details about this procedure Korn, E. and Graubard, B., Estimating variance components by using survey data. *Journal of the Royal Statistical Society: Series B (Statistical Methodology).* 2003, 65(1): pp. 175–190; Carle, A.C., Fitting multilevel models in complex survey data with design weights: Recommendations. *BMC Medical Research Methodology.* 2009, 9(49).

TABLE 10.1

Models for Testing for Race Group Differences (N = 16,109 White; 4,072 Black; 4,819 Hispanic) in Alcohol Dependence Accounting for Different Levels of Income and Educational Attainment Using 2001–2002 NESARC Data

	Additional Constraints Across Race Groups (As Compared to Previous Model in Nested Series)	Results
Model 1		Established invariance of initial MG-MIMIC model with single factor structure
Model 2	Direct effects of income and educational attainment on each of the 27 items used for alcohol dependence	14 equality constraints led to misfit and relaxed (Model 2b) before fitting Model 3
Model 3	Factor loadings	5 equality constraints led to misfit and relaxed (Model 3b) before fitting Model 4
Model 4	Item thresholds	17 equality constraints led to misfit and relaxed before establishing the final model (Model 4b)

to correlate. Multiple constraints were necessary for achieving model identification.[2] This method for developing Model 1 as a configural model for MG-MIMIC analysis for the given constraints was described as the "anchoring" method by Woods et al. [37]. Model 1 fits the data well ([Chi-square test statistic] χ^2 = 2918.43, degrees of freedom (df) = 1151, p < 0.01; RMSEA = 0.014; CFI = 0.98; TLI = 0.98). This provided evidence for internal validity within and across the groups.

10.4.4.2 Evaluating Measurement Bias

Given good fit, analyses proceeded to Model 2, which constrained the direct effects of income and educational attainment on each of the 27 items to zero across all groups. These constraints led to statistically significant misfit ([Chi-Square Difference Test Statistic] $\Delta\chi^2$ = 355.197, df = 156, p < 0.01), indicating bias as a function of income and educational attainment. Iterative item-level analyses using a Benjamini-Hochberg false discovery approach examined the change in fit that occurred when constraining a single item's parameter to equality. These analyses showed that 14 equality constraints led to misfit. Table 10.2, which provides the parameters for the final model, details these differences across the groups. Model 2b relaxed the misfitting constraints.

Model 3 further modified Model 2b to constrain the factor loadings to equivalence across groups. This examined whether the items provided similar reliability and related similarly to alcohol dependence across Whites, Blacks and Hispanics, after accounting for bias due to income and educational attainment. Constraining the loadings resulted in statistically significant misfit ($\Delta\chi^2$ = 94.646, df = 52, p < 0.01) indicating bias as a function of race/ethnicity. Analyses indicated that 5 equality constraints led to the misfit (see Table 10.2). Model 3b relaxed these constraints.

---

[2] Constraints for statistical identification listed here. Fixed the factor mean and variance at one and zero in the WHITE model, while freely estimating factor mean and variance in the BLACK and HISPANIC models. Constraints across all groups: Item intercepts constrained to zero; fixed the direct effect of income and educational attainment on the "usual number of drinks had less effect" item to zero; constrained the factor loading for the "drinks" item to be equal; constrained the threshold for the "drinks" item to be equal; fixed the uniquenesses to one.

TABLE 10.2

Final Partially Invariant Measurement Model (Bolded Values Correspond to Statistically Significantly Different Values Across Groups)

Whites

Item	Loadings	Thresholds	Income's Effect	Education's Effect
Usual number of drinks had less effect	1.301	−2.662	0	0
Needed to drink more to get desired effect	1.975	−4.141	0	0
Drank equivalent of fifth of liquor in one day	1.11	−2.862	0	0
Increased use to get desired effect	2.006	−4.563	0	0
More than once wanted to stop or cut down	1.109	**−2.033**	**−0.067**	0
More than once tried unsuccessfully to stop or cut down	1.253	**−3.49**	0	0
Ended up drinking more than intended	2.033	**−2.86**	**−0.081**	**−0.108**
Kept drinking longer than intended	**2.103**	−3.181	**−0.117**	0
Trouble Falling Asleep when alcohol's effects wore off	**1.083**	−2.563	**−0.129**	**−0.298**
Shook when alcohol's effects wore off	1.52	−3.839	0	**0.008**
Felt anxious or nervous when alcohol's effects wore off	1.666	−3.986	0	0
Nausea when effects of alcohol wearing off	1.262	−2.146	0	**−0.083**
Felt unusually restless when alcohol's effects wore off	1.416	**−3.155**	**−0.064**	0
Sweat/heart beat fast when alcohol's effects wore off	1.268	**−2.997**	**−0.085**	0
See, felt, heard things when alcohol's effects wore off	1.089	−3.809	**0.272**	0
Had fits or seizures when alcohol's effects wore off	1.037	−4.51	0	0
Had bad headaches when alcohol's effects wore off	1.16	**−1.846**	**−0.046**	**−0.172**
Drank or used drugs to get over alcohol's bad effects	1.152	−3.055	0	**−0.108**
Drank or used other drugs to avoid to get over alcohol's bad effects	**1.224**	−3.489	0	0
Spent lot of time drinking	1.633	−3.787	0	0
Spent lot of time getting over drinking's aftereffects	1.466	−4.206	0	0
Gave up or cut down important activities to drink	**2.344**	**−6.215**	0	0
Gave up or cut down pleasurable activities to drink	2.548	−6.949	0	0
Continued to drink though made depressed	1.766	−4.433	0	0
Continued to drink even though causing health problem	1.284	−3.271	0	0
Continued to drink despite prior blackout	1.404	**−3.427**	**−0.063**	0
Found could drink less than before to get desired effect	0.567	−1.369	0	0
Alcohol dependence factor mean	0			
Alcohol dependence factor variance	1			

Black/African-Americans

Item	Loadings	Thresholds	Income's Effect	Education's Effect
Usual number of drinks had less effect	1.301	−2.662	0	0
Needed to drink more to get desired effect	1.975	−4.141	0	0
Drank equivalent of fifth of liquor in one day	1.11	−2.862	0	0
Increased use to get desired effect	2.006	−4.563	0	0
More than once wanted to stop or cut down	1.109	**−1.686**	0	0
More than once tried unsuccessfully to stop or cut down	1.253	**−3.071**	0	0
Ended up drinking more than intended	2.033	**−3.079**	0	0
Kept drinking longer than intended	**1.79**	−3.181	0	0
Trouble falling asleep when alcohol's effects wore off	**1.225**	−3.082	0	0

(Continued)

TABLE 10.2 (*Continued*)

Final Partially Invariant Measurement Model (Bolded Values Correspond to Statistically Significantly Different Values Across Groups)

Item	Loadings	Thresholds	Income's Effect	Education's Effect
Shook when alcohol's effects wore off	1.52	**−4.327**	**0.739**	0
Felt anxious or nervous when alcohol's effects wore off	1.666	**−4.477**	**1.186**	0
Nausea when effects of alcohol wearing off	1.262	−2.146	**0.008**	0
Felt unusually restless when alcohol's effects wore off	1.416	**−3.381**	0	0
Sweat/heart beat fast when alcohol's effects wore off	1.268	−2.997	0	0
See, felt, heard things when alcohol's effects wore off	1.089	−3.809	0	0
Had fits or seizures when alcohol's effects wore off	1.037	−4.51	0	0
Had bad headaches when alcohol's effects wore off	1.16	**−2.193**	0	0
Drank or used drugs to get over alcohol's bad effects	1.152	−3.055	0	0
Drank or used other drugs to avoid to get over alcohol's bad effects	1.224	−3.489	0	0
Spent lot of time drinking	1.633	−3.787	0	0
Spent lot of time getting over drinking's aftereffects	1.466	−4.206	0	0
Gave up or cut down important activities to drink	**3.88**	**−10.325**	0	0
Gave up or cut down pleasurable activities to drink	2.548	−6.949	0	0
Continued to drink though made depressed	1.766	−4.433	0	0
Continued to drink even though causing health problem	1.284	−3.271	0	0
Continued to drink despite prior blackout	1.404	**−3.889**	0	0
Found could drink less than before to get desired effect	0.567	−1.369	0	0
Alcohol dependence factor mean	0.019			
Alcohol dependence factor variance	1.042			

Hispanics

	Loadings	Thresholds	Income's Effect	Education's Effect
Usual number of drinks had less effect	1.301	−2.662	0	0
Needed to drink more to get desired effect	1.975	−4.136	0	0
Drank equivalent of fifth of liquor in one day	1.11	−2.876	0	0
Increased use to get desired effect	2.006	−4.516	0	0
More than once wanted to stop or cut down	1.109	−1.911	0	**0.168**
More than once tried unsuccessfully to stop or cut down	1.253	−3.139	0	**0.285**
Ended up drinking more than intended	2.033	**−3.453**	0	0
Kept drinking longer than intended	2.103	**−3.806**	0	0
Trouble falling asleep when alcohol's effects wore off	1.083	**−2.91**	0	0
Shook when alcohol's effects wore off	1.52	−4.065	0	0
Felt anxious or nervous when alcohol's effects wore off	1.666	−4.213	0	**0.278**
Nausea when effects of alcohol wearing off	1.262	−2.274	0	0
Felt unusually restless when alcohol's effects wore off	1.416	−3.217	0	0
Sweat/heart beat fast when alcohol's effects wore off	1.268	**−3.33**	**−0.126**	0
See, felt, heard things when alcohol's effects wore off	1.089	−3.886	0	0
Had fits or seizures when alcohol's effects wore off	1.037	−4.652	0	0
Had bad headaches when alcohol's effects wore off	1.16	−1.928	0	0
Drank or used drugs to get over alcohol's bad effects	1.152	−2.998	0	0
Drank or used other drugs to avoid to get over alcohol's bad effects	**1.224**	**−3.574**	0	0

(*Continued*)

TABLE 10.2 (*Continued*)

Final Partially Invariant Measurement Model (Bolded Values Correspond to Statistically Significantly Different Values Across Groups)

Item	Loadings	Thresholds	Income's Effect	Education's Effect
Spent lot of time drinking	1.633	−4.1	**−0.15**	0
Spent lot of time getting over drinking's aftereffects	1.466	−4.286	**−0.163**	0
Gave up or cut down important activities to drink	**2.344**	**−6.21**	0	0
Gave up or cut down pleasurable activities to drink	2.548	−6.874	0	0
Continued to drink though made depressed	1.766	−4.485	0	0
Continued to drink even though causing health problem	1.284	−3.388	0	0
Continued to drink despite prior blackout	1.404	−3.667	0	0
Found could drink less than before to get desired effect	0.567	−1.546	0	0
Alcohol dependence factor mean	**−0.18**			
Alcohol dependence factor variance	1.022			

Model 4 modified Model 3b to constrain the thresholds to equality across Whites, Blacks and Hispanics. This examined whether affirmative item endorsements had similar likelihoods across race and ethnicity. Constraining the thresholds resulted in statistically significant misfit ($\Delta\chi^2$ = 280.608, df = 52, p < 0.01), indicating bias. Analyses showed that 17 equality constraints led to misfit (see Table 10.2). The final model (Model 4b) relaxed these constraints. Summarily, analyses revealed statistically significant bias across race, ethnicity, income and education.

10.4.4.3 Adjusting for Measurement Bias

The presence of significant bias indicates that one should not use unadjusted scores to measure alcohol dependence. Rather, one should instead consider using model-based estimates of alcohol dependence levels to mitigate systematic error. Analyses compared model-based estimates that resulted from the final model incorporating measurement differences to estimates that resulted from a model with all of the measurement parameters equivalent across groups and ignored the evidence for bias.

Under the model ignoring bias, Whites served as the reference group and had a mean of zero on the latent construct for alcohol dependence (for statistical identification). Both Blacks and Hispanics had greater factor means $\left(M_{\text{Black}} = -0.07 : z = -2.86; M_{\text{Hispanic}} = -.211 : z = -8.88 \right)$ than Whites where negative values reflect more use. Here z equals the factor mean divided by the factor mean standard error. However, under the model mitigating bias, Blacks no longer differed significantly from Whites ($M_{\text{Black}} = 0.019 : z = 0.28$), and while Hispanics still had greater alcohol dependence levels $\left(M_{\text{Hispanic}} = -0.18 : z = -2.325 \right)$, the disparity was somewhat smaller.

10.4.5 Discussion

This study provides an example of how measurement models can provide an empirically informed method of meeting some of the challenges facing health survey research methodologists. It aimed to show how to use an SEM-based model (MG-MIMIC) to evaluate internal validity. And, it aspired to show the importance of empirically evaluating measurement bias. Additionally, it sought to demonstrate how bias can influence analytic results and how model-based techniques can mitigate this.

In the current example, results supported the notion that one can create a summary score of severity from these questions. Individuals lower on this score will have greater levels of alcohol use behavior related to dependence. Second, income, educational attainment, and race and ethnicity all directly influenced alcohol dependence measurement. Without accounting for this bias, one would conclude that Hispanics and Black demonstrate significantly greater amounts of alcohol dependence behavior than Whites. However, after using model-based estimates that corrected for bias, model-based estimates clarified that only Hispanics demonstrate greater amounts of alcohol dependence behavior in comparison to Whites and that Blacks do not differ significantly from Whites. These findings highlight that research must consider whether group differences (or similarities) reflect true differences or result from bias. And, they highlight that measurement models can effectively address measurement bias when it occurs, allowing users to include biased items in a survey by estimating scores using the partially invariant measurement model.

10.5 Analysis of Overlapping Symptoms of Co-occurring Conditions

One particular problem in the use of multi-item patient-reported scales (as well as many other multi-item scales) is the potential inflation or deflation of scoring due to overlapping symptoms when individuals suffer from co-occurring conditions. For example, multiple sclerosis (MS) and depression are co-occurring conditions. Individuals with MS may experience fatigue, cognitive impairment and functional impairment. These symptoms may also be symptoms of depression. Items for fatigue, cognitive impairment and functional impairment in a multi-item PRO for depression may be endorsed based on level of MS-related symptoms. As a result, the PRO may not correctly measure the intended dimensions of the scale (i.e. self-report depression) in persons with MS.

MIMIC modeling can be used to evaluate relationships between co-occurring conditions. We describe a theoretical example of a basic MIMIC model with a DIF path for analysis of overlapping symptoms of co-occurring conditions (Figure 10.3).

In Figure 10.3, a1, a2 and a3 are three reflective indicators of latent trait A that describe condition A. The observed variable B describes a symptom of a co-occurring condition. The level of B has an influence on the factor mean of A.

However, we hypothesize that the multi-item scale used for measuring latent trait A may be inaccurate due to systematic measurement error. That is, while we hypothesize that a_2

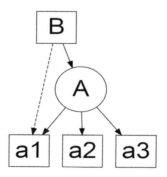

FIGURE 10.3
Application of MIMIC model for analysis of overlapping symptoms of co-occurring conditions.

and a_3 may accurately measure a_2 and a_3 in the study population, we hypothesize a_1 may not measure a_1 alone, but may also be influenced by a subject's level of B. The regression path of a_1 on B represents overlap via a DIF path. *The model represented by Figure 10.3 allows one to measure the latent trait A after accounting for the influence of B on a_1.*

Symptoms of co-occurring conditions might be assumed to occur simultaneously in many studies. Thus, a modification of the MIMIC model for this analysis might assume an association between A and B, but no causal ordering. This model can be extended and revised to reflect nuanced relationships between several or more conditions that overlap (with multiple observed variables, latent constructs and DIF paths) [39]. We will evaluate one such model in an MS-depression illustrative example with multiple DIF paths using a four-step process (see Box 10.1).

BOX 10.1

In analysis of overlapping symptoms, when specifying multiple DIF paths, the procedure for developing a final model can be summarized in four steps:

1. Specify the initial model.
2. Compare the initial model to a model with all DIF paths constrained to zero to evaluate if there is overlap. If there is no overlap, then precede no further.
3. Given that there is overlap, make model revisions as indicated to constrain individual DIF paths to zero that do not estimate meaningful overlap.
4. Perform invariance testing to evaluate for group differences. Incorporate any group differences in the final model.

10.5.1 Overlapping Symptoms of Multiple Sclerosis and Depression

We used data for the study population of 3,507 MS patients who underwent PHQ-9 depression screening as well as assessments of MS-related fatigue, cognitive impairment and functional impairment. We used a unidimensional depression construct with three correlated residuals (Chapter 6 on Model Specification). For step 1, a multidisciplinary panel of expert MS clinicians and methodologists developed a conceptual model depicting potential relationships between single observed variables describing MS-related complications and individual PHQ-9 items. This conceptual model was then translated into a formal structural equation model (see Figure 10.4).

Corresponding to Figure 10.4, observed variables for fatigue and cognitive impairment and functional impairment are all MS-related measures. Level of hand and mobility impairment (via the objective performance measures timed 25-foot walk and 9-hole peg test) are assumed to collectively measure functional impairment. That is, functional impairment is defined by these two correlated objective performance measures and we did not consider models which adjust for only one of the two functional impairment measures to be feasible in this application [39,40]. In practice, we modeled DIF paths e_1 and f_1 for hand impairment and e_2 and f_2 for mobility impairment. For DIF path e (i.e. e_1 and e_2) to be meaningful and significant for the model, then the model estimate of either e_1 or e_2 had to be of at least a small effect size (standardized estimate ≥ 0.10). We either retained both e_1 and e_2 or neither in the modified model. A similar process was used for evaluating DIF path f.

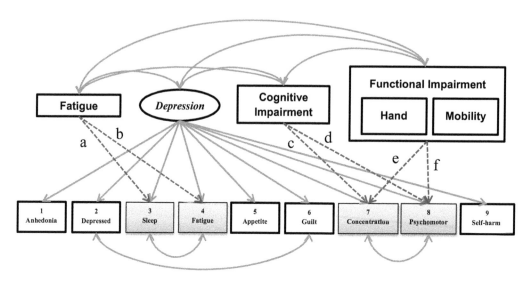

FIGURE 10.4

Hypothesized overlap of depressive symptoms with other symptoms for persons living with MS ($N = 3{,}507$).

Model fit for modified model (with $e = 0$) was acceptable to excellent: chi-square = 479.13 (50), $p < 0.001$; RMSEA = 0.049 (90% CI = 0.045, 0.054); CFI = 0.966; TLI = 0.951; SRMR = 0.029.

Observed covariates for Fatigue (Fatigue domain of the Performance Scales©), Cognitive Impairment (Cognitive domain of the Performance Scales©) and Functional (Hand and Mobility) Impairment (9-Hole Peg Test and Timed 25-Foot Walk) are all MS-related measures. The nine PHQ-9 items describe symptoms of depression.

Adapted with some modification from Gunzler, D., et al., Disentangling multiple sclerosis & depression: an adjusted depression screening score for patient-centered care. *Journal of Behavioral Medicine*, 2015. 38: pp. 237–250.

For a description of the Performance Scales© see Schwartz CE, Vollmer T, Lee H. Reliability and validity of two self-report measures of impairment and disability for MS. North American research consortium on multiple sclerosis outcomes study group. *Neurology*, 1999. 52(1): pp. 63–70.

The model estimates associations between MS-related fatigue, functional impairment and cognitive impairment and *depression* while also determining and correcting for the overlap of MS-related fatigue, cognitive impairment and functional impairment and PHQ-9 items for sleep problems, fatigue, poor concentration and psychomotor symptoms via DIF effects *a, b, c, d, e* and *f*. We used the MLR option in MPlus for performing this analyses.

For step 2, model comparisons can be made using multiple indices and statistics (e.g. chi-square, CFI, TLI, RMSEA, SRMR) and the chi-square difference test. The unconstrained model with all DIF paths as represented in Figure 10.4 has an acceptable to excellent fit, while the model with all "unknown" paths (i.e. DIF paths *a* through *f*) in Figure 10.4 constrained to zero had a relatively poor fit; the chi-square difference test (corrected for the MLR estimator) was significant ($p < 0.001$) [39,40]. Thus, we established meaningful overlap.

For step 3, one can begin with the model with all DIF paths constrained to zero and add in each DIF path one at a time as indicated according to modification indices in determining a modified model. The DIF paths in the modified model to exhibit clinically relevant overlap should be of at least a small standardized path coefficient [39]. In comparing the modified model to the model with all DIF paths constrained to zero, factor loadings will change in magnitude. A positive DIF path estimate will decrease the respective item factor loading. The size of the decrease will be larger with larger magnitude of overlap.

After analysis of modification indices in the modified model, path estimate e in Figure 10.2 was constrained to be zero. In this modified model, there was a large effect for the path (impact of overlap) between MS-fatigue and PHQ-9-fatigue ($b = 0.52$); a moderate effect for the path between MS-cognitive impairment and PHQ-9-concentration ($c = 0.38$); a small to moderate effect for the paths among MS-fatigue and PHQ-9 sleep ($a = 0.21$) and MS-cognitive impairment and PHQ-9-movement ($d = 0.23$); and a small effect for the path between MS-functional impairment and PHQ-9-movement ($f_1 = 0.11$, $f_2 = 0.00$).

For step 4, a researcher can perform multigroup analysis (e.g. MG-MIMIC) to determine if there are potential factors of non-uniform DIF. The grouping variables were all dichotomized in our analyses and tested one at a time in separate models: age (threshold is mean age = 46), sex (male or female), race (White or other), MS type (relapsing or progressive) and time since symptom onset (less than or equal to, greater than 10). The modified model (with $e = 0$) was extended into the MG-MIMIC framework [6]. Multigroup analyses was performed comparing a model freely estimating all parameters across groups to a model constraining DIF paths, factor loadings and item intercepts to be equal across groups. As described in this chapter, we used chi-square difference testing and CFI criteria for testing measurement invariance between models. We used a Bonferroni correction to control the family-wise error rate in the chi-square difference testing (i.e. alpha = 0.05/5 = 0.01). No group differences were found. Thus, the modified model (with $e = 0$) was the final model.

A practical application is to predict an adjusted patient-reported scale score (i.e. scale score accounting for overlapping symptoms of co-occurring conditions) for each individual using the model. Factor scores were predicted for *depression* from the final model and transformed using the probability integral transformation approach (Chapter 7). These MS-adjusted PHQ-9 scores did vary meaningfully in magnitude from the original PHQ-9 for many individuals in the study sample. External validation of this adjusted scale is a necessary future step. See Gunzler, Perzynski et al. [40] and Gunzler and Morris [39] for more details regarding this illustrative example.

10.6 Conclusions

Health and medical research faces a number of challenges with respect to measurement quality. Given the number of potential directions in which measurement quality analyses can lead, it is difficult to describe exact step-by-step procedures to evaluate measurement quality. However, one can make some high-level suggestions. First, survey developers should carefully consider the constructs they intend to measure. Do they expect responses to the questions to measure one or more constructs? Once one has identified a hypothetical measurement model, one should conduct analysis (e.g. CFA) to test the validity of the proposed measurement model. The results will either support the proposed measurement model, or they will prove useful in guiding the development of a modified, empirically based and theory-driven alternative model. After identifying a model that appears valid, one should then test for measurement bias across particular groups of relevance for a study using methods described in this chapter such as MIMIC, MG and MG-MIMIC modeling. These analyses will address whether one can use an instrument such as a scale or questionnaire equivalently across individuals of different backgrounds, or whether additional steps are needed to achieve an appropriate scoring system given measurement bias before comparing people of different backgrounds.

As one can see, the methods described in this chapter provide a powerful conceptual and analytical framework for addressing these challenges. They provide an empirical scaffold for addressing the validity of creating summary scores based on item responses and for evaluating the extent to which measurement bias influences efforts to evaluate health statuses across subpopulations. Importantly, these methods offer a tool to mitigate DIF if it occurs. Hopefully, future work will see these methods more frequently integrated in health survey research.

References

1. Carle, A.C., Assessing the adequacy of self-reported alcohol abuse measurement across time and ethnicity: Cross-cultural equivalence across Hispanics and Caucasians in 1992, non-equivalence in 2001–2002. *BMC Public Health*, 2009. 9: p. 60.
2. Carle, A.C., Tolerating inadequate alcohol dependence measurement: Cross-cultural invalidity of alcohol dependence across Hispanics and Caucasians in 2001 and 2002. *Addictive Behaviors*, 2009. 34: pp. 43–50.
3. Widaman, K.F., E. Ferrer, and R.D. Conger, Factorial invariance within longitudinal structural equation models: Measuring the same construct across time. *Child Development Perspectives*, 2010. 4(1): pp. 10–18.
4. Woods, C.M. and K.J. Grimm, Testing for nonuniform differential item functioning with multiple indicator multiple cause models. *Applied Psychological Measurement*, 2011. 35(5): pp. 339–361.
5. Montoya, A.K. and M. Jeon, MIMIC models for uniform and nonuniform DIF as moderated mediation models. *Applied Psychological Measurement*, 2020. 44(2): pp. 118–136.
6. Immekus, J.C., K.E. Snyder, and P.A. Ralston, Multidimensional item response theory for factor structure assessment in educational psychology research. *Frontiers in Education*, 2019. 4(45): pp. 1–15.
7. Paek, I., et al., Estimation of an IRT model by mplus for dichotomously scored responses under different estimation methods. *Educational and Psychological Measurement*, 2018. 78(4): pp. 569–588.
8. Tsaousis, I., G.D. Sideridis, and A. Al-Sadaawi, An IRT–Multiple Indicators Multiple Causes (MIMIC) approach as a method of examining item response latency. *Frontiers in Psychology*, 2018. 9(2177). doi: 10.3389/fpsyg.2018.02177
9. Nguyen, T.H., et al., An introduction to item response theory for patient-reported outcome measurement. *The Patient*, 2014. 7(1): pp. 23–35.
10. Sudano, J.J., et al., Measuring disparities: Bias in the SF-36v2 among Spanish-speaking medical patients. *Medical Care*, 2011. 49(5): pp. 480–488.
11. Byrne, B.M., *Structural equation modeling with Mplus: Basic concepts, applications, and programming*. 2013, Abington: Routledge.
12. Luk, J.W., et al., Measurement invariance testing of a three-factor model of parental warmth, psychological control, and knowledge across European and Asian/Pacific Islander American youth. *Asian American Journal of Psychology*, 2016. 7(2): pp. 97–107.
13. Putnick, D.L. and M.H. Bornstein, Measurement invariance conventions and reporting: The state of the art and future directions for psychological research. *Developmental Review: DR*, 2016. 41: pp. 71–90.
14. Kueh, Y.C., et al., Testing measurement and factor structure invariance of the physical activity and leisure motivation scale for youth across gender. *Frontiers in Psychology*, 2018. 9(1096). doi: 10.3389/fpsyg.2018.01096

15. Timmons, A., Establishing factorial invariance for multiple-group confirmatory factor analysis. KUant Guide, 2010. 22. http://crmda.dept.ku.edu/resources/kuantguides/22. Factorial_Invariance_Guide.pdf

16. Brown, T.A., *Confirmatory factor analysis for applied research*. 2014, New York, NY: Guilford Publications.

17. Bowen, N.K. and R.D. Masa, Conducting measurement invariance tests with ordinal data: A guide for social work researchers. *Journal of the Society for Social Work and Research*, 2015. 6(2): pp. 229–249.

18. Sass, D.A., T.A. Schmitt, and H.W. Marsh, Evaluating model fit with ordered categorical data within a measurement invariance framework: A comparison of estimators. *Structural Equation Modeling: A Multidisciplinary Journal*, 2014. 21(2): pp. 167–180.

19. Wang, J. and X. Wang, *Structural equation modeling: Applications using Mplus*. 2019, Chichester, West Sussex: John Wiley & Sons.

20. Rudnev, M., et al., Testing measurement invariance for a second-order factor: A cross-national test of the alienation scale. *Methods, Data, Analyses: A Journal for Quantitative Methods and Survey Methodology (MDA)*, 2018. 12(1): pp. 47–76.

21. Jones, R.N., Identification of measurement differences between English and Spanish language versions of the mini-mental state examination. Detecting differential item functioning using MIMIC modeling. *Medical Care*, 2006. 44(11 Suppl 3): pp. S124–S133.

22. Carle, A., Mitigating systematic measurement error in comparative effectiveness research in heterogeneous populations. Medical Care, 2010. 48(6): p. S68.

23. Jones, R.N., Racial bias in the assessment of cognitive functioning of older adults. *Aging & Mental Health*, 2003. 7(2): pp. 83–102.

24. Muthén, B.O., Latent variable modeling in heterogeneous populations. *Psychometrika*, 1989. 54(4): pp. 557–585.

25. Grant, B.F., et al., *Source and accuracy statement for wave 1 of the 2001–2002 national epidemiologic survey on alcohol and related conditions.* 2003, Bethesda, MD: National Institute on Alcohol Abuse and Alcoholism.

26. *Diagnostic and statistical manual of mental disorders*, Fourth Edition. 1994, Washington, DC: American Psychiatric Association.

27. Hasin, D. and A. Paykin, Alcohol dependence and abuse diagnoses: Concurrent validity in a nationally representative sample. *Alcoholism: Clinical and Experimental Research*, 1999. 23: pp. 144–150.

28. Grant, B.F., Convergent validity of DSM-III-R and DSM-IV alcohol dependence: Results from the national longitudinal alcohol epidemiologic survey. *Journal of Substance Abuse*, 1997. 9: pp. 89–102.

29. Grant, B.F., Theoretical and observed subtypes of DSM-IV alcohol abuse and dependence in a general population sample. *Drug and Alcohol Dependence*, 2000. 60(3): pp. 287–293.

30. Harford, T.C. and B.O. Muthén, The dimensionality of alcohol abuse and dependence: A multivariate analysis of DSM-IV symptom items in the national longitudinal survey of youth. *Journal Studies* of Alcohol, 2001. 62: pp. 150–157.

31. Grant, B.F., et al., The alcohol use disorder and associated disabilities interview schedule (AUDADIS): Reliability of alcohol and drug modules in a general population sample. *Drug and Alcohol Dependence*, 1995. 39(1): pp. 37–44.

32. Hasin, D.S., B. Grant, and L. Cottler, Nosological comparisons of alcohol and drug diagnoses: A multisite, multi-instrument international study. *Drug and Alcohol Dependence*, 1997. 47: pp. 217–226.

33. Grant, B.F., et al., The alcohol use disorder and associated disabilities interview Schedule-IV (AUDADIS-IV): Reliability of alcohol consumption, tobacco use, family history of depression and psychiatric diagnostic modules in a general population sample. Drug and Alcohol Dependence, 2003. 71(1): pp. 7–16.

34. Grant, B.F., D.A. Dawson, and D.S. Hasin, *The alcohol use disorder and associated disabilities interview schedule-DSM-IV version (AUDADIS-IV).* 2001, Bethesda, MD: National Institute of on Alcohol Abuse and Alcoholism.

35. Cohen, J., et al., *Applied multiple regression/correlation analysis for the behavioral sciences.* Vol. 3rd. 2003, Hillsdale, NJ: Lawrence Erlbaum Associates.
36. Millsap, R.E. and J. Yun-Tein, Assessing factorial invariance in ordered-categorical measures. *Journal of Multivariate Behavioral Research,* 2004. 39: pp. 479–515.
37. Woods, C.M., Empirical selection of anchors for tests of differential item functioning. *Applied Psychological Measurement,* 2009. 33(1): p. 42.
38. Muthén, B.O., Factor analysis of alcohol abuse and dependence symptom items in the 1988 national health interview survey. *Addiction,* 1995. 90(5): pp. 637–645.
39. Gunzler, D.D. and N. Morris, A tutorial on structural equation modeling for analysis of overlapping symptoms in co-occurring conditions using MPlus. *Statistics in Medicine,* 2015. 34(24): pp. 3246–3280.
40. Gunzler, D., et al., Disentangling multiple sclerosis & depression: An adjusted depression screening score for patient-centered care. *Journal of Behavioral Medicine,* 2015. 38(2): pp. 237–250.

11

Latent Class Analysis

11.1 Introduction to Mixture Distributions

Traditionally, subgroup analysis in health and medicine is used to determine whether individuals respond differently to a treatment, or have a different strength of association, based on one or more clinical characteristics [1]. In such analyses, one typically defines the subgroups a priori based on a theory or even the categories of a single observed variable. For example, let us imagine we would like to evaluate the association between length of stay and health care costs in adults with chronic obstructive pulmonary disease (COPD). We hypothesize there may be differences in this association by sex [2]. Historically, COPD had been viewed as a disease that mostly afflicts men, though recent studies have indicated that prevalence and mortality have been on the rise for women [3]. In order to test a hypothesis about male/female differences, we would create subsets of the data for males and females. Then, we could perform traditional stratified linear regression analyses within each subgroup strata. These types of a priori subgroups (e.g. male/female) are used in conducting moderation analysis (Chapter 9) and measurement invariance testing in the multigroup modeling framework (Chapter 10).

In the sex and COPD example, each subgroup strata is defined by a single category of a single variable. However, the same framework can be used to define subgroup strata using a multivariate measure. For example, we could instead choose to define subgroup strata based on quartiles of an individualized risk score for severity of COPD symptoms defined by levels of sex, race, age, smoking status, BMI and socioeconomic status among other clinical risk factors.

In contrast to describing subgroups defined a priori, in this chapter and the subsequent chapter (as well as Chapter 14), we discuss techniques for identifying subgroups (also commonly referred to as subpopulations or clusters) using latent variables. Understanding these latent variable techniques begins with an introduction to a *mixture distribution*. A mixture distribution is a mixture of two or more probability distributions. Random variables are drawn from at least two distinct subpopulations to form a distribution for the study sample.

Consider an example of a mixture distribution. We simulated data on the length of stay of 10,320 subjects who underwent a surgical procedure (i.e. hip replacement). The mean length of stay is 10 days (SD = 2). However, in the distribution of the data (see Figure 11.1), we observe a mixture of two distinct probability distributions.

We consider that the data consists of a mixture of two normal distributions representing *subpopulation A* ($N = 4,128$) and *subpopulation B* ($N = 6,192$) each with a common standard deviation = 1; the mean length of stay in days for *subpopulation A* is 8 and *B* is 12. Thus, on average, we can conclude that simulated individuals from *subpopulation A* have a shorter

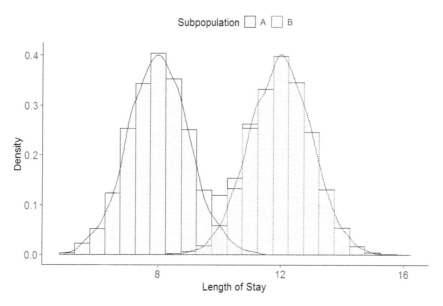

FIGURE 11.1
Histogram overlaid with kernel density curve of simulated length of stay data ($N = 10{,}320$).

length of stay than simulated individuals from *subpopulation B*. While in this example we used a single outcome for a mixture of two univariate distributions, mixed distributions can be a mixture of multivariate distributions.

11.1.1 Finite Mixture Modeling

Finite mixture modeling (FMM) is a set of techniques that uses probabilistic- or regression-based models for identifying unobserved subgroups within a study sample. Synonymously, SEM researchers also use the terms *mixture modeling* or *latent variable mixture modeling*. One considers the distribution of outcomes of interest as a mixture of multiple distributions. These techniques can be applied under the hypothesis that a study sample is comprised of two or more unobserved subgroups [1]. A categorical latent variable is used in a mixture model for representing the unobserved subgroups. In this chapter, along with the forthcoming Chapters 12 and 14, we discuss applications of mixture modeling.

In traditional clustering algorithms such as standard *k*-means or nearest neighbor, clustering is typically based on some form of a distance metric (e.g. squared Euclidean distance). Since a mixture model is a statistical model, one can practically handle missing values and categorical variables in mixture modeling. Even when all items are continuous, unlike the *k*-means clustering approach, the items used in the analysis do not need to have the same scale or equal variances. In addition, mixture modeling allows one to quantify relative fit of a model and statistically test between solutions to help determine the number of subgroups for observed data [4]. The decision to rule in favor of a particular solution for a particular model is thus less subjective than in traditional clustering algorithms [4].

Similar to other SEM techniques, given the large number of parameters in a typical mixture model (especially as the number of subgroups increases), mixture models typically require a large sample size for stable results. Researchers must adhere to distributional assumptions, which if violated can lead to misleading or erroneous results.

11.2 Introduction to Latent Class Analysis

Latent class analysis (LCA) is a multivariate approach for identifying unobserved subgroups using a set of indicators. The subgroups are also termed latent classes. The term LCA implies that each of the indicators is either binary or ordinal. Similar multivariate analysis with continuous indicators (*latent profile analysis*) is described in Chapter 12.

LCA is a person-centered analysis for identifying clusters within a study sample. The general form of the model for LCA is a measurement model in which a latent variable representing the true latent class membership for each individual is not known and must be extrapolated from a set of indicators. Unlike the continuous latent variable used in factor analysis, the latent variable for LCA consists of discrete categories. This categorical latent variable is commonly assumed to come from a multinomial distribution.

Subgroups can be described by the *item-response probabilities* across the multiple indicators within each latent class. Item-response probabilities provide information on the probability of endorsing each category for each indicator within each class [5].

The subgroups identified by LCA are not known a priori but are determined empirically. A one-class solution is specified and then used as a comparison for solutions of increasing class size until the optimal solution is determined. We will discuss later in this chapter how to determine the optimal solution.

Each subgroup should be distinct from the others and provide meaningful information regarding heterogeneity within the study sample. Otherwise, a more parsimonious class solution should be chosen. The choice for the set of indicators and the data quality used for LCA is of upmost importance for obtaining meaningful results.

BRIEF HISTORY OF LATENT CLASS MODELING

Latent class modeling is a diverse set of methods for identifying unobserved subgroups in a study sample. A categorical latent variable is used in a latent class model for representing the subgroups. Latent class modeling was originally derived for categorical observed variables. LCA has its roots in the social and political sciences [6]. Paul Lazarsfeld developed the basic ideas for LCA in the 1950s [7–9] for explaining heterogeneity of survey responses between subjects using dichotomous observed items [9,10]. Another application of latent class modeling with continuous observed variables, latent profile analysis, is commonly used in health and medical research. An early reference for latent profile analysis is Gibson [11]. Latent class models have been developed and extended in many flexible ways over time. For example, observed variables for continuous, survival time, count, categorical or combinations of these types of data can be related to the categorical latent variable. Techniques such as factor mixture modeling (Chapter 12) and a longitudinal extension growth mixture modeling (Chapter 14) use a combination of continuous and categorical latent variables. Nowadays, many applied researchers view the terms latent class modeling, mixture modeling, latent variable mixture modeling and FMM as synonymous.

11.2.1 Local Independence

The standard assumption of LCA, in identifying latent classes, is that within each class each observed indicator is independent of every other observed indicator. This assumption of local independence was discussed previously in Chapter 3. However, now, instead of conditioning on any given value of a continuous latent variable, the conditioning is on membership in a latent class. Again, this assumption leads to a useful interpretation for LCA as the latent variable alone explains why the observed indicators are related to each other [9].

11.2.2 LCA Model for Dichotomous Data

The basic LCA model [5,12] for a set of binary indictors is represented in Figure 11.2.

There are two types of LCA model parameters [5]. The *class probability parameters* specify the relative prevalence (size) of each latent class. The *item parameters* correspond to the item-response probabilities within each latent class.

Suppose we estimate a LCA model. We use a set of M binary indicators $y_1, y_2, ..., y_M$ to identify $k = 1, ..., K$ latent classes. Formally, these K latent classes are represented by the K categories of a nominal latent class variable c.

We express the probability of membership in latent class k as $P(c = k)$, which describes the proportion of individuals in the study sample in latent class k. We assume that

$0 \leq P(c = k) \leq 1$ and $\sum_{k=1}^{K} P(c = k) = 1$. We also express the probability of an observed indicator

y_i, $i = 1, ..., M$ conditional on membership in latent class k as $P(y_i | c = k)$.

Assuming local independence, the joint probability of all the observed indicators is

$$P(y_1, y_2, ..., y_M) = \sum_{k=1}^{K} P(c = k) P(y_1, y_2, ..., y_M | c = k) = \sum_{k=1}^{K} P(c = k) \prod_{i=1}^{M} P(y_i | c = k) \quad (11.1)$$

Equation (11.1) can be used to determine the marginal probability for a certain set of responses on the M indicators. To clarify, the joint probability of a certain set of responses on the M indicators within latent class k will depend on the probability of membership in latent class k and the probability of those responses on the M indicators conditional on membership to latent class k. The marginal probability then of that certain set of responses on the M indicators is the sum of those joint probabilities across the K latent classes. We show a basic example of how to calculate a marginal probability in Box 11.1.

The degrees of freedom for a latent class model are calculated as the number of possible response patterns (i.e. number of cells in the contingency table formed by crossing all observed indicators) minus the number of freely estimated parameters minus one [1]. In many applications, parameters of a mixture model are estimated using maximum likelihood and an EM algorithm. Such approaches can also take advantage of efficient methods for handling missing values.

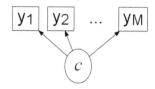

FIGURE 11.2
General latent class analysis model.

BOX 11.1

Example: Consider a LCA model with three binary indicators (each taking on values of 0 or 1) and two latent classes.

We would like to determine the marginal probability that $y_1 = 1, y_2 = 0, y_3 = 1$. Suppose

$$P(c = 1) = .25, P(c = 2) = .75,$$

$$P(y_1 = 1|c = 1) = P(y_2 = 0|c = 1) = P(y_3 = 1|c = 1) = 0.30,$$

$$P(y_1 = 1|c = 2) = P(y_2 = 0|c = 2) = P(y_3 = 1|c = 2) = 0.50.$$

Then, assuming local independence,

$$P(y_1 = 1, y_2 = 0, y_3 = 1)$$

$$= \sum_{k=1}^{2} P(c = k) P(y_1 = 1, y_2 = 0, y_3 = 1 | c = k)$$

$$= \sum_{k=1}^{2} P(c = k) P(y_1 = 1|c = k) P(y_2 = 0|c = k) P(y_3 = 1|c = k)$$

$$= .25 \times .30^3 + .75 \times .50^3 = 0.10$$

11.2.3 Most Likely Latent Class Membership

Individuals are assigned to latent classes based on their *posterior class-membership probabilities*. Posterior class-membership probabilities are computed using Bayes theorem as the probability of belonging to a latent class conditional on the observed data and parameters estimated in the model (i.e. item and class probability parameters). The posterior class-membership probability for any individual across all classes will sum to one. The most likely latent class is the latent class that individual has the highest probability of being a member. For example, consider a two class model. Subject 1 has a probability of 1.00 of being in class one and probability of 0.00 of being in class two. Subject 1 is clearly most likely a member of class one. Subject 2, however, has a probability of 0.55 of being in class one and 0.45 of being in class two. Subject 2 is still most likely a member of class one, but there is a high degree of uncertainty in this classification.

11.3 How to Determine the Number of Latent Classes?

11.3.1 Empirical Criteria

To determine the optimal number of latent classes, one should use empirical criteria as well as consider interpretability. In this section, we discuss the empirical criteria. Interpretability, which will be discussed in the next section of this chapter, should be considered in determining both plausible models (i.e. the different models to consider in the analyses) and the optimal model.

Relative fit indices (information-based criteria) are typically evaluated to determine the best solution. These measures include AIC, BIC, aBIC and AICC as described in Chapter 6.

Entropy is a measure of classification accuracy. Entropy is a continuous measure between zero and one. A lower score shows more uncertainty in classification of individuals to their most likely latent class. As a general rule of thumb, an entropy statistic greater than 0.80 shows acceptable overall classification accuracy.

Let α_{jk} be the probability that individual j, $j = 1, ..., N$, is a member of class k. Then, entropy is defined as

$$\text{entropy} = \sum_{j=1}^{N} \sum_{k=1}^{K} \alpha_{jk} \log \alpha_{jk} \tag{11.2}$$

One can begin to discern for the optimal fitting model from a series of LCA models for the observed data (e.g. models of increasing number of latent classes from one to eight classes) by identifying the model with the minimum AIC, BIC, aBIC and AICC and maximum entropy. Typically in health and medicine, these different criterion will lead one to consider multiple potential models. For example, AIC may be minimized for the three class solution, BIC may be minimized for the four class solution and entropy maximized for the five class solution.

Relative fit indices may keep decreasing as more classes are being considered in the set of latent class models (e.g. ten models) under study. Take as an example BIC. A model with k classes provides an improved fit compared to the prior model with $k - 1$ classes if there is a nontrivial decrease in the BIC. However if a model only has a trivially smaller BIC than the prior model (with one less class), then this would not be a meaningful improvement. See Chapter 6 for a review of information criteria such as BIC, AIC, aBIC and AICC for model comparison.

One should also assess the average of posterior probability of membership in each latent class (as discussed earlier). Posterior probabilities are an indicator on a probability scale of correct latent class membership classification [13,14]. The average probability of being a member of each class should be at least 0.80, as a rule of thumb, for a good fitting model.

Class cell sizes summarize the frequency of cases within each latent class based on most likely latent class membership. A commonly used rule of thumb is that the smallest class cell size should contain at least 5% of the sample. However, in studies with large sample sizes, it is certainly possible to have a meaningful latent class with less than 5% of the cases. Thus one should also consider the raw number of cases in the class.

Likelihood ratio tests (LRTs) can also be used for determining the optimal solution. These tests assess the value of including an additional class; that is the current solution with k classes provides a better fit than the prior solution with $k - 1$ classes. The *Vuong-Lo-Mendell-Rubin LRT* (VLMR-LRT) and *Lo-Mendell-Rubin adjusted LRT* (aLMR-LRT) compare the predicted response pattern proportions to the observed response pattern proportions. In practice, these tests may show bias since regularity conditions may not conform to the usual asymptotic null chi-squared distribution [15]. The *bootstrapped LRT* is a fit test using bootstrapping techniques. Nylund et al. [5] found that the bootstrapped LRT was a very consistent indicator of the number of latent classes in different mixture models considered in simulation studies.

Some researchers do support the use of BIC or aBIC alone for determining the best solution in latent variable mixture models. Nylund et al. [5] found that BIC performed the best of information criterion in determining the number of classes in the simulation studies. In the context of GMM, a simulation study performed by Kim [16] found that aBIC performed well under practical conditions, such as low class separation, smaller sample size and/ or missing data. However, no single measure performed well in all conditions [16]. The authors of this textbook favor that, when available, a researcher should consider multiple measures and tests collectively together with substantive and theoretical interpretation rather than rely on the strengths and limitations of a single measure.

11.3.2 Interpretability

A researcher must strongly consider the interpretability of the proposed optimal solution based on empirical criteria before ruling out alternative solutions. Even further, in many applications in health and medicine, empirical criteria alone does not allow a researcher to pinpoint a single best solution; interpretability plays a vital role in the selection of the number of latent classes. As mentioned, different measures (e.g. AIC, BIC, entropy) may lead a researcher to consider multiple solutions. The authors of this textbook convey that in much of our research this type of scenario is more typical than atypical. However, there may be a single solution (or subset of solutions) that stands above the others based on interpretability, in line with theory, logic and prior literature.

Evaluation of the item parameters within each class in such a model should lead one to identify distinct, meaningful subgroups. A low probability of endorsing an item might be just as meaningful as a high probability of endorsing an item in describing a subgroup. For example, suppose we perform LCA on a series of mental health and physical health indicators in a study of participants who experienced childhood trauma. A class with high item-response probabilities on all indicators suggests strong mental health and physical health. This subgroup is found and described as resilient. Another class is characterized by high item-response probabilities on the mental health indicators but low item-response probabilities on the physical health indicators. We described this class in terms of mental health resiliency in spite of poor physical health.

Interpretability could lead one to include an additional latent class in the model. We might find a latent class with a strong substantive interpretation, such as the resilient subgroup as described earlier, that is not part of the best-fitting solution based on empirical criteria alone.

On the other hand, interpretability could lead one to exclude a completely nonsensical latent class from the solution. Two classes in a solution may have slightly different item-response probabilities, but the substantive interpretation of the classes is identical or near identical. As a result, the optimal solution could combine these two classes as one.

Note that the order of the classes in a solution is not fixed and one can relevel the classes with no change to the fit of the model. If there is a plausible natural order to the classes (e.g. three class solution with classes characterized by poor outcomes, average outcomes and good outcomes), then one can label classes in this order to help clarify the findings.

For binary indicators, graphical displays of the probability of endorsement of each of the indicators can be helpful in assigning meaning to the latent classes. This can be done using a line graph or bar plot. A stacked bar plot could be used as a graphical display to summarize the probability of endorsement of each category for each of the indicators for LCA with ordinal variables or a mixture of binary and ordinal variables. We will showcase these graphical displays later in this chapter with illustrative examples.

11.4 LCA with Covariates and Distal Outcomes

Covariates and *distal outcomes* can be added to the LCA model. Observed covariates may influence latent class membership. Distal outcomes are observed outcomes predicted from the latent class variable [17]. Observed covariates and distal outcomes are also commonly referred to as *auxiliary variables* since they are not part of the main measurement model [18,19].

In Figure 8.3, we include seven methods of smoking (little cigars, traditional cigars, e-cigarettes, waterpipes or hookah, tipped cigarillo, untipped cigarillo, cigarettes) as categorical indicators of latent class membership [20]. Sex, age and race are covariates hypothesized to predict latent class membership. The latent class variable is hypothesized to influence the distal outcome of nicotine dependence. The covariates are also hypothesized to influence the distal outcome in Figure 11.3. When all these paths are specified as "known" paths according to Figure 11.3 (covariates directly influence the distal outcome, indirectly influence the distal outcome via the latent class variable), then the latent class variable is a mediator of the relationship between the covariates and distal outcome. Analysis for this illustrative example will be discussed later in this chapter.

Multinomial regression can be used for regressing a nominal latent class variable on the covariates. Note that when the latent class variable has only two classes, this regression is binary logistic regression. Regression analysis can either be performed at the same time as latent class specification or at a later stage. However, one may not arrive at the same conclusion with both approaches.

In a *one-step approach*, simultaneously, latent classes are extracted and the associations between the most likely class variable and observed covariates are examined [21]. The covariates can shift the probability of being a member of each latent class.

Traditionally, a researcher using a one-step approach determines the number of latent classes first using the measurement model only. Then, the researcher includes the covariates under the preferred class solution. It is also possible to determine the number of latent classes under the conditional model with the covariates. An advantage of the one-step approach is that including covariates at the same stage as latent class extraction may improve the model fit and/or interpretation of the latent classes.

There are also several disadvantages of this one-step approach. The listed advantage is also a potential disadvantage; the single-step approach may weaken the model fit and/or interpretation of the latent classes. It may be impractical to use the one-step approach for a

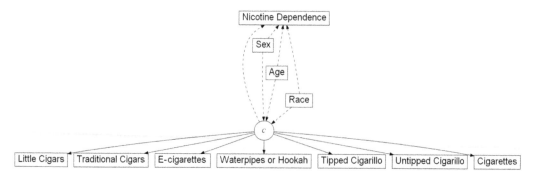

FIGURE 11.3

Latent class analysis model of methods of cigarette smoking with covariates (sex, age and race) and a distal outcome (nicotine dependence).

given data set, especially when the number of explanatory variables is large [22]. The logic of the approach may not fit in with a researcher that wants to understand the meaning of the measurement part of the latent class model separately from any covariates.

In the classic three-step approach, a nominal latent class variable is saved in a data file. Then, the class variable is used as an outcome in multinomial regression with covariates. Recall, the class variable is created based on most likely latent class membership for each individual, which is determined on a probability scale. Therefore, this approach does not correct for measurement error in the latent class variable and can underestimate the strength of associations between latent classes and observed covariates [21].

Currently, many researchers prefer to use a *corrected three-step approach* as discussed by Vermunt [22] and Asparouhov and Muthén [19] to perform regression of the latent class variable on covariates. We use this terminology "corrected" to distinguish three-step regression procedures that correct for uncertainty (measurement error) in the assignment of latent classes.

In these approaches, covariates are introduced to the model at a different stage than latent class extraction. The uncertainty rate is computed using classification probabilities and then fixed and pre-specified for the most likely latent class variable in the regression analysis. See Asparouhov and Muthén [18,19] for an overview of the three steps for the regression procedure.

These aforementioned corrected three-step approaches do not resolve the problem of shifting classes completely [18]. In some situations when the auxiliary variable is included in the final stage, the latent class variable can still shift substantially and invalidate the results [18].

One-step and three-step approaches (classic or corrected) can also be used to evaluate the relationships between distal outcomes and latent class membership [18,19,21]. A researcher is typically interested in assessing differences in the mean of a continuous distal outcome across classes. The within-class variances can be constrained to be equal or freely estimated for the distal outcome. Different types of distal outcomes (e.g. categorical, survival) can be readily evaluated as well.

The *BCH method* was proposed as a corrected three-step approach with continuous distal outcomes [18]. "BCH" is named after the authors who first outlined the approach Bolck, Croon and Hagenaars [23]. The approach uses group specific weights for each observation that are computed during the latent class model estimation [18]. Covariates can be included in analysis using the BCH method. The BCH method avoids shifts in latent class in the final stage. One of the main drawbacks of the BCH method is that in some situations with low entropy, negative values in the BCH weights can lead to inadmissable model estimates [18].

In MPlus, there are automatic procedures to implement an auxiliary model for different corrected three-step approaches or the BCH method with *either* covariates *or* distal outcomes. A manual approach to conducting three steps (implementing each of the steps one at a time) must be done (as of MPlus Version 8.2) for more complex models that include both covariates and distal outcomes [18,19]. This manual approach is flexible in allowing the user to specify the relationships between covariates, distal outcomes and latent classes in line with specific hypotheses of interest.

The analyses discussed thus far with auxiliary variables assumes these variables are part of the theorized causal model (e.g. Figure 8.3). A researcher may want to understand outside of the theorized causal model instead the association between a set of variables and subgroup membership using the extracted nominal variable for most likely latent class membership. That is, how a set of clinical characteristics and factors differ across classes. For continuous variables, a researcher could report within-class means and standard deviations and use ANOVA, if assumptions are met. Class differences could be visual depicted using violin plots or box plots. For categorical variables, a researcher could report within-class the number and percentage of cases and use a chi-square test, if assumptions are met.

While we do not have the book space to go into this topic in any depth, one can also test for measurement invariance across groups for the parameters in the latent class model using multigroup analysis given different equality constraints. See Collins and Lanza [24] for a more in depth introduction of this topic.

11.5 Some FAQs with LCA in Health and Medical Studies

11.5.1 Can I Assume Local Dependence among Indicators within Class?

A researcher assumes local independence in traditional applications of LCA. Depending on the context, one may assume that not all indicators are locally independent of each other. There are applications of latent class models using categorical data where a researcher will explicitly test the local independence assumption [25,26]. Typically, in these applications, a researcher will make the standard local independence assumption up front in determining the best solution for the number of latent classes. Then, the researcher will assess the value under the proposed solution of specifying any dependencies among pairs of indicators. These local dependencies can be either assumed for every latent class in the solution or only within certain classes.

Empirical evidence for adding in a local dependency includes a high value of a standardized bivariate residual between two indicators. There is no absolute criterion for what constitutes a high value of a standardized bivariate residual. However, some researchers assign a value of greater than two as a high value, which would signify greater than two standard deviations from the mean. This criterion should be considered in conjunction with prior theory that a local dependency is meaningful. One should limit the number of local dependencies tested to only a few and should never conduct such analyses solely for the benefit of improved model fit. The interested reader can refer to Oberski [27] for discussion on local dependence in binary data latent class models.

11.5.2 I Can Justify Multiple Solutions, Which Do I Choose?

Addressing this question can be challenging. Empirical results are mixed so a researcher expects to be able to choose the optimal solution based on interpretability in conjunction with the empirical results. However, often enough, two or more solutions become justifiable based on both empirical results and interpretability. Two additional questions can be asked to help decide upon a single solution (without loss of generality, we consider two competing, plausible solutions).

1. Which classes from the lower class solution have the same interpretation in the higher class solution?

2. Do classes only present in the higher class solution provide unique information in relation to auxiliary variables of interest?

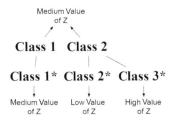

FIGURE 11.4
Hypothetical relationships between proposed two (class 1 and class 2) and three class (class 1*, class 2* and class 3*) solutions and the level of a distal outcome Z.

To elaborate, we consider a hypothetical example. We compare two (class 1 and 2) and three class (classes 1*, 2* and 3*) solutions for the same observed data. Both solutions are plausible based on empirical criteria and interpretability. We can begin choosing between these two solutions by addressing the first question. Class 1 remains the same in class 1*. Class 2 breaks up into class 2* and class 3* (see Figure 11.4).

Now, we can look to address the second question. In the hypothetical example, we observe that class 2* and class 3* have distinct relationships with distal outcome Z (assume a standard deviation of one for Z in every class). The mean value of Z within the three classes is different (medium for class 1*, low for class 2* and high for class 3*). Class 1 and class 2 have similar relationships with Z, where the mean value of Z within both of these classes is of a medium value.

One should note the possibility of two classes that are fairly similar on the surface (small shift in the item-response probabilities between two classes) but have different relationships with auxiliary variables. Rather than rule in favor of a more parsimonious solution, we might decide that each of these two classes provides distinct, meaningful information regarding heterogeneity within the study sample.

11.5.3 Can I Incorporate Nominal Variables as Covariates in a Latent Class Model?

Yes! Nominal variables can be recoded as a set of dummy variables to be readily incorporated as covariates. For example, we have a nominal race variable (African-American, Caucasian and Other). Assume there are no small cell frequencies for any of the three categories. The race variable can be recoded as three dummy variables (African-American vs. Caucasian or Other, Caucasian vs. African-American or Other, Other vs. African-American or Caucasian). Due to linear dependency, we can add any two of the three dummy variables as covariates in the latent class model.

11.5.4 Should One Hold Out a Portion of the Sample as a Validation Sample or Use the Whole Sample?

Many epidemiologists use the tactic of withholding a portion of the sample in analysis for purposes of testing model performance when using unsupervised learning methods. See Hastie, Tibshirani and Friedman [28] and the *R* companion written by James, Witten, Hastie and Tibshirani [29] for a more comprehensive view of this topic.

We have discussed LCA as exploratory data analysis to identify unobserved subgroups with observed categorical data. Model selection criteria discussed in this chapter can be used to help identify the optimal solution from the available observed data among the plausible solutions under consideration. Commonly in research with LCA, one analyzes the entire sample in conducting exploratory data analysis.

The reproducibility of findings in other settings is an important step toward external validation for a LCA model. In confirmatory LCA, one uses previous theory to test hypotheses about latent classes using model constraints [30,31]. These model constraints may include fixing the number of classes and certain parameters (e.g. item parameters) within all or some of the classes in the confirmatory latent class model. Parameters may be set to be equal or inequal across classes, as appropriate. Similar confirmatory data analysis can be conducted for other latent class models.

11.6 Application of LCA with Binary Indicators: Hepatitis C Transmission Awareness Example

Hepatitis C is a widespread, communicable disease that may lead to cirrhosis and sometimes cancer of the liver. More than 170 million people, 3% of the world's population, are infected with the hepatitis C virus (HCV). The goal of a study of 3,092 subjects was to use LCA to identify groups based on level of knowledge of hepatitis C virus (KSHCV) transmission as well as describe and explain the influence of sociodemographic variation in group lay knowledge and understanding of HCV [32]. This study used secondary data from the 2002 Behavioral Risk Factor Surveillance System (BRFSS), a cross-sectional, telephone survey. Further details on the BRFSS sampling design as well as more general procedures are available in the BRFSS User's Guide (CDC, 2005). The hepatitis C module administered in Arizona was a state-added module and not part of the standard or rotating BRFSS cores.

Table 11.1 presents the seven transmission vectors asked about in the survey and the percent answering yes to each binary item. Overall knowledge was poor, with less than 50% knowing that HCV can be spread through contact with the blood of an infected person.

Figure 11.5 graphically depicts the latent class measurement model for these seven indicators. Also shown in Figure 11.5 are five covariates (education, income, race/ethnicity, age and gender) hypothesized to influence latent class membership.

We used the MLR option in MPlus with the EMA algorithm, an accelerated EM algorithm, to perform LCA in this study [33]. To simplify the process in this first example, we

TABLE 11.1

Knowledge of How Hepatitis C Virus(HCV) Is Spread in the Arizona BRFSS[a]

$N = 3,902$		95% CI	
Can HCV Be Spread Thru?	**% Stating Yes**	**Lower**	**Upper**
Sneezing or coughing	15.2	13.9	16.6
Kissing	20.7	19.3	22.1
Unprotected sex	66.3	67.7	68.0
Food or water	19.7	18.3	21.1
Sharing needles to inject street drugs	50.3	49.7	51.6
Using the same bathroom	11.8	10.7	13.0
Contact with the blood of an infected person	48.0	46.3	49.8

[a] Italicized items are ways in which HCV is known to be spread.

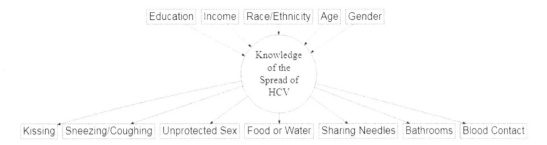

FIGURE 11.5
LCA model of knowledge of the spread of HCV (KSHCV) with covariates (N = 3,902).

TABLE 11.2

Model Fit Comparison for LCA of Knowledge of Spread of HCV (N = 3,902)

# Profiles	BIC	VLMR-LRT	Entropy
1	18443.82		
2	17477.15	<0.001	0.882
3	17494.69	<0.001	0.888
4	17502.04	0.501	0.889
5	17537.31	0.015	0.890
6	17537.31	0.082	0.903
7	17573.90	0.008	0.882

focus our model fit evaluation on BIC, entropy and the VLMR-LRT. Table 11.2 displays the results of the solutions with one through seven classes. From Table 11.2, the three category model of knowledge of the spread of HCV is the preferred model using the LRT criteria; in addition, the BIC is near-minimum and the entropy is near-maximum out of the models tested. The LRT shows that the three class model provides a significantly better fit than the prior solution with two classes ($p < 0.001$), but the four category model does not provide a better fit than the three class model (p = 0.501). While the LRT is again significant in some of the subsequent models (i.e. five vs. four category model and seven vs. six category model), one conducts the test based on the first time criterion is satisfied [5].

Figure 11.6 graphically presents the estimated probability of correctly knowing how HCV is spread on the seven indicators within each class.

LCA allows researchers to assign individuals to the class for which they have the highest probability of membership. In Figure 11.6, the smallest group, comprising 601 individuals (15.4% of the total sample), consists of those who have a high probability of responding that "yes" HCV can be spread through all seven of the vectors in the survey. The largest group consists of those who have the opposite view; 2,143 individuals (54.9% of the total sample) think that "no" HCV cannot be spread through any of the vectors in the Arizona BRFSS questionnaire. The knowledge of the third group of 1,158 individuals (29.7% of the total sample) is the most consistent with scientific understandings of how HCV is spread.

The diagram in Figure 11.6 provides visual confirmation that the three classes are indeed distinct and interpretable and that the model meets the assumption of conditional independence. Individuals in the *HCV Is Nowhere* class (circles) have a very low probability of a scientifically supported response to the questions about unprotected sex, sharing needles

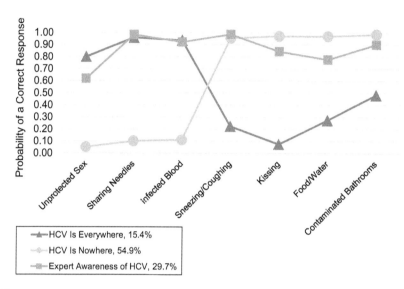

FIGURE 11.6
Estimated item probabilities of KSHCV responses by latent class membership.

and infected blood, but a very high probability of a scientifically supported response to the questions about whether HCV can be spread thru sneezing/coughing, kissing, food/water and contaminated bathrooms. The *HCV Is Everywhere* class (triangles) shows an opposite pattern of response probabilities, while the *"Expert" Awareness* class (squares) has a high probability of a scientifically correct response on all seven survey questions.

11.6.1 LCA for Hepatitis C Transmission Awareness with Covariates

Mean age in the sample was 48.5 (SD = 18.1) and 59% of the subjects were female. Ordinal response categories were used for education (four category) and income (five category); the median categories were "some college" and "$25,000–$35,000." For race/ethnicity, 75.8% were non-Hispanic White, 2.3% were African American, 4.4% were Native American and 17.5% were Hispanic.

In order to include a nominal variable for race in the model, the variable was coded into four dummy variables. Due to linear dependency, the dummy variable for non-Hispanic White was not included in the model. As a result, non-Hispanic White is the reference group in each of the three dummy variables for African American, Native American and Hispanic included in the model.

Table 11.3 presents odds ratios with 95% confidence intervals for the sociodemographic covariates (education, income, race/ethnicity, age, gender) using a corrected three-step regression procedure.[1] In using this corrected three-step approach most likely class of membership definitions remained the same for the subjects. There are two sets of coefficients in the table. The first set compares the *HCV Is Everywhere* form of KSHCV to the *"Expert" Awareness* form of KSHCV. The second set compares the *HCV Is Nowhere* form to the *"Expert" Awareness* form of KSHCV.

---

[1] R3STEP statement in the AUXILIARY option in the VARIABLE command in MPLUS to implement the three step procedure automatically for covariates.

TABLE 11.3

Odds Ratios with 95% Confidence Intervals in Multinomial Regression

Effects of Covariates on Membership in the HCV Is Everywhere Class vs. the "Expert"Awareness of HCV Class			
Covariate	**Odds Ratio**	**95% Lower**	**95% Upper**
Education	0.82	0.70	0.97
Income	0.91	0.82	1.01
African American	3.66	1.45	9.26
Native American	4.32	1.97	9.48
Hispanic	3.30	2.20	4.94
Age	1.01	1.01	1.02
Female	0.79	0.59	1.06
Effects of Covariates on Membership in the HCV Is Nowhere Class vs. the "Expert" Awareness of HCV Class			
Education	0.84	0.75	0.94
Income	0.92	0.86	0.99
African American	2.04	0.93	4.46
Native American	3.45	1.82	6.55
Hispanic	2.17	1.58	2.97
Age	1.02	1.01	1.02
Female	0.96	0.78	1.17

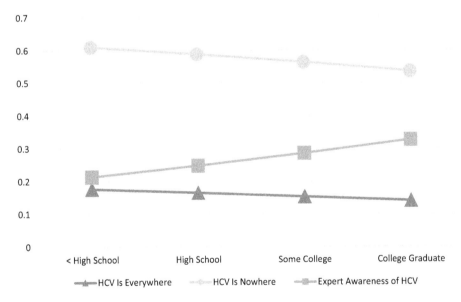

FIGURE 11.7

Relationship between education level and the probability of latent class membership.

Figure 11.7 displays how education affects KSHCV. Higher educated individuals are more likely to have the "Expert" Awareness form of KSHCV. As education increases, so does the likelihood of having the "Expert" Awareness form of knowledge. Individuals with higher education levels are increasingly likely to have the *"Expert" Awareness* form of KSHCV as opposed to the *HCV is Everywhere* or *HCV Is Nowhere* forms. Persons with lower education had lower probabilities of having the *"Expert" Awareness* form of KSHCV.

Generally, individuals of a lower education, lower income, older age and racial and ethnic minority group had lower probabilities of having the *"Expert" Awareness* form of KSHCV. Gender was not associated with KSHCV. For nearly all of the variables in the model, the *Everywhere* and *Nowhere* forms of knowledge had similar relationships with the *"Expert" Awareness* form of KSHCV.

11.7 Application of LCA with Binary and Ordinal Indicators: Methods of Tobacco Use Example

The goal of a study of 1,089 subjects[2] who currently smoke cigarillos was to measure nicotine dependence among users of cigarillos, little cigars, traditional cigars, cigarettes, e-cigarettes and waterpipe/hookah [20]. The study had interest in adolescent and young adult behavior and all participants were between the ages of 14–28. LCA corresponding to the measurement part of Figure 11.3 was performed to identify subgroups based on tobacco use [20]. The LCA involved both binary (no use or any use) and three category ordinal (no use, low amount of use, moderate or high amount of use) indicators.

We again used the MLR option in MPlus with the EMA algorithm [33]. Empirical model selection criteria included BIC, aBIC, AIC, AICC, entropy, VLMR-LRT, aLMR-LRT, bootstrapped LRT, assessment of posterior probabilities and class cell sizes. We identified the seven class solution as the optimal solution. The solution had the minimum AIC and AICC. The solution also still had a significant bootstrapped LRT ($p = 0.024$), whereas the bootstrapped LRT for the eight class solution was not significant. The seven class model was also chosen based on interpretability after careful deliberation with an expert panel. In Figure 11.8, we display the seven classes using stacked barplots. We provide a brief description of each class within the stacked barplot based on the level of endorsement of the different methods of tobacco use.

The BCH method was used for evaluating predictors (age, race and sex) of subgroup membership and differences in nicotine dependence across subgroups (see Figure 11.3). In using this corrected three-step procedure, most likely class of membership definitions remained the same for the subjects. A manual coding approach was used in MPlus to perform this analyses and simultaneously estimate parameters in the model with both covariates and a distal outcome. See the MPlus web note by Asparouhov and Muthen [18] available on the statmodel.com website for coding on how to implement such a model using the BCH method.

Dummy variables were created for the four categories of race (Caucasian, African-American, Hispanic or Other) The three dummy variables for African-American, Hispanic and Other were included in the model making Caucasian the reference category. Age was dichotomized to under 21 or 21 and older in recognition of laws (see https://tobacco21. org/) which prohibit sales of tobacco product to individuals under the age of 21.

We use a subgroup characterized by light tobacco use (class 2: light tipped) as the reference group.[3] The odds ratio for class 1 is higher for male compared to female (OR = 6.58, 95% CI 1.42, 30.50) and lower for African-American compared to Caucasian (OR = 0.16,

---

[2] **NIH NCI/FDA R01CA190130.**
[3] While there are many interesting results of this analyses using other subgroups as reference groups, in the interest of space for this textbook we omit these results.

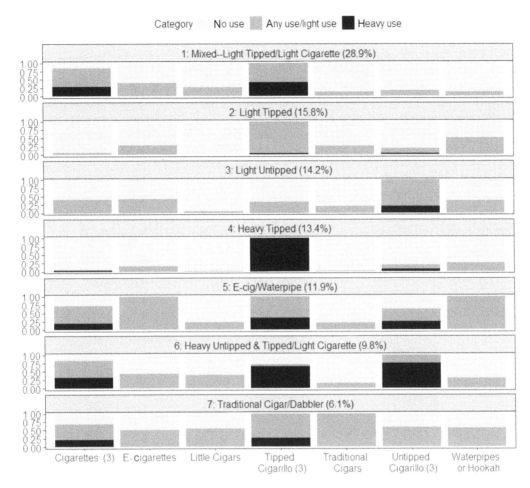

FIGURE 11.8
Stacked barplots of expected probability by category and class for methods of tobacco use (N = 1,089).

The expected probability of the categories within each bar add up to 1.00. Indicators with three categories of use (cigarettes, tipped cigarillo and untipped cigarillo) are denoted in parenthesis (3). Adapted with some modification from supplemental figure from Ishler KJ, Flocke SA, Albert EL, Trapl E, Gunzler D. Cigarillo and multiple tobacco product use and nicotine dependence in adolescents and young adults. *Addictive Behaviors* 2020, doi: 10.1016/j.addbeh.2020.106537.

95% CI 0.03, 0.93). The odds ratio for class 3 is lower for under 21 compared to 21 and older (OR = 0.39, 95% CI 0.16, 0.95) and higher for being Hispanic compared to Caucasian (OR = 3.16, 95% CI 1.15, 8.71). The odds ratio for class 4 (OR = 0.31, 95% CI 0.17, 0.55), 5 (OR = 0.24, 95% CI 0.09, 0.66) and 6 (OR = 0.37, 95% CI 0.17, 0.82) is lower, while class 7 (OR = 4.79, 95% CI 1.92, 11.98) is higher for African-American compared to Caucasian. No other covariates had 95% confidence intervals that did not contain one for this analysis.

We can conclude that there are important predictors that influence membership into the light tipped group (more likely to be under 21 and less likely to be Hispanic as compared to Caucasian) compared to the light untipped group. Similarly, members of the light tipped group are more likely to be female and African-American (vs. Caucasian) compared to the mixed – light tipped/light cigarette group. Members of the light tipped group are more likely to be African-American (vs. Caucasian) compared to members of the heavy tipped, e-cig/waterpipe and heavy untipped and tipped/light cigarette groups. However, members of the light tipped group are less likely to be African-American (vs. Caucasian) compared to members of the traditional cigar/dabbler group.

In the study sample, nicotine dependence score was standardized and the mean equaled 50 (SD = 10), with higher scores indicating higher nicotine dependence [20]. We found groups with more sources of tobacco use, including light or heavy cigarette use (classes 1, 5, 6 and 7), had higher than average nicotine dependence as estimated using the latent class model with covariates and distal outcome (Figure 11.9). Class 4 also had higher than average nicotine dependence and was characterized by heavy use of tipped cigarillo.

Most prominently, the average nicotine dependence score in class 6 was over a standard deviation above the mean. Classes 2 and 3 had below average nicotine dependence and were characterized, respectively, by light use of tipped and untipped cigarillo.

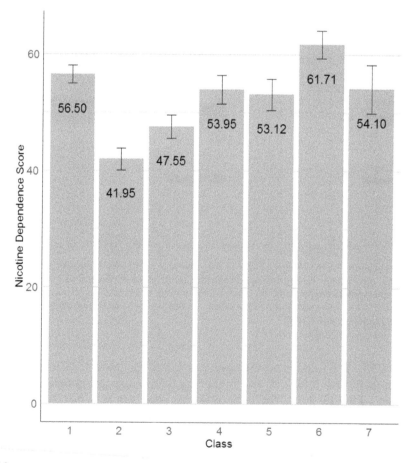

FIGURE 11.9
Within-class means for nicotine dependence score for methods of tobacco use (*N* = 1,089).

95% confidence interval bar drawn on figure. Adapted with some modification from Ishler KJ, Flocke SA, Albert EL, Trapl E, Gunzler D. Cigarillo and multiple tobacco product use and nicotine dependence in adolescents and young adults. *Addictive* Behaviors 2020, doi: 10.1016/j.addbeh.2020.106537.

The regression of the distal outcome on the covariates can be handled using different constraints depending on the research intent of the study and a priori assumptions. In some studies, there may be no interest in performing this regression as one only would like to evaluate the regression of the distal outcome on the latent classes and latent classes on the covariates. Other options include constraining the regression coefficients to be equal across classes or freely estimated within each class. In this example we were interested in the overall effect of sex, age and race on nicotine dependence (equality constraint across classes). Across subgroups, nicotine dependence was significantly lower for males (vs. females) (Estimate = −4.083, 95% CI −5.284, −2.881). No other covariates were significantly associated with nicotine dependence.

11.8 Extensions of Latent Class Analysis with Longitudinal Data

Many data sets in health and medicine include repeated measures data on a group of individuals followed over time. A set of categorical indicators primed for use in a latent class model may have been collected only at baseline or at multiple waves. If data on the set of indicators is only collected at baseline, one could begin by conducting LCA. Subsequently, one could use individualized scores on the nominal latent class variable[4] as fixed values across all the repeated observations in longitudinal data analysis. However, there are several modeling opportunities if data for the indicators is collected across multiple waves.

A special application of the latent class approach is *longitudinal latent class analysis (LLCA)*. This is a longitudinal extension of LCA also called a *repeated measures LCA*. In the repeated measures LCA, the latent classes represent trajectories across multiple waves of data for a given set of indicators [24]. In LLCA change over time is discrete.

Latent transition analysis (LTA) is a longitudinal variation of LCA used to examine membership changes in the subgroups over time [24]. LTA examines both the prevalence of the latent classes and the probability of changing from one latent class to another class at later time points. The rate and paths of change can be different for different individuals. Since latent classes are not stable over time in LTA, these are often referred to as *latent statuses* instead [24]. The interested reader should refer to the textbook by Collins and Lanza [24] for an overview of LLCA and LTA.

11.9 Conclusions

Mixture modeling is a multivariate technique for describing unobserved subgroups in a study sample. Mixture modeling is probabilistic in nature, where subgroups are described based on empirical evidence and interpretability. A categorical latent variable is used for representing the unobserved subgroups. LCA is a useful application of mixture modeling with select categorical indicators. We have presented some of the basic theory of LCA and incorporated covariates and distal outcomes in applied examples in health and medical studies.

---

[4] Note, as mentioned previously, if we simply assign members to their most likely subgroup in defining the nominal latent class variable, a limitation is that uncertainty is not accounted for in the classification approach.

References

1. Lanza, S.T. and B.L. Rhoades, Latent class analysis: An alternative perspective on subgroup analysis in prevention and treatment. *Prevention Science*, 2013. **14**(2): pp. 157–168.
2. Collins, L.M., J.J. Graham, and B.P. Flaherty, An alternative framework for defining mediation. *Multivariate Behavioral Research*, 1998. **33**(2): pp. 295–312.
3. DeMeo, D.L., et al., Women manifest more severe COPD symptoms across the life course. *International Journal of Chronic Obstructive Pulmonary Disease*, 2018. **13**: p. 3021.
4. Schreiber, J.B. and A.J. Pekarik, Using latent class analysis versus K-means or hierarchical clustering to understand museum visitors. *Curator: The Museum Journal*, 2014. **57**(1): pp. 45–59.
5. Nylund, K.L., T. Asparouhov, and B.O. Muthén, Deciding on the number of classes in latent class analysis and growth mixture modeling: A Monte Carlo simulation study. *Structural Equation Modeling*, 2007. **14**(4): pp. 535–569.
6. Heinen, T., *Latent class and discrete latent trait models: Similarities and differences*. 1996, London: Sage Publications, Inc.
7. Lazarsfeld, P.F., Stouffer, S.A., Suchman, E.A., Devinney, L.C., Star, S.A., Williams, R.M., The logical and mathematical foundation of latent structure analysis. Studies in Social Psychology in World War II Vol. IV: Measurement and Prediction, 1950. Princeton, NJ: Princeton University Press, pp. 362–412.
8. Lazarsfeld, P.F., Evidence and inference in social research. *Daedalus*, 1958. **87**(4): pp. 99–130.
9. Lazarsfeld, P.F. and N.W. Henry, *Latent structure analysis*. 1968, New York: Houghton, Mifflin.
10. Magidson, J. and J. Vermunt, Latent class models, in *The Sage Handbook of Quantitative Methodology for the Social Sciences*, D. Kaplan, Editor. 2004, Thousand Oaks, CA: Sage Publications, Inc., pp. 175–198.
11. Gibson, W.A., Three multivariate models: Factor analysis, latent structure analysis, and latent profile analysis. *Psychometrika*, 1959. **24**(3): pp. 229–252.
12. Bartholomew, D.J., M. Knott, and I. Moustaki, *Latent variable models and factor analysis: A unified approach*. Vol. 904. 2011, Chichester, West Sussex: John Wiley & Sons.
13. Schwarz, G., Estimating the dimension of a model. *The Annals of Statistics*, 1978. **6**(2): pp. 461–464.
14. Muthén, B. and K. Shedden, Finite mixture modeling with mixture outcomes using the EM algorithm. *Biometrics*, 1999. **55**(2): pp. 463–469.
15. McLachlan, G.J., On bootstrapping the likelihood ratio test statistic for the number of components in a normal mixture. *Applied Statistics*, 1987, **36**: pp. 318–324.
16. Kim, S.-Y., Determining the number of latent classes in single- and multi-phase growth mixture models. *Structural Equation Modeling: A Multidisciplinary Journal*, 2014. **21**(2): pp. 263–279.
17. Lanza, S.T., X. Tan, and B.C. Bray, Latent class analysis with distal outcomes: A flexible model-based approach. *Structural Equation Modeling: A Multidisciplinary Journal*, 2013. **20**(1): pp. 1–26.
18. Asparouhov, T. and B. Muthén, Auxiliary variables in mixture modeling: Using the BCH method in Mplus to estimate a distal outcome model and an arbitrary secondary model. *Mplus Web Notes*, 2014. **21**(2): pp. 1–22.
19. Asparouhov, T. and B. Muthén, Auxiliary variables in mixture modeling: Three-step approaches using M plus. *Structural Equation Modeling: A Multidisciplinary Journal*, 2014. **21**(3): pp. 329–341.
20. Ishler, K.J., et al., Cigarillo and multiple tobacco product use and nicotine dependence in adolescents and young adults. *Addictive Behaviors*, 2020. **111**: p. 106537.
21. Feingold, A., S.S. Tiberio, and D.M. Capaldi, New approaches for examining associations with latent categorical variables: Applications to substance abuse and aggression. *Psychology of Addictive Behaviors*, 2014. **28**(1): p. 257.
22. Vermunt, J.K., Latent class modeling with covariates: Two improved three-step approaches. *Political Analysis*, 2010. **18**(4): pp. 450–469.

23. Bolck, A., M. Croon, and J., Hagenaars, Estimating latent structure models with categorical variables: One-step versus three-step estimators. *Political Analysis*, 2004. **12**(1): pp. 3–27.
24. Collins, L.M. and S.T. *Lanza, Latent class and latent transition analysis: With applications in the social behavioral, and health sciences. Wiley series in probability and statistics.* 2010, Hoboken, NJ: Wiley.
25. Vermunt, J.K., Latent profile model, in *The Sage Encyclopedia of Social Sciences Research Methods*, Michael S., Lewis-Beck, Alan Bryman and Tim Futing L., Editors. 2004, Thousand Oaks, CA: Sage Publications, Inc., pp. 554–555.
26. Nasim, A., et al., Patterns of alternative tobacco use among adolescent cigarette smokers. *Drug & Alcohol Dependence*, 2012. **124**(1): pp. 26–33.
27. Oberski, D.L., Local dependence in latent class models: Application to voting in elections. in Advances in latent variables [sis 2013 conference proceedings]. 2013. Milan, Italy: Vita e Pensiero.
28. Friedman, J., T. Hastie, and R. Tibshirani, *The elements of statistical learning.* 2001. Springer series in statistics. Berlin: Springer.
29. James, G., et al., *An introduction to statistical learning with applications in R.* 2013. Berlin: Springer.
30. Niileksela, C.R. and J. Templin, Identifying dyslexia with confirmatory latent profile analysis. *Psychology in the Schools*, 2019. **56**(3): pp. 335–359.
31. Schmiege, S.J., K.E. Masyn, and A.D. Bryan, Confirmatory latent class analysis: Illustrations of empirically driven and theoretically driven model constraints. *Organizational Research Methods*, 2018. **21**(4): pp. 983–1001.
32. Perzynski, A.T., *Between facts and voices: Medical and lay knowledge of the spread of Hepatitis C - CORE.* 2008, Cleveland, OH: Case Western Reserve University.
33. Muthén, L.K. and B.O. Muthén, *Mplus: The comprehensive modeling program for applied researchers: User's guide. Eighth edition,* 1998–2017, Los Angeles, CA: Muthén & Muthén.

12

Latent Profile Analysis

12.1 Introduction to Latent Profile Analysis

Latent profile analysis (LPA) relates a set of observed continuous indicators to a set of latent profiles (underlying subgroups). Broadly, LPA differs from LCA (Chapter 11) in using continuous indicators as opposed to categorical indicators. For example, suppose a researcher was interested in assessing whether scores on a set of clinical outcome measures, such as systolic blood pressure, diastolic blood pressure, body mass index, triglycerides, high-density lipoprotein and hemoglobin A1c tended to cluster together in specific ways. There are patients that do poorly on all of these outcomes or well on all of these outcomes, whereas others do well on some but not others. Then, LPA would be appropriate.

It is also possible to perform a mixed latent class/profile analysis with both categorical and continuous variables. While we refer to the subgroups as latent profiles when performing LPA in this textbook, some researchers will use latent class as an umbrella term for the subgroups as identified using any mixture model (or latent class model).

In performing LPA, we use similar criteria for selecting the optimal solution as LCA. We have discussed this model selection criteria in the context of LCA in the previous chapter. While not necessary to have all measures on the same scale with similar variances, standardizing all measures for LPA is a common practice that may help with model convergence and stability [1]. One can also graphically display the estimated means across a set of standardized indicators on a single plot for ease of interpretability. That is, the scale of all the continuous indicators is the same after standardization. Estimated means of zero across the standardized indicators can be construed as average within the study sample.

12.2 LPA Model

First, we present the basic mathematical model [2,3] for LPA. Reconsider Chapter 11, Figure 11.2 with M continuous indicators $y_1, y_2, ..., y_M$ in place of the binary indicators. Let $\mathbf{y}_i$ be the vector of response for individual i on the set of observed continuous indicators.

The joint density function for $\mathbf{y}_i$,

$$f(\mathbf{y}_i) = \sum_{k=1}^{K} P(c = k) f(\mathbf{y}_i | \boldsymbol{\mu}_k, \boldsymbol{\Sigma}_k) \tag{12.1}$$

Here $f\left(\mathbf{y}_i|\mathbf{\mu}_k,\mathbf{\Sigma}_k\right)$ is typically assumed to be the multivariate normal probability density function for the M continuous indictors which is conditional on latent profile membership. Each latent profile has its own mean vector and variance-covariance matrix [4].

12.3 Assumptions Regarding the Variance-Covariance Matrix in LPA

The standard assumptions for LPA include (a) local independence and (b) equal error variances across classes. The specification for LPA under these standard assumptions is similar to K-means clustering [4].

Under the assumption of local independence, within-class covariance terms are set to zero in LPA. Thus, the within-class covariance matrices are diagonal. The error variance terms can still be either freely estimated or constrained across classes. Different assumptions regarding restrictions on the covariance terms across profiles are possible with local dependencies [4]. See Vermunt [4] for a brief description of these additional assumptions.

In a standard application of LPA, the main objective is recovering underlying profiles that differ with respect to their means [5]. Researchers examine the varied patterns of higher or lower values that exist across profile groups. Under the assumption of equal and diagonal covariance matrices across profiles the profiles only differ with respect to their means. The assumption allows one to perform analysis in which results can be interpreted in line with this objective. It is important to note that analysis with less restricted covariance matrices for each profile (especially as the number of profiles increases) may require a very large sample size.

In many applications of LPA, imposing restrictions on the covariance matrices across profiles may be less than reasonable. For example, a subgroup with few medical conditions may have a smaller variance on indicators of physical health than a subgroup with a multitude of different medical conditions. A researcher could compare the fit of the model restricting the within-profile variance to be equal vs. freely (or partially) estimated. However, as noted, restrictions on the covariance matrices across profiles are often used in analysis for the benefit of interpretability and parsimony.

12.4 Outliers in LPA

Latent profiles are described based on estimates of the within-profile means and variances/covariances. Outliers can affect these estimates. Thus, when one conducts LPA without careful handling of univariate and multivariate outliers, potentially

- within-profile means and variance/covariances may shift, changing the substantive interpretation of the profiles
- certain profiles that do exist within the study sample may not be detected given the observed data
- small profiles with only a handful of cases or that have no clear or meaningful interpretation may be detected

We have previously discussed approaches to deal with potential influential observations (both univariate and multivariate outliers) prior to conducting analysis in Chapter 4.

12.5 Application of LPA in Adults with Serious Mental Illness and Diabetes

Care for adults with serious mental illness and diabetes is complicated by clinical and psychosocial heterogeneity [6]. We present an LPA of 200 adults with comorbid diabetes and serious mental illness (DM-SMI) differentiating between patient subgroups that were characterized on the basis of selected dimensions within a biopsychosocial framework: self-efficacy, treatment expectation, social support and depression (see Figure 12.1). The C variable on the diagram represents the discrete latent variable that is used to relate the five observed indicators to latent profiles. We discuss the LPA model with covariates and distal outcomes for this applied example later in this chapter.

The DM-SMI participants in this study were enrolled in a randomized controlled trial from November 2011 through April 2014, in a safety net setting, testing a novel self-management intervention vs. treatment as usual.[1] Within the sample, most subjects were moderately to severely depressed with poor diabetes control [7]. These individuals faced multiple challenges that could impede diabetes self-management [7]. LPA results, given a select controlled trial sample, could lack external validity for a more general population of DM-SMI adults.

Depression symptom severity was measured with the Montgomery-Asberg Depression Rating Scale (MADRS) [8]. Social support was measured with the Multidimensional Scale of Perceived Social Support (MSPSS) [9]. Perceived therapeutic efficacy for diabetes treatment was measured with the Perceived Therapeutic Efficacy Scale (PTES) [10]. Self-efficacy for managing diabetes was measured with the Perceived Diabetes Self-Management Scale (PDSMS) [11]. Self-efficacy for serious mental illness management was measured with a modified template the Perceived Mental Health Self-Management Scale (PMHSMS) [6]. We standardized these five measures prior to performing LPA.

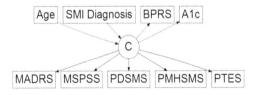

FIGURE 12.1
Mixture model with covariates and distal outcomes for the analysis of adults with serious mental illness and diabetes.

MADRS = Montgomery-Asberg Depression Rating Scale; MSPSS = Multidimensional Scale of Perceived Social Support; PDSMS = Perceived Diabetes Self-Management Scale; PMHSMS = Perceived Mental Health Self-Management Scale; PTES = Perceived Therapeutic Efficacy Scale; SMI = Serious Mental Illness; BPRS = Brief Psychiatric Rating Scale.

[1] 1R01MH085665.

12.5.1 Descriptive Analysis

Pairwise Spearman correlations between these five measures ranged from 0.10 to 0.49 in absolute value. Thus, no pairwise correlations appeared to be so high (e.g. greater than 0.80) as to cause concerns regarding of multicollinearity.

Univariate and multivariate tests and graphical displays (e.g. boxplots) for detecting potential outliers (Chapter 4) indicated extreme values for four cases. We removed these four cases (2% of the cases) from the data.

12.5.2 LPA Results

In Table 12.1, we report the relative fit indices and test results for LPA ($N = 196$). We also graphically depict the results for the fit indices in Figure 12.2.

In evaluating Table 12.1 (and Figure 12.2), along with consideration of interpretability as we will discuss below, we narrowed down the optimal solution to either the three or five profile solution. To avoid any confusion of which solution we are discussing in the text, we label the profiles in the three profile solution with an asterisk (*).

We could favor the three profile solution based on the VLMR-LRT and aLMR-LRT (last solution with significant test results) with BIC close to the minimum. We could favor the five profile solution using the bootstrapped LRT while noting empirically it strongly balances attempting attempting to minimize aBIC, AIC, AICC and BIC and maximize entropy. The three profile solution had a reasonably high proportion of the cases within each profile (profile 1* 23%; profile 2* 18%; profile 3* 59%) and reasonably high average latent classification probabilities (profile 1* 0.899; profile 2* 0.820; profile 3* 0.864) for most likely latent profile. The five profile solution had a reasonable proportion of the cases within each profile (approximately, profile 1 5%; profile 2 21%; profile 3 7%; profile 4 39%; profile 5 29%) and reasonably high average latent classification probabilities (profile 1 0.881; profile 2 0.829; profile 3 0.816; profile 4 0.839; profile 5 0.871) for most likely latent profile. (Selected and Modified MPlus Output in Box 12.1).

A researcher might also consider the six or seven profile solutions as plausible given the empirical results. However, upon evaluation (in consideration of empirical results and interpretability) we found the three and five profile solutions to be "better" fitting. We omit further discussion of these other solutions here so as not to confuse the problem and limit it to two models (three and five profiles).

TABLE 12.1

Fit Indices and Test Results of LPA of Adults with a Serious Mental Illness and Diabetes ($N = 196$)

# Profiles	AIC	BIC	aBIC	AICC	Entropy	VLMR-LRT	aLMR-LRT	BLRT
1	2562.64	2595.42	2563.74	2563.83				
2	2447.69	2500.14	2449.46	2450.73	0.726	0.002	0.003	<0.001
3	2428.40	2500.52	2430.83	2434.25	0.703	0.037	0.042	<0.001
4	2415.43	2507.21	2418.51	2425.15	0.729	0.756	0.762	0.007
5	2404.21	2515.67	2407.96	2419.00	0.760	0.107	0.110	0.013
6	2395.35	2526.47	2399.76	2416.51	0.769	0.707	0.712	0.050[a]
7	2390.05	2540.84	2395.12	2419.07	0.792	0.202	0.206	0.197
8	2388.60	2559.06	2394.33	2427.15	0.788	0.325	0.330	0.577

[a]BLRT is slight greater than 0.05 when going out four decimal places (0.0502). AIC = Akaike Information Criterion; BIC = Bayesian Information Criterion; aBIC = Sample-Size Adjusted BIC; AICC = Corrected AIC for Small Sample Sizes; VLMR-LRT = Vuong-Lo-Mendell-Rubin Likelihood Ratio Test (LRT); aLMR-LRT = Lo-Mendell-Rubin Adjusted LRT; BLRT = bootstrapped LRT.

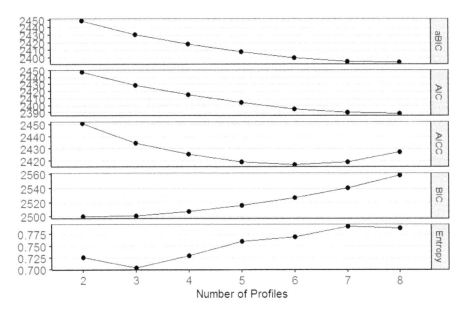

FIGURE 12.2
Facetted plot of AIC, BIC aBIC, AICC and Entropy (*N* = 196).

AIC = Akaike Information Criterion; BIC = Bayesian Information Criterion; aBIC = Sample-Size Adjusted BIC; AICC = Corrected AIC for Small Sample Sizes.

BOX 12.1   CLASSIFICATION OF INDIVIDUALS BASED ON THEIR MOST LIKELY LATENT CLASS MEMBERSHIP

Class Counts and Proportions for Three Profile Solution		
Latent Classes		
1*	45	0.22959
2*	36	0.18367
3*	115	0.58673

Class Counts and Proportions for Five Profile Solution		
Latent Classes		
1	9	0.04592
2	41	0.20918
3	14	0.07143
4	76	0.38776
5	56	0.28571

We also studied graphical displays (Figure 12.3) to compare and contrast the substantive meaning of the three and five profile solutions.

Interpreting the three profile solution was straightforward (see Figure 12.3 Panels A and B). A low score on depression and a high score on the other four variables indicate good psychosocial health within this study sample. A high score on depression and a

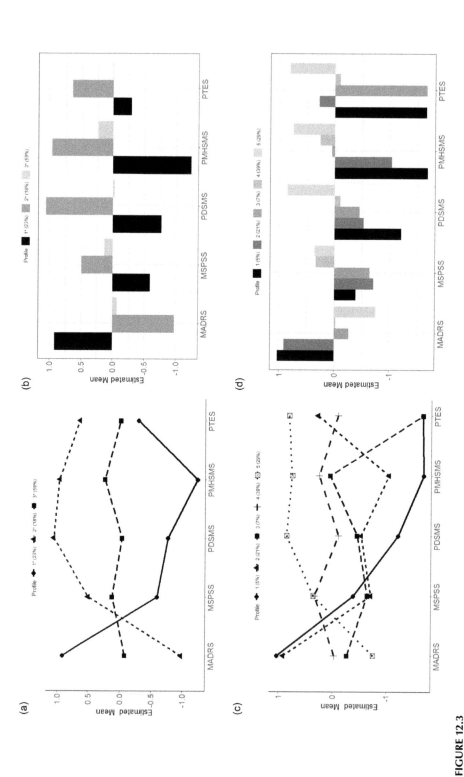

FIGURE 12.3

Graphical displays of the three and five profile solutions (*N* = 196). (a) Line graph for three profile solutions (b) Bar plot for three profile solution (c) Line graph for five profile solution (d) Bar plot for five profile solution.

Standardized estimate results (StdYX option in MPlus), depicted in a mean line graph and similarly in a bar plot. To avoid any confusion, we label the profiles in the three profile solution with an asterisk (*).

low score on the other four variables indicate poor psychosocial health within this study sample. Standardized mean scores around zero of all five variables indicates average psychosocial health within this study sample.

THREE PROFILE SOLUTION

- Profile 1* Poor Psychosocial Health
- Profile 2* Good Psychosocial Health
- Profile 3* Average Psychosocial Health

In the five profile solution, two additional profiles emerged (labeled below in italics as profiles 2 and 3). We now interpret the five profile solution (see Figure 12.3 Panels C and D).

FIVE PROFILE SOLUTION

- Profile 1 Poor Psychosocial Health
- *Profile 2 Optimistic About Treatment*
- *Profile 3 Pessimistic About Treatment*
- Profile 4 Average Psychosocial Health
- Profile 5 Good Psychosocial Health

We can maintain some of the same profile names as profile 1* and profile 1 are somewhat similar, as are profile 2* and profile 5, and profile 3* and profile 4. We refer to profile 2 with the nomenclature "Optimistic About Treatment," since this group has an above average expectation about treatment in spite of generally poor psychosocial health. We use the nomenclature "Pessimistic About Treatment" to refer to profile 3 since this group has a very low treatment expectation. This group has below average depression, social support and diabetes self-management and average mental health self-management. The description of these groups hereafter as "Optimistic" and "Pessimistic" indicates the level of expectation about treatment.

The two completely newly identified profiles in the five profile solution (profiles 2 and 3, the Optimistic and Pessimistic groups) have a reasonable interpretation according to study team experts in psychology. The Optimistic group appears to be a split off from the Poor Psychosocial Health group of individuals, but with better self-efficacy and treatment expectations. One interpretation is that this profile may consist of individuals whose depression could be attributed to overwhelming situation pressures. They, perhaps, stay similar to the Poor Psychosocial Health group on social support because this depression is largely a matter of the reality of external life. The Pessimistic group may be a split from the neutral group (Average Psychosocial Health group). Individuals classified as members of the Pessimistic group may have less self-efficacy for dealing with mental health problems and diabetes and somewhat lower social support. Perhaps as a consequence, members of this group have a very low belief of treatment expectations. Thus, we could further hypothesize that this profile may consist of the individuals in the study who have psychosis or mania rather than depression.

We can also note that in the five profile solution, compared to the three profile solution, more individuals were classified into the Good Psychosocial Health group (29% vs. 18%). In evaluating Figure 12.3, the within-profile mean is slightly higher on depression and lower on the other variables for this group in the five profile solution compared to the three profile solution. Thus, this group in the five profile solution is more inclusive for this study sample, holding a slightly broader interpretation (broader range of values on the five measures).

12.5.3 LPA with Auxiliary Variables Using the Five Profile Model

Both the three and five profile solutions had plausible interpretations. The next step in the analyses was to evaluate for differences across the profiles in relation to auxiliary variables. Of great interest was to evaluate for unique relationships between the Optimistic and Pessimistic group (not observed in the three profile model) and the auxiliary variables. If there were no meaningfully unique aspects of these profiles in relation to covariates and distal outcomes, then the five profile solution might not hold a practical advantage over the three profile solution. That is, if a subgroup does not have a significantly or meaningfully different relationship with clinical variables of interest, one might not gain any useful information in studying that subgroup separately. We are making the assumption that we have not omitted any important auxiliary variables in the model. This assumption is likely not reasonable in practice. In acknowledging this limitation, we could describe other variables we might assess in future studies with a larger sample size.

Due to the sample size used in this analysis, we separately assessed covariates and distal outcomes (see Figure 12.1). We also simplified the analysis by limiting the number of variables to two covariates and two distal outcomes.

We evaluated if covariates for age and SMI diagnosis influenced latent profile membership. SMI diagnosis (depression, bipolar disorder or schizophrenia) was coded into a single binary variable for depression vs. the other two categories. Next, we evaluated if the latent profiles influenced both a mental health and physical health measure. The two distal outcomes were global symptom severity, measured using the Brief Psychiatric Rating Scale (BPRS) [12], and hemoglobin A1c. We used corrected three-step regression procedures to perform LPA with these auxiliary variables.[2] A future study with a larger sample would be necessary to also evaluate other covariates such as race/ethnicity, sex, BMI and diabetes knowledge, and distal outcomes such as functional impairment and assess all the relationships simultaneously.

We found that members of the Optimistic group (Odds Ratio = 4.028, 95% CI 1.363, 11.906) and Average Psychosocial Health group (Odds Ratio = 3.947, 95% CI 1.403, 11.103) were more likely to have a depression diagnosis (compared to other SMI diagnosis categories) than members of the Good Psychosocial Health group. No other pairwise comparisons between profiles for SMI diagnosis were significantly different. There were no significant differences by age across profiles with the overall sample mean age = 52.7 (SD = 9.5).

Some effects could be masked since the Poor Psychosocial Health group and the Pessimistic group especially have a limited number of individuals. Thus, in secondary analysis, we evaluated the number (percentage) of subjects in each profile that have psychosis or mania rather than depression diagnosis (Table 12.2).

The Pessimistic group consists of a high proportion of individuals in the study who have psychosis or mania rather than depression. The Optimistic group had a lower proportion of such individuals. This was in line to our hypothesis about differences in the make-up of these two profiles. These proportions in Table 12.2 may also help explain why members of

---

[2] AUXILIARY command and options for R3STEP for covariates and DU3STEP for distal outcomes (in separate programs) in MPlus.

TABLE 12.2

Number (Percentage) of Subjects in Each Profile in the Five Profile Solution with Schizophrenia or Bipolar Disorder Diagnosis Rather Than Depression Diagnosis ($N = 196$)

Profile	Poor Psychosocial Health	Optimistic About Treatment	Pessimistic About Treatment	Average Psychosocial Health	Good Psychosocial Health
N	9	41	14	76	56
Schizophrenia or bipolar disorder diagnosis	7 (78%)	17 (41%)	9 (64%)	33 (43%)	38 (68%)

TABLE 12.3

Mean (Standard Error) for Hemoglobin A1c and Brief Psychiatric Rating Scale (BPRS) ($N = 196$)

Profile	A1c	BPRS
Poor psychosocial health	9.187 (0.636)	42.691 (2.128)
Optimistic about treatment	9.348 (0.675)	48.239 (1.835)
Pessimistic about treatment	7.051 (0.219)	37.469 (1.133)
Average psychosocial health	9.427 (1.089)	44.658 (2.940)
Good psychosocial health	7.828 (0.505)	36.845 (1.525)

the Poor Psychosocial Health group had lower self-efficacy for managing diabetes and treatment expectation as opposed to the Optimistic group. The majority of subjects in the Good Psychosocial Health group had psychosis or mania rather than depression diagnosis; this is the group characterized by the most positive responses in the sample on the five indicators used for LPA (though still below average compared to the general population). These results are in need of reproducibility in a larger study in different settings before these interpretations are taken as anything more than exploratory.

We now focus on the analyses of the distal outcomes in Figure 12.1. We report the mean (standard error) A1c and BPRS in each profile in Table 12.3.

In tests of the means being equal across profiles conducted in MPlus, there were significant pairwise differences in A1c across the Poor Psychosocial Health group and the Pessimistic group ($p = 0.001$), Pessimistic group and Average Psychosocial Health group ($p = 0.031$) and Optimistic group and Pessimistic group ($p = 0.001$). Further, as shown in Table 12.3, the Pessimistic About Treatment and Good Psychosocial Health profiles (which also happen to have the lowest overall MADRS depression scores) had the two lowest average A1c values.

There were significant pairwise differences in BPRS across the Poor Psychosocial Health group and Pessimistic group ($p = 0.035$), Poor Psychosocial Health group and Good Psychosocial Health group ($p = 0.024$), Optimistic group and Pessimistic group ($p<0.001$), Optimistic group and Good Psychosocial Health group ($p<0.001$), Pessimistic group and Average Psychosocial Health group ($p = 0.026$) and Average Psychosocial Health group and Good Psychosocial Health group ($p = 0.019$). A higher BPRS score indicates more severe psychiatric symptoms.

As shown in Table 12.3, the groups for Pessimistic About Treatment and Good Psychosocial Health had the two lowest mean BPRS. Thus membership in these two groups may lead to better outcomes for physical health (lower A1c) and less severe psychiatric symptoms (lower BPRS) compared to other groups. On the contrary, membership in the Optimistic group and Average Psychosocial Health group may lead to worse outcomes on A1c and BPRS. We should also keep in mind that, in general, all of these A1c and BPRS scores can be considered reasonably high and indicative of poorly controlled diabetes and serious symptomatic mental disorder.

A1c values and BPRS scores are high in Poor Psychosocial Health group (but not significantly different from the Optimistic group and Average Psychosocial Health group). This group may show the select sample for this randomized controlled trial; members have high depression, low psychosocial measures, poor diabetes control and severe psychiatric symptoms but are still active trial participants.

12.5.4 Is the Five Profile Model Optimal?

We can now infer from analysis of auxiliary variables that there are unique aspects to the Optimistic and Pessimistic groups. If the Optimistic group is a split from the Poor Psychosocial Health group, then subjects with depression diagnosis (and slightly higher A1c and BPRS) are more likely to be members of the Optimistic group compared to the Poor Psychosocial Health group. Further, if the Pessimistic group is a split from the Average Psychosocial Health group, then subjects in the Pessimistic group were less likely to have depression diagnosis and had better outcomes for physical health and severity of psychiatric symptoms compared to the Average Psychosocial Health group. Thus, with interest in studying subpopulations with distinct relationships with clinical outcome variables, we choose the five profile model over the three profile model as the working model. The working model should go through some rigorous testing in future studies.

12.5.5 Local Dependencies in LPA for DM-SMI Adults

We assumed local independence and did not test for local dependence, given the sample size. More generally, one could test for local dependencies in an iterative process by freeing up one residual correlation at a time (within certain profiles or across all profiles) between the observed indicators used for LPA. A significant difference test ($p<0.05$) using the log-likelihood for a revised model including a local dependence compared to a model with that local dependence constrained to zero would signify an improvement for the revised model. One could then include meaningful and significant local dependencies with a plausible interpretation in the final model. For example, it might be reasonable to assume depression and mental health self-management and/or diabetes self-management and perceived treatment efficacy are additionally related to each other (besides through the latent variable) through their error terms within profiles. Note that one should limit the number of local dependencies tested to only a few of a theoretically meaningful nature and should never conduct such analyses solely for the benefit of improved model fit.

12.6 Factor Mixture Models

We briefly conclude our material on cross-sectional latent variable mixture models by describing a *hybrid latent variable model* [13]. A hybrid latent variable model includes both continuous and categorical latent variables. *Factor mixture models* [13,14] are a combination of latent class and common factor models. That is, factor mixture models assume a mixture model and then impose a factor model on the within-class mean vector and covariance matrix [15]. For this section, we use the term latent class as an umbrella term to describe clusters regardless of the metric of the indicators (e.g. continuous, categorical).

BASIC FACTOR MIXTURE MODEL FOR A SET OF CONTINUOUS INDICATORS

$$\mathbf{y}_{ik} = \mu_k + \Lambda_k \eta_{ik} + \varepsilon_{ik}$$
$$\eta_{ik} = \alpha_k + \zeta_{ik}$$

(12.2)

For the ith individual in the kth, where $k = 1,...,K$ latent classes and $i = 1,...,n$ individuals. η_{ik} is a vector of factor scores measured by a vector of the observed indicator variables $\mathbf{y}_{ik}$ and ε_{ik} is a vector of error terms. The measurement equations include within-class vectors of intercepts μ_k and matrices of factor loadings Λ_k. α_k is a vector of intercepts of the factors (factor means) for class k. Finally, ζ_{ik} is a vector of error terms for the ith individual in the kth class.

In factor mixture models, due to the within-class factor variable, some of the covariance between observed indicators is explained by common within-class covariation. Thus in factor mixture models covariation between observed indicators is decomposed into class mean differences and continuous factors within class.

In Figure 12.4, we graphically display a path diagram for a representation of one specification of a factor mixture model. A latent construct η accounts for within-class measurement error in the observed indicators $(y_1, y_2,...,y_M)$. A latent class variable c is used to relate the latent construct to a set of latent classes. Class mean differences on the latent construct can be evaluated using this model.

There are several specifications of the factor mixture model differing in the relationship between the latent construct η, latent class variable c and observed indicators $(y_1, y_2,...,y_M)$. See Muthen [13] for an overview of different cross-sectional hybrid models.

One can iteratively fit models of both increasing number of within-class factors and classes to determine the optimal solution for the number of within-class factors and classes. In a typical application, one may assume the within-class factor structure (e.g. assumed due to item content analysis) and then determine the optimal solution for the number of classes.

Just as in LCA and LPA, researchers can incorporate covariates and distal outcomes in factor mixture models. Invariance in the factor structure across classes can be evaluated using constraints of equality. One may also load some or all of the observed items

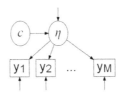

FIGURE 12.4
Factor mixture model.

directly onto the latent class variable. See Lutke and Muthén [14] and Muthén [13] for a more detailed introduction to factor mixture models. We will dedicate a whole chapter (Chapter 14) to another hybrid latent variable model, a longitudinal extension of the factor mixture model called the *growth mixture model*. The growth mixture model can be applied in health and medical research to evaluate heterogeneity in health outcome trajectories.

12.7 Conclusions

LPA is a useful multivariate technique for describing subgroups in study samples based on select continuous indicators. This technique is probabilistic in nature where profiles are described based on empirical evidence and interpretability. Having gone over many of the basic foundations of mixture modeling and in particular LCA in the previous chapter, we focused on an application of LPA in a research study. LPA was conducted using randomized controlled trial participants with a serious mental illness and diabetes. We explored differentiation between subpopulations that were characterized on the basis of selected dimensions within a biopsychosocial framework. We carefully made assumptions and interpreted results in line with theory, logic and prior findings.

More generally, a researcher should explicitly state the assumptions being made in an application of mixture modeling. Researchers in reproducibility replication studies can then either follow the same approach or deduce that different assumptions and model constraints may be necessary.

References

1. Muthén, L.K. and B.O. Muthén, *Mplus: The comprehensive modeling program for applied researchers: User's guide. Eighth edition*, 1998–2017, Los Angeles, CA: Muthén & Muthén.
2. Bartholomew, D.J., M. Knott, and I. Moustaki, *Latent variable models and factor analysis: A unified approach*. Vol. 904. 2011, London, UK: John Wiley & Sons.
3. Nylund, K.L., T. Asparouhov, and B.O. Muthén, Deciding on the number of classes in latent class analysis and growth mixture modeling: A Monte Carlo simulation study. *Structural Equation Modeling*, 2007. **14**(4): pp. 535–569.
4. Vermunt, J.K., Latent profile model, in *The Sage Encyclopedia of Social Sciences Research Methods*, Michael S., Lewis-Beck, Alan Bryman and Tim Futing L., Editors. 2004, Thousand Oaks, CA: Sage Publications, Inc., pp. 554–555.
5. Vermunt, J.K. and J. Magidson, Latent class cluster analysis. *Applied Latent Class Analysis*, 2002. **11**: pp. 89–106.
6. Gunzler, D., et al., Psychosocial features of clinically relevant patient subgroups with serious mental illness and comorbid diabetes. *Psychiatric Services*, 2016: **68**(1): pp. 96–99.
7. Sajatovic, M., et al., Clinical characteristics of individuals with serious mental illness and type 2 diabetes., *Psychiatric Services*, 2015. **66**(2): pp. 197–199.
8. Montgomery, S.A. and M. Åsberg, A new depression scale designed to be sensitive to change. *The British Journal of Psychiatry*, 1979. **134**(4): pp. 382–389.
9. Zimet, G.D., et al., Psychometric characteristics of the multidimensional scale of perceived social support. *Journal of Personality Assessment*, 1990. **55**(3–4): pp. 610–617.

10. Zheng, Y., et al., Psychometric properties of the perceived therapeutic efficacy scale for adhering to a cholesterol-lowering diet. *Journal of Cardiovascular Nursing*, 2014. **29**(3): pp. 257–263.
11. Wallston, K.A., R.L. Rothman, and A. Cherrington, Psychometric properties of the perceived diabetes self-management scale (PDSMS). *Journal of Behavioral Medicine*, 2007. **30**(5): pp. 395–401.
12. Overall, J.E. and D.R. Gorham, The brief psychiatric rating scale. *Psychological Reports*, 1962. **10**(3): pp. 799–812.
13. Muthén, B., Latent variable hybrids: Overview of old and new models. *Advances in Latent Variable Mixture Models*, 2008. **1**: pp. 1–24.
14. Lubke, G.H. and B. Muthén, Investigating population heterogeneity with factor mixture models. *Psychological Methods*, 2005. **10**(1): p. 21.
15. Tueller, S. and G. Lubke, Evaluation of structural equation mixture models: Parameter estimates and correct class assignment. *Structural Equation Modeling*, 2010. **17**(2): pp. 165–192.

13

Structural Equation Modeling with Longitudinal Data

13.1 Introduction to the Repeated Measures Data and Longitudinal Structural Equation Modeling

In health and medicine, the routine care of patients at a health care institution typically involves some form of longitudinal or repeated measurement. *Longitudinal (or repeated measures) data* refers to data recorded on a study sample across different points in time. For example, vital signs such as heart rate, temperature, respiration rate and blood pressure could be measured at each outpatient visit during a year, many times within a day during an inpatient stay or over many years during the life of a person. Height and weight are measured at a typical clinical visit, regardless of the reason for the visit.

Observational studies and experimental studies alike use longitudinal measurements to test hypotheses of interest by making comparisons among different individuals (between-subject analysis) and across time, within the same individual (within-subject analysis). As a result, longitudinal models may need to account for (1) the correlation structure of a repeated measures outcome across time points and (2) missing data and dropouts. We have previously discussed the different mechanisms for missing data in Chapter 4 and how SEM estimation techniques such as FIML (under the assumption of MAR or MCAR) can be used to handle missing data.

A linear *mixed effects model* in traditional longitudinal data analysis extends the linear regression model for repeated measures outcomes by including both *fixed* and *random effects*. Fixed effects are study population characteristics assumed to be shared by all individuals, while random effects are subject-specific effects assumed to be unique to a particular individual and vary across the population.

Multilevel (or *hierarchical models*) are also mixed effects models. Parameters in multilevel models vary at more than one level. For example, in a basic two-level model for longitudinal data in level 1 the within-subject variation is measured, while in level 2 the between-subject variation is measured. The interested reader should refer to the textbooks by Fitzmaurice et al. [1], Singer and Willett [2] and Snijders and Bosker [3] for an overview of mixed effects models and multilevel models.

Intra-individual patterns of change over time which may involve multiple transitions are regularly referred to as *trajectories*. The mixed effects model (and multilevel model) described earlier for longitudinal data can be used to assess outcome trajectories.

Longitudinal relationships between variables and growth trajectories can be assessed using SEM. Variables in longitudinal SEMs can be latent, observed or a combination of latent and observed variables and may be hypothesized by the researcher to be causally related. *Latent growth modeling* (LGM; also termed *latent growth curve modeling*) is an application of SEM for longitudinal data to estimate growth trajectories [4,5]. *Autoregressive modeling* in SEM is an application of path modeling to evaluate relationships between variables across time points. We will discuss these two modeling approaches in detail (as well as consider several other SEM approaches for longitudinal data) in this chapter.

Longitudinal SEMs allow for the analysis of multiple repeated measures outcomes simultaneously and inclusion of both *time-invariant* and *time-varying covariates*. Time-invariant covariates have a single value for each individual in a data set and do not depend on the exact time of observation. Time-varying covariates have values that change across time. Race and sex at birth are typically treated as time-invariant variables in all models (cross-sectional or longitudinal). However, systolic blood pressure has a single value in a cross-sectional data set, but would likely have different values across multiple repeated measures for a single individual.

A notable feature of using SEM for longitudinal applications in health and medicine is that the models can be adapted to many different types of data collected over time and analyses can be performed in line with a hypothesis of interest [6]. There are a variety of approaches and models to evaluate longitudinal data in the SEM framework; choosing an appropriate model will depend, in part, on the goal of the analysis, research questions of interest, available data and clinical and statistical assumptions for a given study. In this chapter, we introduce common types of longitudinal SEMs and provide some applied health and medicine examples. A longitudinal application for evaluating subpopulation trajectories using finite mixture modeling techniques combining categorical and continuous latent variables, growth mixture modeling, is provided later in Chapter 14.

Note that in addition to measurement and data concerns involved with conducting within-subject analysis, longitudinal SEM analysis still includes many of the same measurement and data concerns involved in cross-sectional SEM analysis. For example, researchers need to attend to the measurement level and distribution of variables across time (e.g. continuous and normal or continuous and non-normal or categorical). Longitudinal SEMs often involve many parameters and require very large sample sizes (>200 participants and ideally many more than that). However, fewer participants are typically required in a longitudinal study than a cross-sectional study under similar methods. For example, if a cross-sectional and longitudinal study both were undertaken given the same expected mean difference between treatment groups and sample standard deviation, the longitudinal study would require a smaller sample size to achieve 90% power under alpha=0.05 due to having more observations with the repeated measures data on each individual.

13.2 Basic Longitudinal Path Analysis Models in Health and Medicine

The basic framework for structural models can be extended to the analysis of longitudinal data. That is, in place of time-invariant variables for cross-sectional analysis, variables recorded across repeated measures can be used instead.

We can specify a simple longitudinal structural equation model using observed variables that is structurally identical to a basic path analysis model. For example, using a cross-sectional data set of individual patients, the relationship between salt intake (independent, exogenous variable) and systolic blood pressure (endogenous, dependent or outcome variable) is measured contemporaneously. In a longitudinal example, systolic blood pressure is measured at 7 AM at waking and later at 10 AM, while salt intake is measured at 9 AM (when it occurs during breakfast). Here, we can explicitly establish temporality between salt intake and systolic blood pressure (recall that temporality is an assumption in hypothesizing causality). Longitudinal data can provide more information regarding the temporal order of variables under study compared to cross-sectional data and can permit stronger causal inferences. Even in this very basic example using only three observed indicators, we are confronted immediately with important longitudinal modeling decisions.

If we are merely interested in the effect of salt intake at 9 AM on systolic blood pressure at 10 AM, we would specify a model that regresses 10 AM systolic blood pressure (Y_2) on 9 AM salt intake (X) as in Figure 13.1. The sequence of the time of measurement of the two variables (salt intake and systolic blood pressure) is the feature of this model that enables us to explicitly model temporality while assuming causality.

However, this model can be elaborated in several important ways depending on the hypothesis of interest. For example, we could instead subtract the waking 7 AM blood pressure (Y_1) reading from the 10 AM follow-up reading (Y_2) and then regress the resulting variable (Y_{2-1}) representing the value of the difference in blood pressure over time on 9 AM salt intake (X). This model (Figure 13.2) is different in that it examines the change in blood pressure rather than simply the blood pressure at the follow-up time point.

The change in blood pressure (between 7 AM and 10 AM) was occurring parallel to when we were measuring salt intake (9 AM) and not temporally after. Thus, we can assume salt intake at 9 AM at breakfast had an influence on the difference in blood pressure over time, specifically (though not captured in the data) altering the blood pressure reading from before 9 AM and after 9 AM. The model incorporates longitudinal information on blood pressure at two time points. If the change in blood pressure increases parallel to higher salt intake, we would likely conclude that, pending inclusion of confounders, higher salt intake has a causal effect of increasing blood pressure. With more measurements of salt intake and blood pressure variables over time, this simple model could be further elaborated

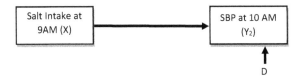

FIGURE 13.1
Basic longitudinal model.

X represents salt intake at 9 AM, while Y_2 represents systolic blood pressure (SBP) measured at 10 AM. D is the error term (disturbance term).

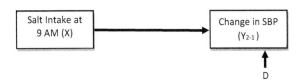

FIGURE 13.2
Basic longitudinal model with difference score.

X represents salt intake at 9 AM, while Y_{2-1} represents the difference between systolic blood pressure (SBP) measured at 7 AM and 10 AM. D is the error term (disturbance term).

and additional questions might be asked about, for instance, changes in blood pressure in response to different levels of salt intake at different meals. In most cases, for health and clinical data involving more than two time points, researchers will want to use one of the additional types of models described in the remainder of this chapter.

13.3 SEM Autoregressive Models

Another type of longitudinal model that can be used for the same salt intake and blood pressure example is termed an *autoregressive model*. Here when we refer to an autoregressive model (other fields use this term differently), we mean a *time series* model that regresses current time point values on values from previous time points for that same time series. A time series is a sequence of data points recorded at intervals, usually regularly, over a period of time. Time series analysis, which can be useful for data collected in a longitudinal study, is often focused on assessing the time-dependency across the data points.

In a basic SEM autoregressive model (see Figure 13.3), blood pressure at 7 AM is a *lagged* value of the observed endogenous variable for blood pressure at 10 AM. The terminology "lagged" is used to describe the relationship between measures across time points; systolic blood pressure at Time 2 is regressed on systolic blood pressure at Time 1. There is a delayed response in a lagged effect in that the level of systolic blood pressure at Time 1 influences the level of systolic blood pressure at Time 2. In addition, there is an indirect effect between blood pressure at 7 AM and 10 AM through salt intake at 9 AM. Salt intake at 9 AM is now an endogenous variable. One can observe that in this example, the longitudinal autoregressive SEM is structurally identical to the basic cross-sectional mediation model in Chapter 7.

As illustrated, the model in Figure 13.3 permits us to evaluate several longitudinal research questions, while controlling for other model relationships:

1) What is the relationship between 7 AM and 10 AM blood pressure? Or alternatively, to what extent does blood pressure on average go up or down between 7 AM and 10 AM? (effect c')

2) What is the relationship between 9 AM salt intake and 10 AM blood pressure? (effect b)

3) What is the relationship between 7 AM blood pressure and 9 AM salt intake? (effect a) For example, it might be hypothesized that individuals with higher blood pressure at 7 AM might decide to eat foods with less salt, and in such an instance the estimate of a would be negative, due to the inverse relationship.

4) What is the indirect relationship between 7 AM and 10 AM blood pressure through 9 AM salt intake (product of effect a and effect b).

We could omit any of the paths in Figure 13.3 (constrain to zero) if theoretically warranted, thus altering the model. For example, omitting the X variable (or if a and b were set to zero), in Figure 13.3, leaves a simple autoregressive longitudinal model of a *lagged effect* for the response variable blood pressure.

In common applications, the autoregressive model can be further extended to include additional time points. For example, perhaps now we have extended our research and

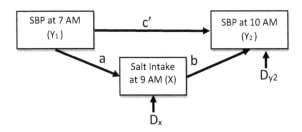

FIGURE 13.3
Basic autoregressive model for the blood pressure example.

Briefly, here a, b and c' are slopes and D_x and D_{y2} are error terms.

repeated blood pressure and salt intake according to the following schedule (*variable representations shown in parentheses*):

   1) Systolic Blood Pressure: 7 AM (Y_1), 10 AM (Y_2), Noon (Y_3), 7 PM (Y_4)
   2) Salt Intake: 9 AM (X_1), 11 AM (X_2), 6 PM (X_3)

The times of data collection can vary greatly for different longitudinal studies, even when studying the same phenomena. Longitudinal studies can be conducted over hours, days, weeks, months or years. Repeated measures data can be collected every second, every minute, hourly, daily, weekly, monthly or yearly, as appropriate for a study.

   In the earlier example, data on indicators (blood pressure and salt intake) was collected separately throughout the day with seven separate time points. The specification of the hypothesized relationships between indicators can take into account the temporal sequence of the data collection.

   Figure 13.4 displays one potential autoregressive, *cross-lagged* effects longitudinal model for the elaborated salt and blood pressure data structure [7]. The terminology "cross" is used to describe the relationship across measures (i.e. systolic blood pressure and salt intake). There are several lagged effects in this model. For example, the effect of systolic blood pressure at 10 AM to the previous time point of 7 AM or to salt intake at 9 AM is due to lagged effects.

   Notice that the model specified in Figure 13.4 has several important features. First, the model is not fully saturated. Recall, a fully saturated model is just-identified and has zero degrees of freedom. Here some paths are omitted from the model. For example, there is no path drawn from X_1 to Y_3 nor is there a path from X_1 to Y_4. This suggests that we are hypothesizing that 9 AM salt intake has no direct effect on noon or 7 PM blood

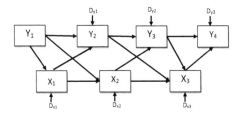

FIGURE 13.4
Autoregressive cross-lagged effects model for extended blood pressure example.

$D_{x1}, D_{x2}, D_{x3}, D_{y1}, D_{y2}$ and D_{y3} are error terms.

pressure. These additional direct effects along with others could be added to the model (and visually depicted with additional corresponding arrows in the diagram) if theoretically warranted. Due to the number of potential effects that can be specified in an autoregressive, cross-lagged effects model, one should pay close attention to the sample size relative to the number of parameters. Further, potential model specification issues would need to be considered such as model equivalence or non-identifiability or misspecification. Therefore, determining a clinically meaningful autoregressive model may involve careful consideration of available data and which causal paths to include or omit.

Different units of time can lead to a different interpretation of an estimate in the model results for an autoregressive model. For example, hourly as compared to yearly data collection can lead to an interpretation of a path estimate between blood pressure at successive time points as change in blood pressure over an hour as opposed to change in blood pressure over a year. Different spacing of time points might be built into the interpretation too. For example, if data on blood pressure is collected at day 1, 2, 3 and 17. Then the time between the first three measures is daily while the time between the final two time points is 2 weeks.

An important aspect of autoregressive, cross-lagged effects models is that there are many paths in the model for which interpretations can quickly become challenging or cumbersome. Each arrow drawn in Figure 13.4 can be thought of as representing a test for which there is the possibility of making an inference of temporal causality. The path effect for $X_2 \rightarrow Y_3$ displayed in Figure 13.4 can be used as a test of the hypothesis that salt intake at time 2 influences systolic blood pressure at time 3, while accounting for other previous model relationships in the time series (e.g. time-varying relationship that blood pressure has with itself between time 2 and time 3, indirect effect of blood pressure between time 1 and time 3). In any such autoregressive model, it is critical that researchers have a clear understanding of both how their data is structured and how this data structure is represented in an autoregressive path diagram.

Autoregressive models can be used to model feedback loops by taking advantage of a temporal sequence in the relationships between reciprocal variables. The complexity involved in specifying and analyzing an autoregressive model as the number of variables and time points increases makes them less ideal for certain studies. These models are often best used in practice with only a few waves of data (e.g. around three to five waves), only a few variables (e.g. two or three) and a large data set.

13.4 Longitudinal CFA

Longitudinal CFA can be conducted with repeated measures data on multiple items to be treated as surrogates of a latent construct(s). One may aim to evaluate equivalence of measurement across time (i.e. longitudinal invariance) using such a longitudinal measurement model. The latent constructs as the effects of reflective items recorded across time may be hypothesized to be associated with each other. There are many possible alternative specifications for a longitudinal measurement model, according to the hypothesized relationships across observed and unobserved repeated measures. For example, one could hypothesize the latent construct at each time point influences the latent construct at the next time point in a structural model. An items' uniquenesses across multiple time points can be correlated [8]. The interested reader should refer to Widaman et al. [9] or Little [10] for an overview of longitudinal measurement models.

13.5 Latent Growth Models

Latent Growth Modeling (LGM; also termed *latent growth curve modeling*) is a latent variable application for longitudinal data to estimate growth trajectories [4,5]. LGM approaches are useful techniques for understanding change over time in longitudinal outcomes (e.g. health outcomes and behaviors) in health and medicine. Latent growth and related models have been used to estimate growth trajectories in prior studies of maternity [11], childhood and adolescence [12], adolescence through young adulthood [13], response to antidepressants among adults [14,15], disability among older adults [16], patients who have had a cardiovascular event [17,18] and many other studies in health and medicine.

LGM is also an application of CFA for repeated measures data [5]. Factor loadings are specified in LGM using constraints to reflect hypothesized time trends in the data and treated as regression coefficients.

13.5.1 Path Diagram for a Basic Linear Latent Growth Model

The diagram in Figure 13.5 depicts a linear latent growth model with four observed variables, or indicators, Y_1, Y_2, Y_3 and Y_4 with one square box for each of the 4 days on which the outcome was measured. These four indicators are endogenous to two latent variables, I and S, where I is the intercept (estimated baseline level) of the latent growth function and S is the slope (estimated linear change over time). A covariance (curved, double-headed arrow) is drawn between the intercept (I) and the slope (S), such that the value of the intercept has an association with the slope. Also shown in the diagram are four error terms (e_1, e_2, e_3 and e_4) and eight manually specified path coefficients (i.e. factor loadings).

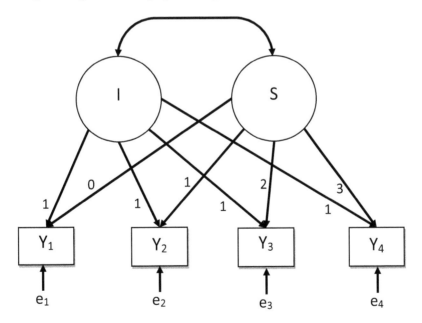

FIGURE 13.5
Latent growth model.

I=level of Y_1 (at time 0); S=linear rate at which outcome changes. Y_1, Y_2, Y_3 and Y_4 are four repeated measures for each individual at each time point (0, 1, 2 and 3). e_1, e_2, e_3 and e_4 are error terms.

The path coefficients from the intercept (*I*) to each of the repeated outcome measurements are all constrained to equal 1. The time points are equally spaced at fixed time points 0, 1, 2 and 3 (e.g. measurements for an outcome recorded at baseline time 0 and at each of three follow-up days). Note that the same model could be estimated for data where the outcome is measured over months or years with the units of measurement changing, and the spacing between measured time increments does not have to be equal (e.g. data could be collected at time 0, 1 year, 5 years and 10 years).

Covariances between each of the error terms are assumed to be zero in the model represented by this path diagram. We do not suppose residual covariance, since the same outcome is assumed to be measured in the same manner across all the time points (e.g. days) [19]. Thus the latent growth factors are assumed to explain how the observed indicators are related to each other in the growth model. However, when time-varying covariates that influence repeated measures of the outcome have been omitted from the model, it is reasonable to assume that some or even all of the errors do co-vary [19].

The linear latent growth model in Figure 13.5 is a measurement model with two latent variables and cross-loading between the latent variables and observed indicators. One can extend the linear latent growth model to include a quadratic term for nonlinear growth. This can be accomplished through an additional latent variable, and specifying the factor loadings as the square (for a quadratic model) of the slope factor loadings for each item. Further nonlinear growth, such as a cubic term, is sometimes modeled as well.

Latent growth models often include covariates and distal outcomes in order to evaluate the antecedents and consequences of the growth curve for an outcome of interest over time. That is, one can evaluate if the covariates influence growth in the outcome of interest over time and/or growth in the outcome of interest over time influences distal outcomes. Time-invariant or time-varying variables can be included in the model as appropriate for a given study and observed data.

13.5.2 Mathematical Form of a Linear Latent Growth Model

The latent growth model is equivalent to a multilevel random effects model; in the latent growth model, the random effect intercept and slope are latent variables [20]. For an outcome Y_{it}, the general form of a linear latent growth model as a two-level model at repeated measures index *t*, 1,..., *T*, for subject *i*, *i* = 1,..., *n* is:

Level-1 Within-Subject Model:

$$Y_{it} = I_i + S_i \tau_{it} + e_{it} \tag{13.1}$$

Level-2 Between-Subject Model:

$$I_i = \alpha_0 + \varsigma_{0i}$$
$$S_i = \alpha_1 + \varsigma_{1i} \tag{13.2}$$

I_i is the latent intercept for subject *i*, and S_i is the latent slope for subject *i*. One typically assumes a normal distribution with zero means for e_{it}, the error term for subject *i* at time *t* and the between-subject residual terms ς_{0i} and ς_{1i}. α_0 and α_1 are the mean between-subject intercepts and slopes. τ_{it} is the time-related variable (i.e. time scores for study days 0–3). The independence of I_i and S_i from e_{it}, ς_{0i} and ς_{1i} are assumed. However, ς_{0i} and ς_{1i} can be correlated, although these residual terms are assumed to be uncorrelated with e_{it}.

LGM can be performed taking into account features of real-world data. For example, when estimating a latent growth model, missing data can be handled using a FIML procedure. In addition, the intercept and slope terms in a latent growth model, as latent variables, account for measurement error in the outcome at baseline and growth of the outcome over time. Modeling this uncertainty is useful for many measures in health and medicine in which some within-subject variation across visits can be due to error. For example, patient ratings or biometric measurements such as blood pressure often are assumed to be measured with error at any given visit. Further, one can account for individually varying follow-up appointments and irregular follow-up time in a latent growth model [21]. For an individually varying time point τ_{it} in (13.1) is modified for $1 \leq t \leq T$. If for an individual the number of observed repeated measures $t = T^*$ and if $T^* < T$, then the last $T - T^*$ repeated measures will be considered missing. This represents a typical case with hospital observational data (such as EHR-based data from typical clinical visits) where appointment days vary by individual.

Note that the model represented in Figure 13.5 with fixed time points across individuals is a special case of our depiction of the more general within-subject model with individually varying times of measurement. Formally, in the model in Figure 13.5, $\tau_{i1} = 0, \tau_{i2} = 1, \tau_{i3} = 2$ and $\tau_{i4} = 3$.

13.5.3 Quadratic Latent Growth Model with a Time Invariant Covariate

We extend the model described earlier to include both a quadratic (nonlinear) growth term for subject i (Q_i) and a time invariant covariate for subject i (X_i). The covariate (X_i) is specified to influence each of the latent growth terms (I_i, S_i, Q_i).

Level-1 Within-Subject Model:

$$Y_{it} = I_i + S_i \tau_{it} + Q_i \tau_{it}^2 + e_{it} \tag{13.3}$$

Level-2 Between-Subject Model:

$$I_i = \alpha_0 + \gamma_0 X_i + \varsigma_{0i}$$

$$S_i = \alpha_1 + \gamma_1 X_i + \varsigma_{1i} \tag{13.4}$$

$$Q_i = \alpha_2 + \gamma_2 X_i + \varsigma_{2i}$$

One typically assumes a normal distribution with zero means for e_{it}, the error term for subject i at time t and the between-subject residual terms ς_{0i}, W and ς_{2i}. α_0, α_1 and α_2 are the mean between-subject intercepts and slopes, while γ_0, γ_1 and γ_2 are the parameters for the association between the covariate and each latent growth term. τ_{it}^2 is the square of the time-related variable (e.g. time scores for study days 0, 1, 2 and 3 squared are, respectively, 0, 1, 4 and 9). The independence of I_i, S_i and Q_i from e_{it} and ς_{0i}, ς_{1i} and ς_{2i} are assumed. However, ς_{0i}, ς_{1i} and ς_{2i} can be correlated, although these residual terms are assumed to be uncorrelated with e_{it}.

The model can be further extended to include a cubic term or additional time-invariant covariates. Further extension allows one to include time-varying covariates as well. Time-varying covariates are included in the Level-1 Within-Subject Model. That is, at each time point, the time-varying covariate directly influences the observed outcome at that time point. See the textbook by Singer and Willet [2] for a description of these extensions.

13.5.4 Applications of Latent Growth Models in Health and Medicine

Applications of latent growth models are commonly performed under a set of basic requirements. Typically, these requirements include: (1) a dependent variable measured at three or more consecutive time points; (2) consistency of measurement units across time; and (3) record of the time structure of observations in the data or known sequence and spacing of the measurements for each research participant.

Typically, latent growth models are applied to continuous measured outcomes under distributional assumptions (e.g. residuals are assumed to be normally distributed) at each time point. Latent growth models can be applied to categorical data [22]. Multiple examples of such models with categorical outcomes exist in the research literature in health and medicine [23,24]. Latent growth models are typically applied to raw individual level data. Individual level data is typically necessary for a FIML procedure, and missing data and dropouts are common in longitudinal studies.

We have thus far discussed the univariate latent growth model (i.e. model for a single repeated measures outcome). *Associative latent growth models* are multivariate latent growth models [4]. One can evaluate the correlations between growth parameters for two or more repeated measures outcomes using associative latent growth models. The interested reader can refer to the textbook by Duncan et al. [4] for an overview of associative latent growth models.

We have also only discussed observed repeated measures outcomes in latent growth models. One can also model growth in latent variables rather than observed scores (*second-order latent growth curve model*). See the textbook by Newsom [25] for an overview of second-order latent growth curve models.

13.5.5 Modeling the Trajectory of Depression in Persons Living with HIV

The PHQ-9 total score was recorded in a database for 416 people living with HIV in a collaborative care program[1] who had screened positive for depression (PHQ-9 total score ≥ 10) with at least two repeated measure outcomes up to 15 months between June 29, 2015, and December 31, 2017 [26]. The collaborate care model is an evidence-based integrated care model for treating depression in primary care settings, while relatively new to HIV settings [26]. Follow-up times after the first visit in the study time period were individually varying times of observations.

The study objective was to describe the average growth of depression over time for people living with HIV participating in an intervention (see Figure 13.6). We were also interested in evaluating if covariates for sex and reported trauma influence growth of depression. Self-reports of abuse or trauma were based on detailed notes from behavioral health care managers, medical case managers and physician notes.

Data was in the wide format. We assumed nonlinearity in the trajectory of depression over time by including a quadratic term in the latent growth model [27,28]. We used the MLR option in MPlus to perform model estimation. The model handled missing data following a MAR assumption via FIML. The intercept and linear and quadratic slopes were regressed on sex and reported trauma.

Model fit statistics and indices (i.e. Chi-Square Test Statistic, CFI, TLI, RMSEA and SRMR) are readily available for an application of latent growth model with fixed repeated measures (e.g. measurements at 0, 1, 2, 3 days). Recall, the follow-up times were individually

---
[1] This study was possible because of research funding by the Health Resources and Services Administration (H97HA27429-01-00)

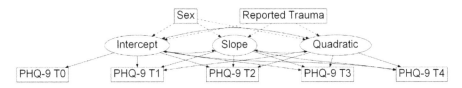

FIGURE 13.6
Latent growth model for people living with HIV screening positive for depression (PHQ-9≥10) at baseline (T_0) in the collaborative care study.

PHQ-9 is the PHQ-9 total score. $T0$ is the baseline time point for each subject. $T1 – T4$ are individually varying follow up times over 15 months for each subject. Reported Trauma (46% Yes)=self-reported history of trauma under a patient chart review as described by sexual, physical or emotional abuse. Sex (28% Female)=Female (vs. reference Male).

varying times of observations in the HIV example. Mplus currently provides the number of parameters, log-likelihood value (with a scaling correction factor for MLR), AIC, BIC and sample-size adjusted BIC for this analysis. Thus, model fit cannot readily be evaluated for this example, given no comparison to a competing model (e.g. independence and saturated models).

The model results in Box 13.1 show that there is a significant decrease in depression growth over time as estimated by the slope and quadratic terms (see Model Results in Box 13.1 under "Intercepts" heading). The average baseline PHQ-9 total score of approximately 16 represents moderately severe depression.

BOX 13.1   SELECT AND MODIFIED MPLUS INPUT AND OUTPUT:

```
USEVARIABLES are
!Individually varying times of measurement (baseline and four
!follow-up times)
  T0 T1 T2 T3 T4
!PHQ-9 scores at each time of measurement
P0 P1 P2 P3 P4
!covariates for reported trauma (TRAUMA) and sex
TRAUMA SEX;
!code to signify time scores are individually varying
Tscores =  T0-T4;

!type must be random with the individually varying time scores
  ANALYSIS: type = random;

!generate 100 different random starting values for the parameters;
!use parameter estimates with the best 20 likelihood values as
!starting values for optimization using the MLR estimator
  STARTS = 100 20;
  ESTIMATOR=MLR;

 MODEL:
!latent growth model with intercept (I), slope (S) and quadratic (Q)
!term
  I S Q | P0-P4 AT T0-T4;
!regress I, S and Q on TRAUMA and SEX
  I S Q ON TRAUMA SEX;
```

```
!include means, variances and covariance of TRAUMA and SEX for FIML
procedure
[TRAUMA SEX];
TRAUMA SEX;

MODEL RESULTS
```

			Estimate	S.E.	Est./S.E.	Two-Tailed P-Value
I	ON					
	TRAUMA		1.654	0.476	3.479	0.001
	SEX		-0.649	0.507	-1.279	0.201
S	ON					
	TRAUMA		0.018	0.239	0.076	0.940
	SEX		-0.214	0.245	-0.874	0.382
Q	ON					
	TRAUMA		0.006	0.022	0.275	0.783
	SEX		0.015	0.022	0.694	0.488
S	WITH					
	I		1.018	0.709	1.436	0.151
Q	WITH					
	I		-0.067	0.059	-1.152	0.249
	S		-0.113	0.035	-3.228	0.001
SEX	WITH					
	TRAUMA		-0.002	0.011	-0.220	0.826
Means						
	TRAUMA		0.329	0.023	14.087	0.000
	SEX		0.724	0.022	32.997	0.000
Intercepts						
	I		15.760	0.476	33.130	0.000
	S		-0.975	0.223	-4.376	0.000
	Q		0.044	0.020	2.196	0.028

See Figure 13.7 for a visual depiction of the decline in average self-report depression total score over time in months in this study population.

Regarding the relationships between the covariates and the growth terms, only the effect of reported trauma on the intercept is statistically significant ($p=0.001$) with a positive estimate (see Box 13.1). Thus, at baseline, those individuals in this sample with reported trauma have a higher PHQ-9 total score than individuals in this sample with no reported trauma. However, the subsequent growth of depression (including slope and quadratic terms) under the intervention program is not influenced by reported trauma.

13.6 Multilevel (Hierarchical) Models for Longitudinal Data

Multilevel regression and SEMs can be used for analysis of individual and group level effects by assuming both within-subject (individual level) and between-subject (group level) variation and covariation. We have described how LGM is a multilevel model for longitudinal data. Software for SEM such as MPlus can be used to analyze many different

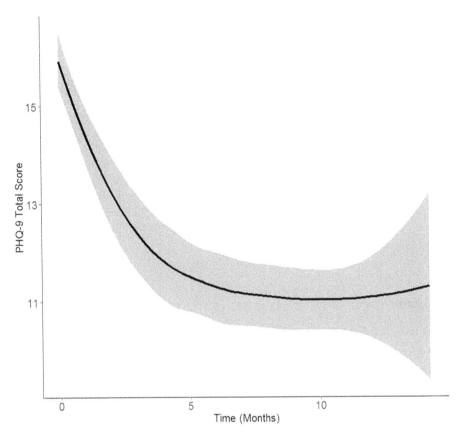

FIGURE 13.7

Local regression smoothing plot of average depression screening trajectory over time in people living with HIV screening positive for depression (PHQ-9≥10) in the collaborative care study (N=416).

Shaded region represents a 95% Confidence Interval.

specifications of longitudinal hierarchical SEMs with data in either the wide or long format. Latent variables can be included in multilevel SEM as endogenous and exogenous variables. The interested reader can refer to the chapter by Hox [29] for an introduction to multilevel SEM analysis.

13.7 Longitudinal Mediation

The methods that we have described in Chapter 9 for mediation analysis can be applied to longitudinal data, given a single measure is used for each variable within a mediation model. For example, given a study with data collected at baseline and two follow-up visits, one could use data for an independent variable recorded at baseline, mediator recorded at the second visit and outcome recorded at the third visit [30].

While we do not have the space in this book to present this topic in detail, SEM can be used for evaluating mediating relationships using longitudinal data within a single framework [5]. The longitudinal techniques introduced in this chapter can all be used for mediation analysis with repeated measures data. LGM shows great flexibility in evaluating mediating relationships between multiple time-varying measures [5,31]. Separate growth curves can be modeled for the repeated measures data in the independent variable, mediator and outcome. The LGM framework then assumes a temporal relationship between the growth of the independent variable, growth of the mediator and growth of the outcome.

Autoregressive modeling techniques, *latent difference scores* and multilevel SEM have all been used for longitudinal mediation analysis [32]. Latent difference score models [29] incorporate latent variables (that can be measured without error unlike observed differences) for representing change scores between adjacent observed values across time in longitudinal data. The interested reader can refer to the textbook by MacKinnon [32] for an overview of longitudinal mediation analysis.

13.8 Survival Analysis

Survival (time-to-event) outcomes can be integrated into the SEM framework [33–35] within, for example, path models and multilevel models (see www.statmodel.com for starting references and code on this topic). Survival time can be measured in either discrete or continuous values. Non-parametric, semi-parametric or parametric regression models are all used for analyzing the effect of covariates (e.g. risk factors) on survival time. The Cox proportional hazards (regression) model is a semi-parametric model (i.e. the hazard function is estimated from the data, but the functional form of the covariates is parametric). It is also the most commonly used model for the analysis of survival data.

Censoring is a characteristic that distinguishes survival analysis from other types of statistical analysis. Censoring occurs when incomplete information is available about the survival outcome for some of the individuals in a study. For example, one is examining a survival outcome over a pre-specified time interval using a large electronic health registry from a single institution. Typical reasons for censoring may include an individual may (1) not have experienced the event within the time interval, (2) have moved and be lost to follow-up, or (3) have received care at a different institution for the event. Some individuals may be observed over a shorter time interval than other individuals (depending on when data for an individual is first recorded in the registry), giving less of a time frame for the event to occur.

Survival variables can be used as outcomes in joint models with other types of longitudinal outcomes. For example, one can analyze a latent growth model for a repeated measures continuous PRO and a Cox model for a time to event outcome jointly, while accounting for the association between the two data types [36]. Discrete-time survival outcomes can also be combined with mixture model analysis, so that one can account for unobserved heterogeneity in survival [34]. In this mixture analysis, different latent classes have different hazard and survival functions [34]. Survival outcomes can also be distal outcomes in latent variable mixture models.

13.9 Cohort Sequential Modeling Techniques

In a longitudinal, age-related developmental study, a group of individuals of the same age (single cohort) are followed over time. An *accelerated longitudinal design* (also termed *cohort sequential design*) instead takes multiple single cohorts, each one starting at a different age [37]. There is tremendous growth and development that occurs as a child and adolescent ages; therefore, it is important to accurately model this development in a study in which different subjects enter the study at different ages. For example, Figure 13.8 visualizes a basic accelerated longitudinal design for adolescents aged 14–17 for a study of how social norms influence risky health behavior trajectories over time. The age at baseline for different participants was either 14 or 15. Adolescents are divided into two cohorts according to their age at the first assessment (14 or 15). These individuals are then followed for 3 years.

Multiple group multiple cohort LGM has been used to investigate such differential cohort effects using a cohort sequential design. In the approach, one extends the latent growth model in the multiple group framework, where individuals are nested within a cohort (grouping variable).

One can use this study design and approach to test the hypothesis that a common developmental trajectory exists across all ages studied [38]. The ages evaluated within each cohort group model contribute a different section of an overall growth curve. There will be overlap between ages across cohort group models. For example, for the design in Figure 13.8, measurements for age 15 are recorded at the second visit for Cohort A, while they are recorded at the first visit for Cohort B. In total, Cohort A includes adolescents aged 14-16 while Cohort B includes adolescents aged 15–17. One can build a complete growth curve (e.g. common intercept and slope means) using information across the cohort group models. Thus, using data for the design in Figure 13.8, we can estimate parameters representative of the growth curve from ages 14 to 17. Specific model parameters for observed values that involve a similar age across the cohort group models are constrained to be equal. The interested reader should refer to Duncan et al. [4,38] for applications of cohort-sequential latent growth models.

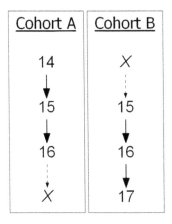

FIGURE 13.8
Cohort sequential design with two cohorts for a developmental study of adolescents aged 14-17.

13.9.1 Age-Period-Cohort Analysis

The analysis to study age-related development using multiple group multiple cohort LGM as discussed earlier can be viewed as a special case of *age-period-cohort (APC)* analysis. APC models are used to study the variability in trajectories of change over time and include *age, period* and *cohort effects*. Age effects have been described as phenomena associated with growing older; period effects as general influences that vary through time or epochs; and cohort effects as phenomena associated with individuals born around the same time [39].

The influence of events varies depending on the stage of life at which they are experienced. Thus more generally than just in the context of an age-related developmental study, one can evaluate the influence of such events (e.g. historic events) on study samples at different ages by following cohorts over time [40]. For example, infectious disease epidemics of the 20th century (e.g. hepatitis C and human immunodeficiency viruses) influenced lives and health outcomes differently for distinct birth cohorts. Similarly, technological and therapeutic innovations can have considerably different influences on the lives of different cohorts in different time periods.

A major impediment exists to APC research called the "identification problem" in that chronological age, time period and birth cohort effects are linearly dependent [41,42]. That is, mathematically *age = period – cohort* [41,42]. In other words, given any two of these three characteristics one can calculate the third.

In the multiple group multiple cohort latent growth model, cohort is treated as a grouping variable. One uses the model to estimate parameters (e.g. slope mean) that are representative of the growth trajectory in an outcome across a range of ages and time periods. However, one does not separately consider age and time period in the model. Thus, these techniques are able to work around the "identification problem."

Several solutions have been proposed to address the "identification problem" in the APC literature while attempting to estimate age, period and cohort effects separately [40,41,43]. For example, a widely known solution in the APC literature, Yang and Land [41] proposed the Hierarchical APC (HAPC) model to resolve identifiability. The proposed mixed effects modeling approach described in Yang and Land [41] uses repeated measures data across individuals and includes fixed effects for linear and quadratic age and random effects for cohort and period. However, more generally, proposed methods to address the "identification problem" and estimate age, period and cohort effects separately rely on consequential assumptions and require researchers to impose implicit constraints on the model parameters that may fail to recover the underlying APC effects. Studies have shown these methods can be sensitive to different model parameterizations [42,44–48].

In addition, these prior frameworks for APC analysis assume that all individuals at a given age have the same risk of outcome (e.g. mortality) when holding period and cohort fixed. Aging is a process that does not happen uniformly, linearly or sometimes even monotonically, over time. Health behaviors, functional status, comorbid illnesses, genetic and epigenetic markers, environmental and neighborhood-level exposures, medication use and other effects may introduce substantial heterogeneity in outcome risk for persons of a given chronological age. Estimates of a "biological age" incorporating many of these factors have been shown to be a better predictor of mortality than chronological age [49].

13.9.2 Risk-Period-Cohort Approach

The *risk-period-cohort (RPC) approach* was developed by two of the authors of this textbook (Gunzler and Perzynski) along with colleagues (2019) as a practical approach that does not attempt to solve the "identification problem", but rather employs a measure of *age-related risk* in place of chronological age [39]. In this alternative framework for considering effects relating to age, period and birth cohort, age-related risk is the accumulation of physiological, lifestyle, environmental, sociological and other contextualizing risks as a representation of how the process of aging is affecting an individual [50,51].

Age-related risk can be quantified for an individual in a given study by computing a *risk score*. A *risk score* is a calculated value that reflects the severity of a risk due to some factors. For example, the Framingham risk score is a well-known risk score to forecast 10-year risk of heart attack [52]. An online calculator for the Framingham risk score[2] asks an individual to enter age, sex, smoker status, total cholesterol, HDL cholesterol, systolic BP and if one is being treated with an antihypertensive and will output a risk score. The Framingham risk score is an example in which an external prognostic model is used to calculate the risk score.

Risk scores can also be calculated using an internal prognostic model [53–56] fit on available data from a study sample. A risk score for age-related risk can be manifested as a predicted value in a regression model, for example after regressing an outcome of interest at baseline on chronological age and other age-related risk factors (e.g. smoking, area deprivation index, sex). Another way to conceptualize age-related risk using an internal risk model is as a predicted chronological age after accounting for biological and sociological factors that influence the aging process. Predicted chronological age can be quantified by modeling baseline chronological age as a function of other risk factors (e.g. using multivariable linear regression). In the context of SEM, age-related risk can be quantified as a formative latent construct using chronological age as well as other risk factors.

Multilevel SEM can be used with the RPC approach with individual-level data [39]. One can regress a repeated measures health outcome on age-related risk and include random effects for period and cohort. See the textbook on APC by Yang and Land [41] for an in-depth introduction to APC models and the use of hierarchical modeling for APC analysis. See Gunzler et al. [39] for an introduction to the RPC approach.

13.10 Conclusions

This chapter presented applications of SEM for longitudinal data by incorporating time-varying variables in place of cross-sectional analogues. We described methods for how SEM longitudinal models can be used to study both within-subject and between-subject differences in an outcome trajectory over time. Special attention was given to autoregressive modeling and LGM. Briefly, we discussed extensions of LGM as well as longitudinal mediation analysis, longitudinal CFA, multilevel modeling, survival analysis, cohort-sequential modeling and APC analysis.

Longitudinal SEMs are extremely flexible, but this flexibility can quickly lead to considerable complexity of model specification and interpretation. Fortunately, there are many excellent methodology volumes devoted to the description of longitudinal SEMs [4,5,10,31,57,58]. An exhaustive description of the many possible configurations and versions of longitudinal SEM is beyond the scope of this volume. Little [10] provides a careful and comprehensive text for readers looking to gain an in depth understanding of longitudinal SEM. Duncan et al. [4] provide an introduction to latent growth curve modeling.

---

[2] https://www.mdcalc.com/framingham-risk-score-hard-coronary-heart-disease#use-cases

References

1. Fitzmaurice, G.M., N.M. Laird, and J.H. Ware, *Applied longitudinal analysis.* 2012, Hoboken, NJ: John Wiley & Sons.
2. Singer, J.D. and J.B. Willett, *Applied longitudinal data analysis: Modeling change and event occurrence.* 2003, Oxford: Oxford University Press.
3. Snijders, T.A. and R.J. Bosker, *Multilevel analysis: An introduction to basic and advanced multilevel modeling.* 2011, Thousand Oaks, CA: Sage.
4. Duncan, T.E., S.C. Duncan, and L.A. Strycker, *An introduction to latent variable growth curve modeling: Concepts, issues, and application.* 2013, Abingdon: Routledge.
5. Preacher, K.J., A.L. Wichman, N.E. Briggs, and R.C. MacCallum, *Latent growth curve modeling.* 2008, Thousand Oaks, CA: Sage.
6. Duncan, T.E. and S.C. Duncan, The ABC's of LGM: An introductory guide to latent variable growth curve modeling. *Social and Personality Psychology Compass,* 2009. **3**(6): pp. 979–991.
7. Kearney, M.W., Cross lagged panel analysis. *The SAGE Encyclopedia of Communication Research Methods,* M. Allen, Editor. 2017, Thousand Oaks, CA: Sage, pp. 312–314.
8. Roesch, S.C., G.J. Norman, E.L. Merz, J.F. Sallis, and K. Patrick, Longitudinal measurement invariance of psychosocial measures in physical activity research: An application to adolescent data. *Journal of Applied Social Psychology,* 2013. **43**(4): pp. 721–729.
9. Widaman, K.F., E. Ferrer, and R.D. Conger, Factorial invariance within longitudinal structural equation models: Measuring the same construct across time. *Child Development Perspectives,* 2010. **4**(1): pp. 10–18.
10. Little, T.D., *Longitudinal structural equation modeling.* 2013, New York: Guilford Press.
11. Drozd, F., S.M. Haga, L. Valla, and K. Slinning, Latent trajectory classes of postpartum depressive symptoms: A regional population-based longitudinal study. *Journal of Affective Disorders,* 2018. **241**: pp. 29–36.
12. Meadows, S.O., J.S. Brown, and G.H. Elder, Depressive symptoms, stress, and support: Gendered trajectories from adolescence to young adulthood. *Journal of Youth and Adolescence,* 2006. **35**(1): pp. 89–99.
13. Olino, T.M., S.J. Bufferd, L.R. Dougherty, M.W. Dyson, G.A. Carlson, and D.N. Klein, The development of latent dimensions of psychopathology across early childhood: Stability of dimensions and moderators of change. *Journal of Abnormal Child Psychology,* 2018. **46**(7): pp. 1373–1383.
14. Uher, R., et al., Trajectories of change in depression severity during treatment with antidepressants. *Psychological Medicine,* 2010. **40**(8): pp. 1367–1377.
15. Muthén, B., T. Asparouhov, A.M. Hunter, and A.F. Leuchter, Growth modeling with nonignorable dropout: Alternative analyses of the STAR*D antidepressant trial. *Psychological Methods,* 2011. **16**(1): p. 17.
16. Taylor, M.G. and S.M. Lynch, Trajectories of impairment, social support, and depressive symptoms in later life. *The Journals of Gerontology Series B: Psychological Sciences and Social Sciences,* 2004. **59**(4): pp. S238–S246.
17. Kaptein, K.I., P. De Jonge, R.H. Van Den Brink, and J. Korf, Course of depressive symptoms after myocardial infarction and cardiac prognosis: A latent class analysis. *Psychosomatic Medicine,* 2006. **68**(5): pp. 662–668.
18. Llabre, M.M., S. Spitzer, S. Siegel, P.G. Saab, and N. Schneiderman, Applying latent growth curve modeling to the investigation of individual differences in cardiovascular recovery from stress. *Psychosomatic Medicine,* 2004. **66**(1): pp. 29–41.
19. Muthén, L.K. and B.O. Muthén, *Mplus: The comprehensive modelling program for applied researchers: User's guide.* 2012, Los Angeles, CA: Muthén & Muthén.
20. Muthén, B. Latent variable analysis, in *The Sage handbook of quantitative methodology for the social sciences,* Vol. 345, D. Kaplan, Editor, 2004, p. 368.

21. Gunzler, D., N. Morris, A. Perznski, D. Miller, S. Lewis, and R.A. Bermel, Mediation analysis of co-occurring conditions for complex longitudinal clinical data. *SM Journal of Biometrics and Biostatistics*, 2017. **1**(1): p. 1004.

22. Masyn, K.E., H. Petras, and W. Liu, Growth curve models with categorical outcomes, in *Encyclopedia of criminology and criminal justice*, G. Bruinsma and D. Weisburd, Editors. 2014. New York: Springer, pp. 2013–2025.

23. Muthén, B., Second-generation structural equation modeling with a combination of categorical and continuous latent variables: New opportunities for latent class–latent growth modeling, in Decade of behavior: New methods for the analysis of change, L.M. Collins and A.G. Sayer, Editors. Worcester, MA: American Psychological Association. 2001, pp. 291–322.

24. Yang, C., S. Nay, and R.H. Hoyle, Three approaches to using lengthy ordinal scales in structural equation models: Parceling, latent scoring, and shortening scales. *Applied Psychological Measurement*, 2010. **34**(2): pp. 122–142.

25. Newsom, J.T., *Longitudinal structural equation modeling: A comprehensive introduction*, 2015. Abingdon: Routledge.

26. Gunzler, D., et al., Depressive symptom trajectories among people living with HIV in a collaborative care program. *AIDS and Behavior*, 2019. **24**(6): pp. 1765–1775.

27. Bengtson, A.M., et al., Trajectories of depressive symptoms among a population of HIV-infected men and women in routine HIV care in the United States. *AIDS and Behavior*, 2018, 22: pp. 1–12.

28. Owora, A.H., Major depression disorder trajectories and HIV disease progression: Results from a 6-year outpatient clinic cohort. *Medicine*, 2018. **97**: p. 12.

29. Hox, J.J., Multilevel regression and multilevel structural equation modeling. *The Oxford handbook of quantitative methods*, 2013. **2**(1): pp. 281–294.

30. Gunzler, D., W. Tang, N. Lu, P. Wu, and X.M. Tu, A class of distribution-free models for longitudinal mediation analysis. *Psychometrika*, 2014. **79**(4): pp. 543–568.

31. Cheong, J., D.P. MacKinnon, and S.T. Khoo, Investigation of mediational processes using parallel process latent growth curve modeling. *Structural Equation Modeling*, 2003. **10**(2): pp. 238–262.

32. MacKinnon, D., *Introduction to statistical mediation analysis*. 2012, Abingdon: Routledge.

33. Asparouhov, T., *Continuous-time survival analysis in Mplus*. 2014, Technical appendix Los Angeles: Muthén & Muthén.

34. Muthén, B. and K. Masyn, Discrete-time survival mixture analysis. *Journal of Educational and Behavioral statistics*, 2005. **30**(1): pp. 27–58.

35. Muthén, B., T. Asparouhov, M. Boye, M. Hackshaw, and A. Naegeli, *Applications of continuous-time survival in latent variable models for the analysis of oncology randomized clinical trial data using Mplus*. 2009, Los Angeles, CA: Muthén & Muthén.

36. Wang, P., W. Shen, and M.E. Boye, Joint modeling of longitudinal outcomes and survival using latent growth modeling approach in a mesothelioma trial. *Health Services and Outcomes Research Methodology*, 2012. **12**(2–3): pp. 182–199.

37. Galbraith, S., J. Bowden, and A. Mander, Accelerated longitudinal designs. An overview of modelling, power, costs and handling missing data. *Statistical Methods in Medical Research*, 2017. **26**(1): pp. 374–398.

38. Duncan, S.C., T.E. Duncan, and L.A. Strycker, Alcohol use from ages 9–16: A cohort-sequential latent growth model. *Drug Alcohol Depend*, 2006. **81**(1): pp. 71–81.

39. Gunzler, D.D., A.T. Perzynski, N.V. Dawson, K. Kauffman, J. Liu, and J.E. Dalton, Risk-period-cohort approach for averting identification problems in longitudinal models. *PLos One*, 2019. **14**(7): p. e0219399.

40. O'Brien, R.M., Age period cohort characteristic models. *Social Science Research*, 2000. **29**(1): pp. 123–139.

41. Yang, Y. and K.C. Land, *Age-period-cohort analysis*, Vol. 10, Interdisciplinary Statistics Series. 2013, Boca Raton, FL: Chapman & Hall/CRC, p. b13902.

42. Bell, A. and K. Jones, Another 'futile quest'? A simulation study of Yang and Land's hierarchical age-period-cohort model. *Demographic Research*, 2014. **30**: p. 333.

43. Mason, K.O., W.M. Mason, H.H. Winsborough, and W.K. Poole, Some methodological issues in cohort analysis of archival data. *American Sociological Review,* 1973. **38**: pp. 242–258.

44. Bell, A. and K. Jones, The impossibility of separating age, period and cohort effects. *Social Science and Medicine,* 2013. **93**: pp. 163–165.

45. Bell, A. and K. Jones, Don't birth cohorts matter? A commentary and simulation exercise on Reither, Hauser, and Yang's (2009) age–period–cohort study of obesity. *Social Science and Medicine,* 2014. **101**: pp. 176–80.

46. Luo, L., Assessing validity and application scope of the intrinsic estimator approach to the age-period-cohort problem. *Demography,* 2013. **50**(6): pp. 1945–1967.

47. Luo, L., Paradigm shift in age-period-cohort analysis: A response to Yang and Land, O'Brien, Held and Riebler, and Fienberg. *Demography,* 2013. **50**(6): pp. 1985–1988.

48. Pelzer, B., M. Te Grotenhuis, R. Eisinga, and A.W. Schmidt-Catran, The non-uniqueness property of the intrinsic estimator in APC models. *Demography,* 2015. **52**(1): pp. 315–327.

49. Levine, M.E., Modeling the rate of senescence: Can estimated biological age predict mortality more accurately than chronological age? *The Journals of Gerontology Series A, Biological Sciences and Medical Sciences,* 2013. **68**(6): pp. 667–674.

50. Couoh, L.R. Differences between biological and chronological age-at-death in human skeletal remains: A change of perspective. *American Journal of Physical Anthropology,* 2017. **163**(4): pp. 671–695.

51. Jylhävä, J., N.L. Pedersen, and S. Hägg, Biological age predictors. *EBioMedicine,* 2017. **21**: pp. 29–36.

52. Lloyd-Jones, D.M., et al., Framingham risk score and prediction of lifetime risk for coronary heart disease. *The American Journal of Cardiology,* 2004. **94**(1): pp. 20–24.

53. Burke, J.F., R.A. Hayward, J.P. Nelson, and D.M. Kent, Using internally developed risk models to assess heterogeneity in treatment effects in clinical trials. *Circulation: Cardiovascular Quality and Outcomes,* 2014. **7**: pp. 163-169.

54. Hayward, R.A., D.M. Kent, S. Vijan, and T.P. Hofer, Multivariable risk prediction can greatly enhance the statistical power of clinical trial subgroup analysis. *BMC Medical Research Methodology,* 2006. **6**(1): p. 1.

55. Kent, D.M., A. Alsheikh-Ali, and R.A. Hayward, Competing risk and heterogeneity of treatment effect in clinical trials. *Trials,* 2008. **9**(1): p. 30.

56. Sussman, J.B., D.M. Kent, J.P. Nelson, and R.A. Hayward, Improving diabetes prevention with benefit based tailored treatment: Risk based reanalysis of Diabetes Prevention Program. *BMJ,* 2015. **350**: p. h454.

57. Little, T.D., J.A. Bovaird, and N.A. Card, *Modeling contextual effects in longitudinal studies.* 2007, Abingdon: Routledge.

58. Collins, L.M. and A.G. Sayer, *New methods for the analysis of change.* 2001, Worcester, MA: American Psychological Association.

14

Growth Mixture Modeling

14.1 Introduction to Growth Mixture Modeling

Theories of change over time for a disease or other health outcome are often inconsistent with the assumption that a single growth curve adequately describes the population. Subgroup differences in outcome change over time can exist due to sociodemographic (e.g. cultural, ethnic, regional and gender) or biological differences, or even due to unknown factors. These differences can mask or distort the results of longitudinal studies when researchers fail to adequately model the considerable heterogeneity than can exist.

In this chapter, we describe longitudinal SEM techniques that are well suited to discovering and modeling patterns of change over time in unobserved subgroups within study samples. Recall in Chapters 11 and 12, LCA and LPA are applications of mixture modeling that can be used to identify subgroups *across a set of variables*. *Growth mixture modeling (GMM)* is instead a type of mixture modeling for longitudinal data that can be used to identify subgroups *across time*. The subgroups identified by GMM are also commonly referred to as latent classes, trajectories, subpopulations or clusters.

Growth mixture models (GMMs) are often applied to data for a single observed outcome with three or more repeated measures. The basic structure of GMMs follows logically from that of latent growth models (Chapter 13, Figure 13.5 for a representation of a basic linear latent growth model). GMMs are hybrid models that include a categorical latent variable to represent the subgroup trajectories and continuous latent variables to represent the intercept and slopes. This categorical latent variable is assumed to influence the latent intercept and slopes.

Stated differently, there are underlying, "hidden" subgroups of individuals and membership in one of these subgroups predicts, or causes, variation on the underlying response variables in the model. Similar to LCA/LPA, there may be much uncertainty in the classification of individuals to their most likely latent class in applications of GMM. Individuals are again assigned to latent classes based on their posterior class-membership probabilities.

In Figure 14.1, we represent a basic growth mixture model. The C variable on the diagram represents the latent categorical variable. All other notation was previously described for the basic (unconditional) linear latent growth model represented in Chapter 13, Figure 13.5. Again, since GMM is an extension of LGM, subpopulation trajectories can be nonlinear (e.g. quadratic and cubic).

GMM allows for the investigation of antecedents and consequences of change [1]. Techniques are available that allow researchers to examine the extent to which covariates or predictors influence which persons are members of which latent classes (i.e. what predicts being in a particular type of trajectory of change?). Similarly, GMM can be used

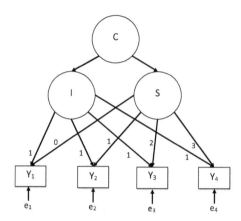

FIGURE 14.1
Growth mixture model.

to examine how being part of a particular latent class (trajectory) is related to a particular distal health outcome. Despite representing subpopulation trajectories, latent class membership within the GMM framework is viewed as time-invariant (unlike, for example LTA as discussed in Chapter 11) [2]. Thus, researchers typically regress a categorical latent variable in a growth mixture model on time-invariant covariates only (and not time-varying covariates). Similar one and three-step regression procedures as discussed in Chapter 11 in the context of LCA can be applied to GMMs with auxiliary variables [1]. As in other applications of mixture modeling, researchers applying GMM methods should follow a sequence of identifying an appropriate research question (and an accompanying suitable longitudinal data resource), specifying models, selecting the most appropriate model and interpreting model results.

We end this introductory section on GMM by emphasizing its basic notion. Techniques that estimate one set of growth parameters for the entire study population assume a single average homogenous distribution from which individuals vary. GMMs are available to evaluate heterogeneity over time in longitudinal change (i.e. Are there empirical subclasses of how people change over time?). Below we describe typical steps and procedures involved in implementing GMMs and share some applied examples. Researchers interested in additional elaboration of the statistical theory behind GMM will find the work of Muthén and Asparouhov [3], and those seeking additional guidance for fitting models should look to Jung and Wickarama's extremely useful introduction [3–5]. Adapting modeling strategies for health and clinical outcomes to be consistent with underlying heterogeneity can uncover trends and relationships that have been heretofore been obscured by the change homogeneity assumption.

14.2 Determining the Optimal Number of Latent Trajectories

Similar criteria for GMM are used as in LCA/LPA to determine the optimal number of latent classes to retain. To briefly review, a series of plausible models are compared until the relative "best" solution is determined. Typically, each model in the series, starting with the single class model, retains a different number of classes. One considers interpretability and statistical criteria (AIC, BIC, aBIC, AICC, posterior probability assessment, class cell sizes and entropy [6,7]) and tests such as aLMR-LRT, VLMR-LRT and bootstrapped LRT [8] in determining the best solution. These criteria are reviewed in the context of LCA in Chapter 11. Again, once the optimal solution for the number of latent classes is identified, individuals can be assigned to their most likely latent class based on their posterior probabilities [7]. A graphical display of the mean trajectories over time within each cluster can help assign meaning to these clusters. We will apply GMM in illustrative examples in this chapter and visualize the mean trajectories in graphical displays.

14.3 Latent Class Growth Analysis

Mixture modeling techniques use probabilistic modeling and make statistical assumptions (Chapter 11). Within-class normality is often (but not necessarily) assumed in GMMs. A FIML procedure can be used such that respondents with missing data can still be included in the analysis, and supplemental methods like bootstrapping are available and can be useful [9–11].

The more general GMM approaches assume each latent class should have its own class-specific, nonzero variances and covariances in the latent growth parameters (i.e. intercept and slopes). *Latent class growth analysis (LCGA)* instead implements a constraint that the variances and covariances of these growth parameters across the latent classes are constrained to be equal (e.g. trivially to zero). Thus, GMM and LCGA are closely related longitudinal latent variable mixture modeling techniques, where LCGA is more restrictive in the variance-covariance matrix for the growth parameters across classes [12–14].

These constraints for LCGA hold the advantage that the different latent classes can be compared to each other solely based on the mean trajectory. Further, the influence of any covariates on the latent classes can be evaluated in terms of mean trajectory for each latent class. As a limitation, these assumptions regarding the variances and covariances in LCGA are often done for statistical expediency and may not be true in practice and lead to model misspecification [15].

14.4 An Applied Example of Latent Class Growth Analysis from the Health and Retirement Study

Many researchers use longitudinal techniques under the assumption of a homogenous study sample. Adapting modeling strategies for health and clinical outcomes that allow for underlying heterogeneity can uncover trends and relationships that have been heretofore been obscured by the homogeneity assumption.

For example, depression is a heterogeneous condition [16]. Depression symptoms may differ in severity and change over time [17–19]. In studies of elderly people, depression can be common and may contribute to adverse health outcomes and can interfere with treatment for other medical problems [20]. In this example, we used LCGA to investigate the potential for multiple distinct depressive symptom trajectories in the Health and

Retirement Study (HRS). HRS is a nationally representative survey and the models presented here properly accounted for the HRS complex sampling design. Data characteristics in HRS are thoroughly described elsewhere [21].

We analyzed 5,195 age-eligible adult respondents from the 1992 HRS cohort who completed interviews in all seven study waves through 2004. Demographic characteristics of this cohort subsample are 60.3% female, 76.4% non-Hispanic White, 14.4% Black, 7.4% Hispanic, 1.8% other racial/ethnic groups; median age = 55; and mean education = 12.4 years (SD = 3.0).

Depressive symptoms were measured at each time point for each individual using an 8-item version of the CES-D (CES-D 8). Each item is dichotomized. Based upon factor analytic results, Kohout et al. [22] concluded that shortened, dichotomized CES-D measures are a valid form of CES-D measurement, reducing respondent burden and study cost. The total number of depressive symptoms for the CES-D 8 can be calculated as the sum of the 8 items (ranging from 0 to 8).

For the sake of simplifying this example, we specify changes in depressive symptoms as being linear within this nationally representative US older study population. There were six repeated measures for each individual recorded biannually over 12 years (1994–2004). These repeated measures were assumed to be equally spaced over time. We compared the fit of mixture models for the total number of depressive symptoms for the CESD-8 ranging from two to eight classes using MPlus. We used the MLR option. Table 14.1 presents the comparison of select model fit criteria used for this example.

The VLMR-LRT suggests that the four trajectory model is best supported by the data due to the change in statistical significance. That is, comparing the three trajectory model with the four trajectory model was significant ($p = 0.015$) and four trajectory model with the five trajectory model ($p = 0.192$) was not significant. The four trajectory model also has excellent classification quality (entropy = 0.925).

The distinct trajectories of depressive symptoms for these four subgroups are displayed in Figure 14.2: (class 1) almost no symptoms throughout = 73.5%; (class 2) decreasing symptoms = 9.6%; (class 3) increasing symptoms = 11.5%; (class 4) many persistent symptoms = 5.4%. Thus the four class solution had a plausible interpretation.

After determining the optimal number of latent class trajectories, we examined the influence of selected covariates on trajectory membership. We specified a conditional latent class model with covariates and used a one-step regression procedure (Chapter 11), as described by Jung and Wickarama [5]. Note that from the unconditional model (with no covariates) the class cell sizes did not change much in the conditional model in

TABLE 14.1

Fit Indices and Test Results for LCGA to Evaluate Depression Symptom Trajectories ($N = 5,195$)

k	LL	BIC	aBIC	Entropy	VLMR-LRT Test Statistic	VLMR-LRT p
2	−56367.49	112983.09	112890.94	0.955	10525.69	0.000
3	−55146.65	110618.41	110497.66	0.922	2410.38	0.000
4	−54652.99	109708.09	109558.74	0.925	974.66	0.015
5	−54357.08	109193.27	109015.32	0.901	519.88	0.149
6	−54090.08	108736.27	108529.72	0.912	397.39	0.354
7	−54079.98	108793.06	108557.91	0.920	97.55	0.392
8	−53895.87	108501.85	108238.10	0.732	307.84	0.314

k, number of latent classes retained; LL, log-likelihood; BIC, Bayesian Information Criterion; aBIC, Sample-Size Adjusted BIC; VLMR-LRT, Vuong-Lo-Mendell-Rubin Likelihood Ratio Test.

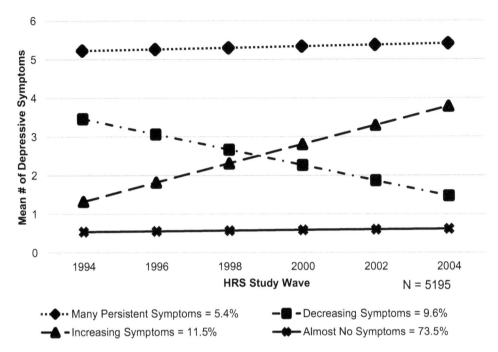

FIGURE 14.2

Four class model for depressive symptom trajectories over 12 years of the HRS.

Results of the latent class growth analysis showing four trajectories of depressive symptoms with differences in the intercept and slope of each trajectory.

this example. However, in other examples this may not be the case. Researchers will want to determine the best approach for inclusion of covariates (or distal outcomes) carefully according to the research question at hand and the characteristics of variables and data and trajectories being modeled. Other techniques such as the corrected three-step method are often appropriate [1].

The covariates included age (in years), sex (male or female), race (Black, Hispanic or non-Hispanic White and Other) and education level in years (reverse coded high to low). Box 14.1 presents example MPlus syntax for this model. For a more complete walkthrough of the code, see Jung and Wickrama [5]. In general, relationships between trajectories and covariates can be thought of as taking the form of a multinomial regression in which likelihood of a given trajectory, as opposed to the reference trajectory is regressed on the covariates.

In Table 14.2, while there are many interesting findings, in the interest of space, we focus on the comparison between the "many persistent symptoms" trajectory and the "almost no symptoms" trajectory. Results show a greater likelihood of the "many persistent symptoms" trajectory as opposed to the "almost no symptoms" trajectory for younger individuals (OR = 0.94, $p = 0.010$), women (OR = 2.19, $p < 0.001$), Blacks (OR = 1.89, $p < 0.001$) and those with lower education (OR = 1.32, $p < 0.001$). The reference category for race/ethnicity is "non-Hispanic White."

This relationship between education and the depressive symptom trajectories is further visualized in Figure 14.3. We stratified the sample according to most likely latent class membership. Then, we graphed out the relationship between the probability of being a

BOX 14.1 EXAMPLE SYNTAX FOR A CONDITIONAL LATENT CLASS GROWTH ANALYSIS (LCGA) WITH COVARIATES OF DEPRESSIVE SYMPTOMS IN THE HEALTH AND RETIREMENT STUDY

```
Data:
  File is HRS_CESD.dat ;
Variable:
  Names are
      id hispan black gender edyrs age
      r2 r3 r4 r5 r6 r7;
  Usevariables are
      hispan black gender edyrs age
      r2 r3 r4 r5 r6 r7;
  CLASSES = c(4);
  Missing are all (-999);
ANALYSIS:
  STARTS = 500 50 ;
  LRTSTARTS = 20 10 25 10;
  LRTBOOTSTRAP = 100 ;
  TYPE IS MIXTURE COMPLEX;
  ESTIMATOR IS MLR;

MODEL: %OVERALL%
i s | r2@0 r3@1 r4@2 r5@3 r6@4 r7@5 ;
i s c#1 c#2 c#3 ON hispan black gender edyrs age ;
i-s@0;
%c#1%
[r2-r7*0];
%c#2%
[r2-r7*-.5];
%c#3%
[r2-r7*0];
%c#4%
[r2-r7*-3];

OUTPUT:  SAMPSTAT TECH1 TECH11 TECH4 CINTERVAL STANDARDIZED;
PLOT:  TYPE=PLOT3;
series is r2 r3 r4 r5 r6 r7 (*);
```

Note for Box 14.1 that the study results reported in Figure 14.3 include an adjustment for the HRS complex sampling design, and that adjustment is omitted from this box to not distract the reader.

member of each subgroup according to years of education. More years of education show a strong positive relationship with having the "Almost no symptoms" trajectory. Individuals with the most years of education are the most likely to be in the group that experiences almost zero depressive symptoms throughout the study period.

Conclusions drawn from LCGA can be very different than with other techniques that ignore "hidden" longitudinal trajectories. As an illustrative comparison, we calculated the bivariate correlation (Pearson's r) between the years of education variable and the number of depressive symptoms in waves 1 and 7 of the HRS. The correlation was −0.30 (95% CI −0.27, −0.33) in HRS Wave 1 and −0.23 (95%CI −0.20, −0.26) in Wave 7. Thus in viewing

TABLE 14.2

Effects of Demographics on Trajectory Type (Latent Class Membership)

	Reference Class = Almost No Symptoms								
	Vs. Many Symptoms			Vs. Decreasing			Vs. Increasing		
	OR	B	p	OR	B	p	OR	B	p
Age	0.94	−0.057	0.010	0.96	−0.043	0.014	1.02	0.016	0.422
Female	2.19	0.785	0.000	1.53	0.428	0.001	1.41	0.346	0.002
Black	1.89	0.635	0.000	1.90	0.641	0.000	1.54	0.429	0.001
Hispanic	1.12	0.113	0.655	1.59	0.461	0.018	1.19	0.178	0.461
Education	1.32	0.274	0.000	0.84	−0.173	0.000	0.90	−0.105	0.000
	Reference Class = Many Symptoms								
	Vs. Almost None			Vs. Decreasing			Vs. Increasing		
Age	1.06	0.057	0.010	1.01	0.014	0.611	1.08	0.074	0.009
Female	0.46	−0.785	0.000	0.70	−0.357	0.009	0.64	−0.439	0.008
Black	0.53	−0.635	0.000	1.01	0.005	0.979	0.81	−0.206	0.301
Hispanic	0.89	−0.113	0.655	1.42	0.348	0.263	1.07	0.064	0.805
Education	0.76	−0.274	0.000	1.11	0.100	0.000	1.18	0.169	0.000

OR, odds ratio; B, log odds ratio.

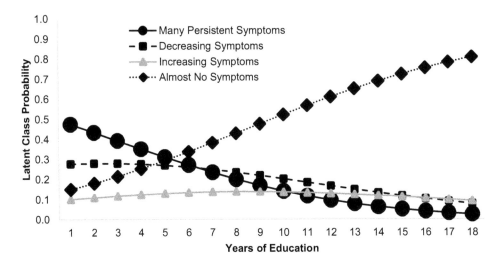

FIGURE 14.3

Relationship between years of education and depressive symptom trajectories ($N = 5,195$).

Results of the conditional latent class growth analysis with covariates indicate the probability of membership in each latent class (trajectory) of depressive symptoms has a strong relationship with years of education; as education increase the likelihood of being in the "Almost No Symptoms" group increases dramatically while the likelihood of being in the "Many Persistent Symptoms" group decreases.

the sample homogenously, the associations do not adequately portray the gradual yet dramatically protective effect of each additional year of education as observed in the plot presented in Figure 14.3. Researchers using a form of longitudinal modeling that does not suppose underlying subpopulations would be unable to observe these important nuances of the relationship between education and depressive symptoms.

In this example, results support a four trajectory typology that can serve as a framework for better understanding depressive symptoms and underscore the importance of gender, race and education for mental health among older adults. Interpretation of these example results is somewhat straightforward. The vast majority of older adults are in the flat "almost no symptoms" trajectory, which suggests in most older adults in this study sample, depressive symptoms remain stable over a long period of time. We found four trajectories overall. If depressive symptom trajectories over time are indeed heterogeneous in this study sample and our model assumptions are met, models in the prior literature that assume a single, average trajectory for the entire sample are misspecified. That is, older adults with almost no symptoms, many persistent symptoms, decreasing symptoms or increasing symptoms should not be lumped together into the same general pattern when analyzing change over time. Such misclassification by ignoring longitudinal heterogeneity could also lead to errors in hypothesis testing of the relationship between depressive symptoms and other variables such as race, education, age and sex.

This example illustrated how LCGA can be implemented to discover variability in how a health outcome changes over the life course. While our example utilized depressive symptoms, it is easy to imagine many innovative applications of GMM and LCGA for other important symptoms and health conditions of interest to population health researchers.

14.5 `MplusAutomation` and `Runmplus`: Useful Tools for Summarizing Results for a Series of Latent Variable Mixture Models

`MplusAutomation`, written by Michael Hallquist, is a R package designed to run MPlus in the R programming environment [23]. `Runmplus`, written by Rich Jones, is a Stata module designed to run Mplus within Stata [24]. `Runmplus` and `MplusAutomation` both provide an interface for formatting data, writing syntax and executing Mplus code. These are useful time-saving tools for users of R and Stata.

An important benefit of `MplusAutomation` and `runmplus` is a streamlining of conducting model comparisons. The user can create a group of related models and then extract useful information and save selected results (e.g. fit indices and/or parameter estimates) across the models. These results can then be summarized in tables and graphical displays allowing for model comparison.

We have used `MplusAutomation` and `runmplus` in practice often to run a series of latent variable models, including mixtures models like LCA, LPA and GMM, in MPlus and extract and tabulate model parameters and fit measures in R [23] and Stata [24], respectively. This procedure is very efficient for the user as (1) a single program with a loop creates and runs the series of models in MPlus and (2) results from the series of models can be extracted into R or Stata and summarized in tables and graphical displays. We now describe an application of `MplusAutomation` for LCGA.

14.5.1 An Applied Example of LCGA for People Living with HIV Using `MplusAutomation`

We revisit the longitudinal data for the PHQ-9 total score in a database for 416 people living with HIV in a collaborative care program (Chapter 13). Recall, follow-up times after

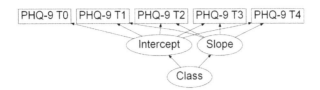

FIGURE 14.4

Mixture model for the PHQ-9 total score in people living with HIV in a collaborative care program.

PHQ-9 is the PHQ-9 total score. *T0* is the baseline time point for each subject. *T1-T4* are individually varying follow up times over 15 months for each subject. We used this mixture model to determine the optimal solution for the number of classes and classify individuals into most likely latent class membership. Description of the within-class trajectories subgroups was subsequently done under no assumption of linearity. Adapted with some modification from Gunzler, D., et al., Depressive symptom trajectories among people living with HIV in a collaborative care program. AIDS and Behavior, 2019. 24(8): pp. 1765–1775.

the first visit in the study time period were individually varying times of observations.[1] The study objective here was to describe the depression trajectories for people living with HIV participating in an intervention. MplusAutomation was used to perform LCGA.

We used the mixture model corresponding to Figure 14.4 under an assumption of linearity, to (1) determine the optimal solution for the number of classes and (2) classify individuals into most likely latent class membership. The assumption of linearity may not be appropriate in this study [25,26]. However, the series of models did not all converge to a global solution when including a nonlinear term (i.e. quadratic term). Description of the within-class trajectories subgroups was subsequently done under no assumption of linearity.

Code was developed in a single MPlus file with a loop to iteratively generate code for eight mixture models of increasing number of classes from one up to eight in MPlus. The eight input files were then created in MPlus using the createModels function in R programming language. The models were run in MPlus using the runModels function in R program and then extracted output into the R environment using the readModels function in R program. We individually extracted each model output into R using this approach. For more examples of the software coding in MplusAutomation, an interested reader can refer to the paper by Hallquist and Wiley [23].

The four class solution was selected after examination of model summaries in a single table in R (concatenated by the MplusAutomation tool) (Table 14.3) and evaluating the model interpretability.

Log-likelihood, AIC, BIC, AICC, aBIC and entropy were printed out in Table 14.3 of model summaries.[2] There was not a clear solution that minimized AIC, AICC, BIC and aBIC while maximizing log-likelihood and entropy. We did conclude the four class solution was the most reasonable. BIC was at a minimum for the four class solution. In addition, the four class solution had a reasonable interpretation over other potential solutions, in line with theory and previous study findings [25,26] (see Figure 14.5).

We identified that two of the four latent classes were characterized by highly responsive (C2; 19.5%) and improving (C4; 58.4% [of participants]) depressive symptoms. Thus, a high proportion of individuals were classified into subgroups marked by improvement.

---

[1] In MPlus, ANALYSIS: TYPE = RANDOM MIXTURE. Options to test the number of latent classes using the aLMR-LRT or VLMR-LRT in TECH11 and the bootstrapped LRT in TECH14 are not available with this type of analysis.

[2] e.g. for the four class solution which we term "m4" and "m4$summaries" in R program outputs the indices.

278

Structural Equation Modeling for Health and Medicine

TABLE 14.3

Model Fit Indices for One through Eight Class Solutions Latent Class Growth Analysis Example Using MPlusAutomation

Number of Classes	Log-Likelihood	DF	Scaling Correction for MLR	AIC	AICC	BIC	aBIC	Entropy
1	−3670.94	7	0.85	7354.39	7354.66	7382.60	7360.39	
2	−3580.96	10	1.15	7181.92	7182.46	7222.22	7190.49	0.720
3	−3567.71	13	1.33	7161.42	7162.33	7213.82	7172.57	0.770
4	−3549.17	16	1.14	7130.33	7131.69	7194.82	7144.05	0.707
5	−3545.66	19	1.11	7129.31	7131.23	7205.90	7145.61	0.608
6	−3542.55	22	0.98	7129.10	7131.68	7217.78	7147.97	0.754
7	−3528.58	25	1.07	7107.16	7110.49	7207.93	7128.60	0.677
8	−3528.58	28	0.95	7113.16	7117.36	7226.02	7137.17	0.697

Source: Table adapted from Gunzler, D., et al., Depressive symptom trajectories among people living with HIV in a collaborative care program. *AIDS and Behavior*, 2019. **24**(8): pp. 1765–1775.

DF, Degrees of Freedom; MLR, maximum likelihood with robust standard errors; AIC, Akaike Information Criteria; AICC, corrected AIC for small sample sizes; BIC, Bayesian Information Criteria; aBIC, sample-size adjusted BIC.

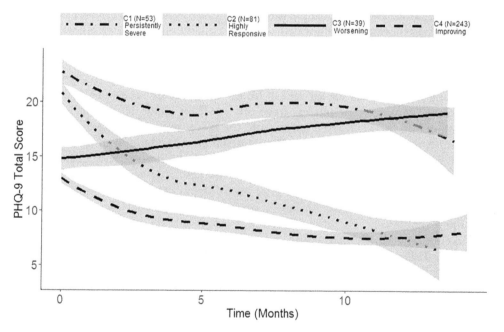

FIGURE 14.5

Four class solution for LCGA in people living with HIV in a collaborative care program ($N = 416$).

Plot of average within-class trajectories based on most likely latent class clustering using local regression smoothing. Shaded region in each plot represents a 95% Confidence Interval. Individuals were classified into most likely class membership using the mixture model represented in Figure 14.4 under the assumption of linearity. Description of these within-class trajectories was done under no assumption of linearity. Adapted with some modification from Gunzler, D., et al., Depressive symptom trajectories among people living with HIV in a collaborative care program. AIDS and Behavior, 2019. 24(8): 1765–1775.

One latent class was persistently severe (C1; 12.7%) in depressive symptoms. One latent class (C3; 9.4%) experienced worsening depressive symptoms over time.

In Figure 14.6, we graph the within-class spaghetti plots to help evaluate individual variation around the estimated within-class mean trajectories.

If we account for the unequal class sizes and different slopes across the subgroups, we might conclude that individual variation around the within-class intercepts and slopes across classes is somewhat similar across plots. This examination of slopes and class sizes is a step for verifying that the assumption of LCGA regarding equality of variance across latent classes is reasonable. We might also note some of the individually plotted lines look as though they could potential fit with more than one of the average trajectory classes.

These same type of plots as in Figures 14.5 and 14.6 can be done using the model results for estimated means rather than a post-hoc analyses using an extracted categorical latent class membership variable to define groups. Here we used the post-hoc strategy for modeling the within-class trajectories since the LCGA with nonlinear growth terms did not converge for all solutions given our sample size.

Gunzler et al. [17] also described clinical characteristics of people living with HIV associated with these depression trajectories. That is, self-reported trauma, posttraumatic stress disorder, lower education and fewer HIV and psychiatry clinic visits were associated with worsening or persistently severe depressive symptom trajectories in group comparisons. Members of the persistently severe group (compared to the improving group) were also less likely to be virally suppressed after 12 months. We conducted this LCGA with auxiliary variables solely in MPlus; the corrected three-step regression procedures available for performing these analyses in MPlus [1] in relating latent classes to covariates and outcomes were described in Chapter 11.

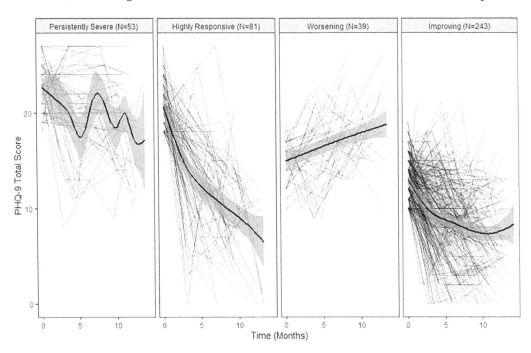

FIGURE 14.6
Facetted plot showing individual within-class variation in four class solution (*N* = 416).

Local regression smoothing plots of average within-class trajectories based on most likely latent class. Shaded region in each plot represents a 95% Confidence Interval.

Recall from Chapter 13 when we applied LGM to this study sample that overall, the average trajectory of self-reported depression started at moderately severe and decreased over 15 months, while still above the threshold for major depression. Thus, in a manner similar to the HRS example among older adults, we might conclude that interventional studies analyzing data in aggregate in people living with HIV fail to observe intrinsic variation in subgroup response for depressive symptoms [17]. Analysis of subgroup depression trajectories in people living with HIV is essential for understanding (1) the progression of depression and (2) for whom the intervention may be effective or ineffective. Four subgroups were a better fit for the data than one homogenous group based on LCGA model fit and interpretation.

14.6 Conclusions

GMM, a technique used to analyze heterogeneous longitudinal data, was discussed in this chapter. GMM is an extension of LGM to identify subpopulation trajectories. Having gone over many of the fundamental properties of FMM techniques as applied in LCA and LPA in Chapters 11 and 12 and LGM in Chapter 13, we focused on applications of LCGA in health and medical research to describe heterogeneous depressive symptom trajectories over time and associated background factors.

There are many creative extensions of GMM that can be useful for applied questions in health and decision science studies. One can apply GMM with ordered-categorical data [27]. The ordinal response for each individual at each time point is made by thresholds imposed on an underlying continuous latent response variable as we have previously discussed in Chapter 7. See for example Pennoni and Romeo [27] for more details on this GMM approach with ordered-categorical data. One can extend the cohort-sequential modeling approaches as discussed in Chapter 13 for GMM. See for example Holmes et al. [28] for an application of cohort-sequential GMM to assess heterogeneity in the patterns of developmental trajectories of language development and academic functioning in children who have experienced maltreatment. There are also second order GMMs [29] and parallel process GMMs [30]. Thus, provided in this textbook is a basic overview of the concepts and usage of GMM. The reader can then apply GMM or an extension of GMM after further readings in a manner appropriate for a given research question and setting.

References

1. Asparouhov, T. and B. Muthén, Auxiliary variables in mixture modeling: Three-step approaches using M plus. *Structural Equation Modeling: A Multidisciplinary Journal*, 2014. **21**(3): pp. 329–341.
2. Muthén, L.K. and B.O. Muthén, *Mplus: The comprehensive modelling program for applied researchers: User's guide.* Eighth edition 1998–2017, Los Angeles, CA: Muthén & Muthén.
3. Muthén, B. and T. Asparouhov, Growth mixture modeling: Analysis with non-Gaussian random effects. *Longitudinal Data Analysis*, 2008: pp. 143–165.

4. Muthén, B., et al., Growth modeling with nonignorable dropout: Alternative analyses of the STAR* D antidepressant trial. *Psychological Methods*, 2011. **16**(1): p. 17.

5. Jung, T. and K.A. Wickrama, An introduction to latent class growth analysis and growth mixture modeling. *Social and Personality Psychology Compass*, 2008. **2**(1): pp. 302–317.

6. Schwarz, G., Estimating the dimension of a model. *The Annals of Statistics*, 1978. **6**(2): pp. 461–464.

7. Muthén, B. and K. Shedden, Finite mixture modeling with mixture outcomes using the EM algorithm. *Biometrics*, 1999. **55**(2): pp. 463–469.

8. Collins, L.M., et al., Goodness-of-fit testing for latent class models. *Multivariate Behavioral Research*, 1993. **28**(3): pp. 375–89.

9. Lubke, G.H. and I. Campbell, Inference based on the best-fitting model can contribute to the replication crisis: Assessing model selection uncertainty using a bootstrap approach. *Structural Equation Modeling: A Multidisciplinary Journal*, 2016. **23**(4): pp. 479–490.

10. Ram, N. and K.J. Grimm, Methods and measures: Growth mixture modeling: A method for identifying differences in longitudinal change among unobserved groups. *International Journal of Behavioral Development*, 2009. **33**(6): pp. 565–576.

11. Dziak, J.J., S.T. Lanza, and X. Tan, Effect size, statistical power, and sample size requirements for the bootstrap likelihood ratio test in latent class analysis. *Structural Equation Modeling: A Multidisciplinary Journal*, 2014. **21**(4): pp. 534–552.

12. Berlin, K.S., G.R. Parra, and N.A. Williams, An introduction to latent variable mixture modeling (part 2): Longitudinal latent class growth analysis and growth mixture models. *Journal of Pediatric Psychology*, 2014. **39**(2): pp. 188–203.

13. Muthén, B., The potential of growth mixture modelling. *Infant and Child Development*, 2006. **15**(6): p. 623.

14. Muthén, B. and L.K. Muthén, Integrating person-centered and variable-centered analyses: Growth mixture modeling with latent trajectory classes. *Alcoholism: Clinical and Experimental Research*, 2000. **24**(6): pp. 882–891.

15. Bauer, D.J. and P.J. Curran, Distributional assumptions of growth mixture models: Implications for overextraction of latent trajectory classes. *Psychological Methods*, 2003. **8**(3): p. 338.

16. Goldberg, D., The heterogeneity of "major depression". *World Psychiatry*, 2011. **10**(3): pp. 226–228.

17. Gunzler, D., et al., Depressive symptom trajectories among people living with HIV in a collaborative care program. *AIDS and Behavior*, 2019. **24**(8): pp. 1765–1775.

18. Gunzler, D.D., et al., Heterogeneous depression trajectories in multiple sclerosis patients. *Multiple Sclerosis and Related Disorders*, 2016. **9**: pp. 163–169.

19. Gomez, R., et al., Growth mixture modeling of depression symptoms following traumatic brain injury. *Frontiers in Psychology*, 2017. **8**: 1320.

20. Blackburn, P., M. Wilkins-Ho, and B.S. Wiese, Depression in older adults: Diagnosis and management. *British Columbia Medical Journal*, 2017. **59**(3): pp. 171–177.

21. Sonnega, A., et al., Cohort profile: The health and retirement study (HRS). *International Journal of Epidemiology*, 2014. **43**(2): pp. 576–585.

22. Kohout, F.J., et al., Two shorter forms of the CES-D depression symptoms index. *Journal of Aging and Health*, 1993. **5**(2): pp. 179–193.

23. Hallquist, M.N. and J.F. Wiley, MplusAutomation: An R package for facilitating large-scale latent variable analyses in Mplus. *Structural Equation Modeling: A Multidisciplinary Journal*, 2018. **25**(4): pp. 621–638.

24. Jones, R., RUNMPLUS: Stata module to run Mplus from Stata. 2013.

25. Bengtson, A.M., et al., Trajectories of depressive symptoms among a population of HIV-infected men and women in routine HIV care in the United States. *AIDS and Behavior*, 2018. **22**(8): pp. 1–12.

26. Owora, A.H., Major depression disorder trajectories and HIV disease progression: Results from a 6-year outpatient clinic cohort. *Medicine*, 2018. **97**(12): p. e0252.

27. Pennoni, F. and I. Romeo, Latent Markov and growth mixture models for ordinal individual responses with covariates: A comparison. *Statistical Analysis and Data Mining: The ASA Data Science Journal*, 2017. **10**(1): pp. 29–39.

28. Holmes, M.R., et al., Promoting the development of resilient academic functioning in maltreated children. *Child Abuse and Neglect*, 2018. **75**: pp. 92–103.

29. Kim, E.S. and Y. Wang, Class enumeration and parameter recovery of growth mixture modeling and second-order growth mixture modeling in the presence of measurement noninvariance between latent classes. *Frontiers in Psychology*, 2017. **8**: 1499.

30. Wu, J., et al., A parallel process growth mixture model of conduct problems and substance use with risky sexual behavior. *Drug and Alcohol Dependence*, 2010. **111**(3): pp. 207–214.

15

Special Topics

15.1 Introduction to Special Topics for SEM for Health and Medicine

Throughout the book, we have introduced and discussed the vocabulary, usages and concepts of SEM. We have focused on applications to health and medicine. The closing chapter of this textbook presents a series of special topics. We discuss both methods and applications. We reiterate that SEM is a flexible set of methods and creatively minded methodologists can surely find new and exciting implementations and innovations to advance a particular research question or hypothesis. References are provided for those readers interested in pursuing any of these topics further.

15.2 Challenges in Using Electronic Health Records

In many of the applications in this textbook, we have used complex and messy observational data such as data extracted from electronic health records. The data was preprocessed in order to handle some of the messiness. For example, identified data errors were modified or removed. Codes and lab values were evaluated for consistencies and inconsistencies in diagnoses in helping to define study samples. Given a reasonably cleaned data set, a researcher has to be extremely prudent about what questions can be asked and answered with the available data (Box 15.1). Taksler and colleagues have provided a helpful introduction to many of these considerations in their manuscript on the challenges of working with electronic health record data [1].

BOX 15.1

In performing SEM using real-world data one should:

- Draw from expert knowledge in identifying research questions of interest that can be answered with available data
- Make reasonable assumptions regarding the study population
- Draw an appropriate sample and make inclusion and exclusion decisions in line with these assumptions
- Use quantitative and subjective criteria in tandem to analyze the data
- Draw reasonable conclusions given the study sample

We have noted that some studies using electronic health record data have samples that do not represent the population of interest well. However, as health informatics and modern technology continue to improve, study samples drawn from data more representative of a population of interest are becoming more readily available. For example, two institutions, public and private, have electronic health records with similar information. A large study sample has been drawn from these two data sources more representative of a wider range on the socioeconomic spectrum.[1] There were many difficult steps in order to merge these data together. For example, incompatible codes from these data bases had to be made compatible and subjects that utilized both institutions could not be double counted.

Determining study sample boundaries is often challenging, especially in longitudinal designs. For example, in a typical retrospective study using a registry at an institution recorded over many years, individuals of interest enter the registry at arbitrary points in time and for different time periods. As a result, individual subjects often have varying follow-up, irregular follow-up and missingness. One might only include individuals in the study with follow-up data after a selected baseline date living in a particular geographic region (e.g. for a higher probability that individuals get most of their care at that institution). One might exclude individuals with a history of conditions that could influence the outcome or who are missing basic data points for the study (e.g. no recorded age, sex or blood pressure measurement). In general, determining inclusion and exclusion criteria must be done very carefully. The addition or subtraction of groups of individuals in a study can alter effect size estimates dramatically.

Further persistent challenges exist in the interpretation of results. For example, a patient may make more frequent appointments (and have more recorded data) if they are having more health problems. Thus estimates of health in a sample characterized by these types of uneven variation in care utilization may be weighted more heavily toward individuals of poorer health, simply due to the fact that they have more data recorded. Contrarily, making more appointments could, in a different sample, be indicative of a subset of individuals pursuing a healthier lifestyle and seeking to maintain wellness through more regular checkups. Variability in health outcomes occurring between visits is often not recorded and a researcher is often only observing snippets of the true outcome trajectory over the study period. Certain recorded measures (e.g. multi-item patient reported scales) are often assumed to be recorded with measurement error, and likely systematic measurement error (Chapter 10), that should be accounted for in statistical analyses.

SEM is a flexible multivariate technique well-suited to examine relationships between variables using real-world data. A researcher, however, when applying SEM using such data should carefully follow points listed in Box 15.1. Many opportunities now exist to draw upon the theory of SEM as discussed in this textbook and creatively apply these methods to specify and analyze complex measurement models, latent variable mixture models, systems-based models and longitudinal models. In health and medicine, such analyses can lead to a more comprehensive evaluation of interventions, health outcomes and disease progression among many other purposes.

[1] NIH-NIA, R01 AG055480-01 (Dalton and Perzynski)

15.3 Genetics

In this textbook, we have focused on studies of environmental influences to health outcomes. *Behavioral genetic research* aims to study the relative contribution of genetic and environmental influences to individual differences in traits (phenotypes) [2,3]. The package Mx allows flexibility in using SEM to model genetically sensitive data [4]. MPlus can also be used for genetics analysis [5].

15.3.1 SEM for Twin Data

A special methodological approach of SEM known as the *twin method* can be used to disentangle the influences of environmental and genetic factors on a measured trait (phenotype) by comparing two groups of twins. Data is used from *monozygotic (MZ)* and *dizygotic (DZ)* twin pairs. MZ twins develop from the same egg and have similar genetic code [3]. DZ twins develop from two different eggs fertilized at the same time; DZ twins share 50% of genetic variation [3]. In the SEM framework, the sources of genetic and environmental variation are represented by latent variables while the phenotype is represented by an observed variable. *Heritability* is the relative contribution of genetic factors to the total phenotypic variance. Twin models can be extended to evaluate multiple measured traits [2].

15.3.2 Genome-Wide SEM

Genome-wide association studies (GWAS) are observational studies to identify genes involved in human disease. Researchers use data from these types of studies to pinpoint genes that influence the risk of developing certain diseases.

The genome is searched for small variations, called *single nucleotide polymorphisms (SNPs)*, that are more likely to occur in people with a certain disease than in people without the disease. Typical GWAS look at many SNPs (e.g. thousands) at the same time. The availability of high quality genomic data has rapidly and greatly increased [6]. However, complex traits are typically determined by multiple variants with very small effect sizes. Therefore, very large sample sizes are necessary to compensate for the low statistical power to detect genetic associations [7].

The genotype is a sequence of alleles along the loci of an individual. Univariate regression is used between a single SNP and continuous phenotype to determine if the genotype at a single SNP predicts the phenotype. In a standard approach, polygenic risk scores are calculated by computing the sum of risk alleles corresponding to a phenotype of interest in each individual, weighted by the effect size estimate of the most powerful GWAS on the phenotype [8].

Multivariate methods such as multivariate regression, MANOVA and principal components analysis have been used for GWAS studies evaluating multiple phenotypes [7]. SEM is well-suited as a multivariate technique to consider relationships between SNPs (and other genetic characteristics) and multiple phenotypes (or subphenotypes).

Figure 15.1 depicts an application of a MIMIC model to estimate the influence of SNPs on a latent antisocial behavior variable [9]. Antisocial behavior is hypothesized to influence multiple observed questionnaire items assessing behavioral and mental health issues (i.e. levels of aggression, lying, violate the law, substance abuse, depression and anxiety). The regression of the latent variable on each SNP is estimated using a single parameter.

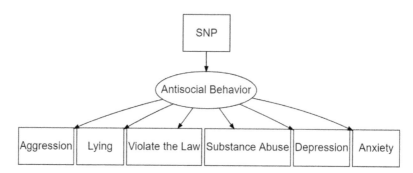

FIGURE 15.1
MIMIC model for influence of SNPs on an antisocial behavior latent variable.

There are many potential extensions of the model corresponding to Figure 15.1 for GWAS. For example, a latent construct can be formed consisting of multiple SNPs (latent genetic variable). Then, a researcher can regress a latent phenotype variable on the latent genetic variable [10].

Relationships between SNPs and specific observed items can also be evaluated by adding in DIF paths to Figure 15.1. Multifactor models can be used to examine comorbidity between phenotypes. LGM and autoregressive modeling can be used for longitudinal data on phenotypes (e.g. repeated measures data on SBP or total cholesterol). Mediation analysis and systems-based modeling can be used to evaluate hypothesized relationships between phenotypes.

The authors of this text are embarking on a new effort to use mediation analysis in an SEM framework to understand the linkages between neighborhood socioeconomic conditions and racial and ethnic disparities in triple negative breast cancer. In this research, we will specify models that examine whether racial differences in novel RNA expression characteristics of breast cancer tumors can be explained by neighborhood socioeconomic circumstances.[2] We anticipate that such novel applications of SEM to transdisciplinary, biosocial research questions will become increasingly common as more researchers become familiar with SEM.

15.4 Bayesian SEM

We have mostly discussed methods and applications using a frequentist viewpoint. That is, we have assumed that the free parameters to be estimated in the modeling approaches are unknown but fixed. In *Bayesian statistical inference,* the free parameters are considered random with a probability distribution that reflects the level of uncertainty about the true value [11]. Bayesian SEM is derived from the principles of Bayes' theorem and these approaches use Bayesian analysis for SEM [11–15]. We provide here a very brief overview of Bayesian analysis and Bayesian SEM.

The *prior probability* is the probability that is assigned before taking into consideration available information. The *posterior probability* is the updated estimate of the probability

[2] Role of Wave3 in the Development and Progression of Breast Cancer, Khalid Sossey Alaoui, Principal Investigator (NIH grant no. 5R01CA226921)

after taking into consideration available information. Using Bayesian statistical inference one can obtain the posterior density, which is proportional to the likelihood function for the data (given the model parameters) multiplied by the prior for the parameters. Summaries of the posterior distribution (e.g. mean, median, mode, variance, quantiles) can be used to provide a description of the distribution and allows one to test hypothesis of interest [11]. As aforementioned in Chapter 4, Bayesian analysis can be performed using powerful computational algorithms referred to as *Markov Chain Monte Carlo (MCMC)* methods [14].

The specification of the prior distribution for the model parameters is a distinguishing feature of Bayesian statistical inference [11]. The prior can be *informative* or *noninformative*. In a simplified sense, an informative prior gives numerical information that has an impact on the posterior distribution. A noninformative prior gives vague information that has minimal impact on the posterior distribution.

Bayesian perspective allows one to form a *credibility interval*. A credibility interval of the quantiles obtained from the posterior distribution of the model parameters has a straightforward interpretation. A 95% credibility interval translates that the probability that the parameter lies in the interval is 0.95. The confidence interval in the frequentist sense is less intuitive, and instead a 95% confidence interval translates to 95% of the confidence intervals formed this way capture the true parameter under the null hypothesis. Additionally, a credibility interval does not assume symmetry and allows for a strongly skewed distribution [14].

Model fit can be assessed for Bayesian SEM using *posterior predictive checking (PPC)* [16]. PPC uses the posterior predictive distribution of replicated data for assessing possible model misspecification [11]. PPC implies that the replicated data should match the observed data closely if we are to conclude a good model fit. In MPlus, PPC uses the likelihood ratio chi-square test as the discrepancy function between the actual data and data generated by the model [5,11]. A posterior predictive *p*-value can then be obtained via the corresponding fit statistic.

The posterior predictive *p*-value does not behave like a classical *p*-value for a chi-square test of model fit. The posterior predictive *p*-value takes into account the variability of the model parameters and does not rely on asymptotic theory. If the posterior predictive *p*-value is small (e.g. using a guideline similar to a classical chi-square test of <0.05), this is an indication of model misspecification. A 95% confidence interval is produced for the difference in the value of the chi-square model test statistic for the observed sample data and that for the replicated data [11,13]. Other Bayesian measures for model selection, as previously discussed, Bayes factor, BIC and DIC (Chapter 6) are useful for choosing among a set of competing models.

Plausible values are imputed values. Plausible values, when grouped as intended, are useful for constructing factor scores estimate for a latent variable [17]. Typically between 100 and 500 such imputed values are drawn to obtain the posterior distribution for the purpose of computing factors scores (and their standard errors). In certain analysis, plausible values may be the only method to estimate factor scores. For example, ML or WLS estimators may yield negative residual variances (i.e. Heywood cases). This can occur in some studies for no other reason than that the sample size is small [17]. A Bayes estimator can construct factor score estimates using plausible values with these data, but frequentist estimation methods will not be able to construct factor score estimates [17]. Plausible values can also be used differentially for obtaining a consistent estimate of population characteristics.

We now outline some general advantages of Bayesian SEM approaches. Aforementioned in Chapter 4, in small data sets, Bayesian approaches to SEM analyses have been shown to perform well on such data [12]. Also aforementioned, Bayesian SEM approaches are well-suited for handling of non-normal parameters (such as the indirect effect of a mediation analysis) as they can deal with asymmetric distributions [18]. Further, analyses can be made less computationally demanding for certain complex models (i.e. categorical outcomes and many latent variables) [14]. Some very complex models can only achieve admissible results (i.e. identifiable solution and plausible values for the parameters) with Bayesian SEM and informative priors [14,18]. However, computational time can also increase for other models due to the iterative sampling techniques such as MCMC used for model estimation [18]. Bayesian methods also allow the researcher to incorporate background information via prior distributions.

A basic limitation to Bayesian SEM approaches includes the possible undue influence of the prior specification, which could be chosen because of opportune reasons [18]. Another critique is that in Bayesian analysis one assumes every parameter has a distribution in the population [18].

In general, there is a wide range of modeling flexibility in using Bayesian SEM approaches [11]. Researchers can analyze multilevel models or GMMs using Bayesian SEM approaches [11]. Bayesian analysis is readily available in MPlus [5,13]. For an introduction to Bayesian SEM, the interested reader can refer to the chapter by Kaplan and Depaoli [11] or the book by Lee and Song [12].

15.5 Partial Least Squares Structural Equation Modeling (PLS-SEM)

In this textbook, we have been discussing methods for covariance-based SEM. Covariance-based SEM uses methods such as maximum likelihood to minimize differences between observed and implied covariance matrices (Chapter 4). We can analyze means as well. *Partial least squares structural equation modeling (PLS-SEM)* provides an alternative approach to covariance-based SEM analysis. PLS-SEM uses an OLS regression-based method for the data with the aim of maximizing the amount of variance explained for the endogenous variables [19]. An iterative algorithm is used.

Indicators are linearly combined to calculate weighted composite variables [20], which serve as proxies for the concepts under investigation (approximations for latent variables) [21]. This is different than covariance-based SEM which considers latent variables as common factors that explain the covariation between their associated indicators [22]. Some critics have stated that the PLS components as a result are not latent variables since they only approximately explain the covariation of their indicators [23].

PLS-SEM is well-suited for prediction and explanation of target constructs given its aim of maximizing the amount of variance explained (i.e. maximizing R^2) [19]. Also, the approach generally makes few distributional assumptions. Therefore, it may be well-suited for small sample sizes. PLS-SEM also provides an approach for including both reflective and formative constructs without the usual strict identification requirements in SEM for estimating latent variables [24,25].

When using PLS-SEM one must use adjunct methods, typically bootstrapping or other resampling techniques, to obtain standard errors for hypothesis testing. Model fit is typically evaluated using R^2-type statistics. Different software options exist for PLS-SEM, such as SmartPLS [26].

Critics of the method claim that, despite having a reputation as a viable technique for very small sample sizes, like other techniques, it still suffers from decreased statistical power and reduced accuracy with small samples sizes [27–29]. PLS-SEM may show problems in reproducibility of results in other settings [30]. It may also show bias in that "poor" measures can appear to be reliable and valid [30]. Another important concern is that approaches to examining and comparing model fit are currently less well developed in PLS-SEM than in other branches of SEM methodology. For an introduction to PLS-SEM, see Hair et al. [19].

15.6 Intensive Longitudinal Data

New technologies like smartphones and tablets have brought about studies involving *intensive longitudinal data*. Intensive longitudinal data are data with many measurements over time. These studies present new possibilities to measure fluctuations in such phenomena as sleep, mood and physical health outcomes such as blood pressure, body temperature and heart rate. Apps can be used to prompt subjects for response on items at short intervals (e.g. daily or multiple times daily). Studies involving ecological momentary assessments (EMAs) have been useful in collecting many repeated measures of self-report outcomes, thus reducing variability in the findings [31]. EMAs assess the experiences, moods and behaviors for a subject in real-time and natural setting. For example, a single question of fatigue at a single time point might not accurately capture a subject's day-to-day fatigue level. However, if prompted multiple times a day to rate one's level of fatigue over a period of several months, we might get a good indication if one's fatigue level is low, moderate, high or varying.

SEM methods have been developed for multilevel time series analysis of intensive longitudinal data [32]. Autocorrelation parameters – quantities that describe the relationship between a current value and prior values across repeated measurements – are used in the models to account for the proximity of observations in intensive longitudinal data. In general, given current developments in technology and these types of studies, the use of SEM methods for intensive longitudinal data is a growing field. See Asparouhov et al. [32] for an introduction to dynamic SEMs for intensive longitudinal data.

15.7 Dashboards for Health and Medical Decision Making: The Future of SEM?

We have discussed throughout this textbook the complex set of decisions a team of researchers may have to make in specifying models, conducting analyses and interpreting results when applying SEM techniques. Summarizing findings to all interested parties can sometimes be very challenging. Interfaces for dynamic visualization may make these methods more accessible for clinicians, nurses, patients and other interested stakeholders.

A *dashboard* is a data-driven decision support tool that presents key performance indicators and/or results in an easy-to-interpret graphical format, often in a fashion visually similar to a car's dashboard [33,34]. The *R* user interfacing package named *Shiny* can help in the development of such interfaces. *Shiny* allows for building flexible and interactive web application and is becoming popular for visualization of biomedical data [35–37].

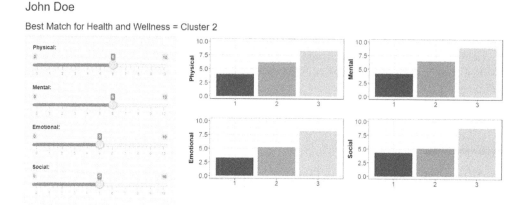

FIGURE 15.2
A basic, single tab mock-up interactive dashboard for visualization of health and wellness clusters.

The style of an interface is very flexible. An interface can have multiple tabs to click through. Data can be analyzed in real time to improve early prediction of the long-term evolution of a condition and identify actionable opportunities for intervention.

In a very basic illustrative example, *Shiny* is used to develop an interface to summarize the results of LPA and apply them for personalized care. In Figure 15.2, the current set of scores on physical, mental, emotional and social domains of a health and wellness scale puts this subject (John Doe) most likely in cluster 2 (e.g. the middle, average cluster) within the study sample.

A single tab is displayed in the figure. One could extend this interface in many ways. For example, effects of being in cluster 2 and potential clinical recommendations for John Doe could be summarized in another tab in the interface.

15.8 Conclusions

In the closing chapter of this textbook, we presented a series of special topics for SEM in health and medicine. The authors' goal in this textbook was to introduce the reader to SEM and discuss the nuances of applications for research studies in health and medicine. We discussed scenarios that researchers will commonly encounter in practice, such as conflicting empirical output for model selection, and gave guidelines on how to proceed with analyses. It is our hope that researchers will use this textbook as a reference to apply SEM in future studies in health and medicine.

References

1. Taksler, G.B., et al., Opportunities, pitfalls and alternatives in adapting electronic health records for health services research. *Medical Decision Making*. In Press.
2. Rijsdijk, F.V. and P.C. Sham, Analytic approaches to twin data using structural equation models. *Briefings in Bioinformatics*, 2002. 3(2): pp. 119–133.

3. Voronin, I., V. Ismatullina, I. Zakharov, G. Vasin, and S. Malykh, Structural equation modeling in the genetically informative study of the covariation of intelligence, working memory and planning. *ITM Web of Conferences*, 2016, Moscow, Russia, EDP Sciences.

4. Neale, M.C., S.M. Boker, G. Xie, and H.H. Maes, *Mx: Statistical modeling*, Department of Psychiatry. 1997, Richmond, VA: Medical College of Virginia.

5. Muthén, L.K. and, B.O. Muthén, BO. *Mplus: The comprehensive modelling program for applied researchers: user's guide*. Eighth edition, 1998–2017, Los Angeles, CA: Muthén & Muthén.

6. Paltoo, D., et al., National institutes of health genomic data sharing governance, C. *Nature Genetics*, 2014. **46**: p. 934.

7. Verhulst, B., H.H. Maes, and M.C. Neale, GW-SEM: A statistical package to conduct genome-wide structural equation modeling. *Behavior Genetics*, 2017. **47**(3): pp. 345–359.

8. Choi, S.W., T.S.H. Mak, and P. O'Reilly, A guide to performing polygenic risk score analyses. BioRxiv, 2018. doi: 10.1101/416545.

9. Bentley, M.J., et al. Gene variants associated with antisocial behaviour: A latent variable approach. *Journal of Child Psychology and Psychiatry*, 2013. **54**(10): pp. 1074–1085.

10. Kim, J.-Y., J.-H. Namkung, S.-M. Lee, and T.-S. Park, Application of structural equation models to genome-wide association analysis. *Genomics and Informatics*, 2010. **8**(3): pp. 150–158.

11. Kaplan, D. and S. Depaoli, Bayesian structural equation modeling, in *Handbook of latent variable and related models*, J. Palomo, D.B. Dunson, and K. Bollen, Editors. 2012, North Holland: Elsevier, pp. 163–188.

12. Lee, S.-Y. and X.-Y. Song, *Basic and advanced Bayesian structural equation modeling: With applications in the medical and behavioral sciences*. 2012, Hoboken, NJ: John Wiley & Sons.

13. Muthén, B., *Bayesian analysis in Mplus: A brief introduction*, 2010. Technical Report. Version 3, http://www.statmodel.com/download/IntroBayesVersion%203.pdf

14. Muthén, B. and T. Asparouhov, Bayesian structural equation modeling: A more flexible representation of substantive theory. *Psychological Methods*, 2012. **17**(3): p. 313.

15. Palomo, J., D.B. Dunson, and K. Bollen, Bayesian structural equation modeling, in *Handbook of latent variable and related models*, Sik-Yum Lee. 2007, Amsterdam: Elsevier, pp. 163–188.

16. Gelman, A., X.-L. Meng, and H. Stern, Posterior predictive assessment of model fitness via realized discrepancies. *Statistica Sinica*, 1996. **6**: pp. 733–760.

17. Asparouhov, T. and B. Muthén, Plausible values for latent variables using Mplus, 2010. Unpublished, http://www statmodel com/download/Plausible.pdf.

18. van de Schoot, R., D. Kaplan, J. Denissen, J.B. Asendorpf, F.J. Neyer, and M.A.G. van Aken, A gentle introduction to Bayesian analysis: Applications to developmental research. *Child Development*, 2014. **85**(3): pp. 842–860.

19. Hair Jr, J.F., G.T.M. Hult, C. Ringle, and M. Sarstedt, *A primer on partial least squares structural equation modeling (PLS-SEM)*. 2016, Thousand Oaks, CA: Sage Publications.

20. Lohmöller, J.-B. *Latent Variable Path Modeling with Partial Least Squares*. 2013, Berlin: Springer Science & Business Media.

21. Rigdon, E. Choosing PLS path modeling as analytical method in European management research: A realist perspective, 2016.

22. Sarstedt, M., J.F. Hair, C.M. Ringle, K.O. Thiele, and S.P. Gudergan, Estimation issues with PLS and CBSEM: Where the bias lies! *Journal of Business Research*, 2016. **69**(10): pp. 3998–4010.

23. McDonald, R.P., Path analysis with composite variables. *Multivariate Behavioral Research*, 1996. **31**(2): pp. 239–270.

24. Chin, W. and G. Marcoulides, The partial least squares approach to structural equation modeling, 1998.

25. Kline, R.B., Principles and practice of structural equation modeling, fourth edition. 2016, New York: Guilford Press.

26. Ringle, C.M., S. Wende, and J.-M. Becker, SmartPLS 3. Boenningstedt: SmartPLS GmbH, 2015. http://www smartpls com.

27. Kock, N. and P. Hadaya, Minimum sample size estimation in PLS-SEM: The inverse square root and gamma-exponential methods. *Information Systems Journal*, 2018. **28**(1): pp. 227–261.

28. Rönkkö, M., C.N. McIntosh, J. Antonakis, and J.R. Edwards, Partial least squares path modeling: Time for some serious second thoughts. *Journal of Operations Management*, 2016. **47–48**(1): pp. 9–27.

29. Goodhue, D.L., W. Lewis, and R. Thompson, Does PLS have advantages for small sample size or non-normal data? *MIS Quarterly*, 2012. **36**: pp. 981–1001.

30. Rouse, A. and B. Corbitt, There's SEM and "SEM": A critique of the use of PLS regression in information systems research. *ACIS 2008 Proceedings*, 2008: p. 81. http://aisel.aisnet.org/acis2008/81.

31. Armey, M.F., H.T. Schatten, N. Haradhvala, and I.W. Miller, Ecological momentary assessment (EMA) of depression-related phenomena. *Current Opinion in Psychology*, 2015. **4**: pp. 21–25.

32. Asparouhov, T., E.L. Hamaker, and B. Muthén, Dynamic structural equation models. *Structural Equation Modeling: A Multidisciplinary Journal*, 2018. **25**(3): pp. 359–388.

33. Karami, M., M. Langarizadeh, and M. Fatehi, Evaluation of effective dashboards: Key concepts and criteria. *The Open Medical Informatics Journal*, 2017. **11**: pp. 52–57.

34. Khairat, S.S., A. Dukkipati, H.A. Lauria, T. Bice, D. Travers, and S.S. Carson, The impact of visualization dashboards on quality of care and clinician satisfaction: Integrative literature review. *JMIR Human Factors*, 2018. **5**(2): p. e22.

35. Badgeley, M.A., et al., EHDViz: Clinical dashboard development using open-source technologies. *BMJ Open*, 2016. **6**(3), p. e010579.

36. Schmidt, S., et al., Improving initiation and tracking of research projects at an academic health center: A case study. *Evaluation and the Health Professions*, 2017. **40**(3): pp. 372–379.

37. Schultheis, H., et al., WIlsON: Web-based Interactive Omics VisualizatioN. *Bioinformatics*, 2018. **35**(6): pp. 1055–1057.

Index

Note: Page numbers in *italics* and **bold** refer to figures and tables.

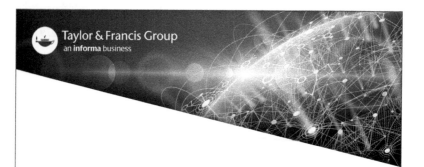

...up UK Ltd.
...024
...00026B/2211